Rare Diseases and Syndromes of the Spinal Cord

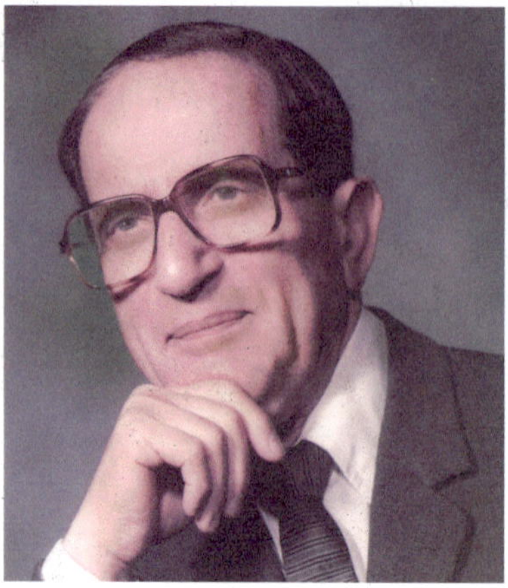

Ibrahim M. Eltorai

Rare Diseases and Syndromes of the Spinal Cord

Springer

Ibrahim M. Eltorai
The Spinal Cord Injury and Disorders Healthcare Group
The Veterans Affairs Long Beach Healthcare System
Long Beach, CA
USA

ISBN 978-3-319-45146-6 ISBN 978-3-319-45147-3 (eBook)
DOI 10.1007/978-3-319-45147-3

Library of Congress Control Number: 2016959045

Printed on acid-free paper

This Springer imprint is published by Springer Nature
The registered company is Springer International Publishing AG Switzerland
The registered company address is Gewerbestrasse 11, 6330 Cham, Switzerland

This book is dedicated to my beloved wife

Salwa

who was my guardian angel, my inspiration, friend, and the light of my life. Her guidance and support, for nearly 60 years, remain in my heart and mind and will never be forgotten.

Acknowledgments

- Department of the Veterans Administration, Long Beach, for their encouragement as a volunteer to continue this research.
- The Spinal Cord Injury Service at the Long Beach V.A. Medical Center, where I worked and conducted my research for nearly four decades.
- My assistant, Leslie K. Shimoda, who was instrumental in doing the meticulous literature research for the updates, bookkeeping, as well as typing the manuscript.
- Many thanks to the Springer Publishing Company staff and to everyone who helped with this book, including each editor individually.
- My grandson, Adam Eltorai, who is an MD/PhD candidate, for facilitating the communications with Springer, since my eyesight is very poor.
- Many thanks to the libraries of the Long Beach VA Medical Center and the University of California, Irvine, for giving me access to the literature research.
- Stanley van den Noort (1930–2009) the former Dean of Medicine at the medical school in Irvine, and chairman of the Neurosciences Department, was a great consultant. He was always following me and my progress on this book. He promised to write a forward to this book, but unfortunately passed away in an accident before the publication of this book.

Contents

Part I Congenital and Familial Causes of Myelopathy

1 **Cervical Myelopathy Due to Exostosis of the Posterior Arch of the Atlas** . . . 3

2 **Myelopathy Due to Congenital Hypoplasia of the Atlas** . . . 7

3 **Congenital Absence of the Posterior Elements of the Axis** . . . 11

4 **Congenital Afibrinogenemia** . . . 13

5 **Anterior Arch Aplasia with OS Odontoideum** . . . 17

6 **Myelopathy in Pediatric Blau Syndrome** . . . 19

7 **Intradural Extramedullary Bronchgenic Cyst** . . . 21

8 **Intramedullary Capillary Hemangioma** . . . 25

9 **Intradural Extramedullary Capillary Hemangioma** . . . 27

10 **Spinal Intradural Cerebellar Ectopia** . . . 31

11 **Cystic Dilatation of the Conus Ventriculus Terminalis** . . . 33

12 **Syringomyelia in Association with Dandy-Walker Syndrome** . . . 37

13 **Myelopathy Due to Duplication of the Laminae** . . . 39

14 **Compression Myelopathy Due to an Intramedullary Cyst Containing Ectopic Choroidal Plexus Tissue** . . . 41

15 **Chiari 1 Malformation and Holocord Syringomyelia in Hunter Syndrome** . . . 43

16 **Myelopathy in Infantile Myofibromatosis** . . . 47

17 **Tetraparesis in Laurence-Moon-Biedl-Bardet Syndrome** . . . 51

18 **Lymphangiomatosis** . . . 53

19 **Ischemic Myelopathy Due to Marfan's Syndrome** . . . 55

20 **Myelopathy in Neurocutatneous Melanosis** . . . 57

21 **Myelopathy in Osteogenesis Imperfecta** 59

22 **Prader-Willi Syndrome** 63

23 **Compression Myelopathy in Proteus Syndrome** 65

24 **Segmental Spinal Dysgenesis** 69

25 **Ischemic Myelopathy Due to Sickle Cell Trait** 73

26 **Sotos Syndrome as a Cause of Compression Myelopathy** 77

27 **Atlantoaxial Instability in Spondyloepiphyseal Dysplasia Congenita** 79

28 **Brown Séquard Syndrome Associated with Sprengel's Deformity** 81

29 **Synovial Chondromatosis** 85

30 **Myelopathy Due to Tourette's Syndrome** 87

Part II Endocrine Causes of Myelopathy

31 **Adrenomyeloneuropathy Causing Spastic Paresis** 93

32 **Copper Deficiency** 97

33 **Diabetic Myelopathy** 101

34 **Cervical Myelomalacia in Laron Syndrome** 105

35 **Compression Myelopathy due to Tophaceous Gout** 109

Part III Iatrogenic

36 **Myelopathy due to Acupuncture** 113

37 **Bronchial Artery Embolization (BAE) for Severe Hemoptysis** 117

38 **Spinal Cord Infarction Following Central Line Insertion** 119

39 **Chemical Myelopathy due to Cervical Myelography** 121

40 **Myelopathy due to Cervical Spinal Manipulation** 125

41 **Paraplegia Following Chemonucleolysis** 129

42 **Spinal Cord Injury After Chest Compressions** 131

43 **Cervical Myelopathy Contrast Injection** 133

44 **Acute Transverse Myelitis in an Infant After Dtap Vaccination** 135

45 **Paraplegia After Endovascular Repair of Abdominal Aortic Aneurysm** 139

46 Spinal Cord Infarction After Endoscopic Esophageal Varix Ligation 141

47 Subacute Combined Degeneration Provoked by Nitrous Oxide Anethesia Patients with Cobalamin Deficiency 143

48 Myelopathy due to Cervical Spine Flexion for Pediatric Tracheal Resection 147

49 Spinal Cord Stimulator Scar Tissue 151

50 Neonatal Paraplegia Through Umbilical Catheterization 153

51 Malfunction of a Ventriculo-Peritoneal Shunt 157

52 Viper Antivenin Induced Brown-Séquard Syndrome 159

Part IV Idiopathic

53 Baastrup's Disease Causing Neurogenic Claudication 163

54 Castleman's Disease 167

55 Cruciate Paralysis 171

56 Myelopathy Due To Gorham's Disease 175

57 Hajdu Cheney Syndrome 179

58 Holocord Myelopathy with Thoracic Stenosis 181

59 Myelitis due to Hypertrophic Dens 183

60 Myelopathy due to Léri's Disease 187

61 Idiopathic Primary Spinal Myoclonus 191

62 Idiopathic Retroperitoneal Fibrosis 193

63 Isolated Spinal Neuro-Behçet Disease 197

64 Subacute Progressive Ascending Myelopathy (SPAM) 203

65 Idiopathic Spinal Cord Herniation 207

66 Spontaneous Spinal Epidural Hematoma 211

67 Tumoral Calcinosis of the Spine 215

68 Transient Cervical Myeloneurapraxia 219

Part V Infectious Cause of Myelopathy

69 Bacterial Meningitis in Adults 225

70 Guillain-Barré Syndrome Following Allogeneic Bone Marrow Transplantation 227

71 **Myelopathy due to *Cladosporium trichoides* or *Cladophialophora bantiana*** 231

72 **Coxsackie Transverse Myelitis** 235

73 **Cytomegalovirus Myelitis** 239

74 **Degos Disease (DD)** 243

75 **Dengue Myelitis** 247

76 **Dental Extraction** 251

77 **Holospinal Epidural Abscess** 253

78 **Imported Vaccine-Associated Paralytic Poliomyelitis** 255

79 **Lemierre's Syndrome** 259

80 **Listeriosis** 261

81 **Melioidosis** 265

82 **Mumps Viraemia** 269

83 **Myelitis due to Sparganosis** 271

84 ***Toxocara canis*** 275

85 **Toxoplasmosis of the Spinal Cord** 279

86 **Trypanosomiasis** 283

87 **Compression Myelopathy due to Typhoid Spondylodiscitis** 287

88 **West Nile Virus Infection** 289

89 **Zoster Myelitis** 293

Part VI Neoplastic Causes of Myelopathy

90 **Adamantinoma of the Spine** 299

91 **Amyloidosis** 301

92 **Acute Paraplegia Secondary to Brown Tumor** 305

93 **Myelopathy due to Chondroblastoma of the Spine** 309

94 **Costal Osteochondroma Causing Compression Myelopathy** 313

95 **Cutaneous Adenocystic Carcinoma** 317

96 **Myelopathy due to Intraspinal Desmoid Tumor** 319

97 **Intramedullary Ectopic Adrenal Cortical Adenoma** 323

98 **Spinal Tanycytic Ependymoma** 325

99 **Follicular Dendritic Cell Sarcoma (FDCS)** 331

100 Left Atrial Papillary Fibroelastoma 335

101 Gliofibroma 339

102 Glioneuronal Tumor 343

103 Myelopathy in Primary Spinal Epidural Mantle Cell Lymphoma 345

104 Malingnant Eccrine Poroma 349

105 Melanoma 353

106 Intramedullary Meningioma of the Cervical Spinal Cord 357

107 Metastatic Retinoblastoma (Pediatric) 361

108 Infantile Myofibromatosis 363

109 Myopericytoma of the Thoracic Spine Causing Myelopathy 367

110 Natural Killer T-Cell Lymphoma of the Cauda Equina 369

111 Myelopathy in Neurocutatneous Melanosis 373

112 Anaplastic Oligodendroglioma 375

113 Oncocytoma in Melanocytoma 379

114 Osteosarcoma 381

115 Myelopathy Due to Spinal Paraganglioma 385

116 Plasma Cell Leukemia (PCL) 389

117 Pleomorphic Xanthoastrocytoma 391

118 Primary Intraspinal Primitive Neuroectodermal Tumor (PNET) . . . 395

119 Intramedullary Schwannoma Associated with Neurofibromatosis 399

120 Secondary Syringomyelia due to Spinal Intramedullary Metastasis 403

121 Spinal Hemangioblastomas in Von Hippel Lindau Disease 407

122 Spinal Artery Steal Syndrome in Paget's Disease of the Bone 411

123 Intramedullary Teratoma 413

Part VII Toxic Causes of Myelopathy

124 Benzene Myelitis 419

125 Myelopathy due to Flexion Drug Overdose 423

126 Myelopathy due to Heroin Addiction 427

127 Myelopathy due to Wasp Sting 431

Part VIII Vascular Causes of Myelopathy

128 Anterior Spinal Artery Syndrome . . . 437

129 Cervical Myelopathy Caused by Bilateral Persistence of the First Intersegmental Arteries . . . 441

130 Myelopathy in Cobb Syndrome . . . 445

131 Eale's Disease . . . 449

132 Ectopic Choroidal Plexus Tissue . . . 453

133 Myelopathy due to Fibrocartilaginous Spinal Cord Embolism . . . 455

134 Intravascular Papillary Endothelial Hyperplasia . . . 459

135 Posterior Spinal Artery Syndrome . . . 463

136 Myelopathy due to Spinal Cord Vasculitis . . . 465

137 Epidural Varix . . . 469

Part IX Miscellaneous Causes of Myelopathy

138 Paraplegia of Cerebral Origin . . . 477

139 Decompression Sickness . . . 481

140 Exertional Myelopathy due to Congenital Kyphosis Type II . . . 485

141 Thoracic Compression Myelopathy due to Facet Joint Osteophyte . . . 487

142 Hysterical Paralysis . . . 489

143 Differential Diagnosis: Hypermagnesemia . . . 493

144 Spinal Epidural Lubricant Grease . . . 495

145 Myelopathy due to Intramedullary Herniated Nucleus Pulposus . . . 497

146 Spinal Cord Injury Without Radiologic Abnormality (Sciwora) . . . 499

147 Surfer's Myelopathy . . . 503

148 Trampoline Spinal Cord Injuries in Pediatrics . . . 507

149 Traumatic Tethering . . . 509

Conclusion . . . 513

About the Author

Dr. Ibrahim Eltorai completed his medical education at Cairo University in Egypt (formerly King Fouad University, affiliated with London University) and then completed postgraduate training in Neurosurgery and Cardiovascular surgery at multiple European institutions. He was appointed Professor of Surgery at the Cairo University School of Medicine. He has published nearly 150 articles in Egyptian and European journals.

When Dr. Eltorai moved to the United States, he joined the Spinal Cord Injury Service at the Veterans Administration Medical Center, Long Beach. Dr. Eltorai worked closely with Dr. Ernst Bors and Dr. A. Estin Comarr on laying the foundations of spinal cord injury treatment as a medical specialty, which was taught not only in the VA system, but also in hospitals nationwide. Dr. Eltorai practiced SCI medicine in Long Beach, California, for more than 30 years until his retirement in 2004. After retirement, Dr. Eltorai served as a SCI medicine consultant and historian. Dr. Eltorai continues to research and document the history and the evolution of SCI medicine until the present.

Dr. Eltorai published numerous clinical articles on SCI medicine and edited a book on emergencies in spinal cord injury patients. He is a founding member and a past President of the American Paraplegia Society, as well as, a Fellow of the International Spinal Cord Society. Dr. Eltorai's research on the evolution of SCI medicine is currently displayed at the Long Beach V.A. Medical Center and will soon be published in a book.

Introduction

My interest in this subject goes back, close to 50 years, when I first emigrated to the United States. At that time, searching for rare diseases I relied on the Index Medicus monthly. I then copied them and currently they are stored at the Historical Archives of SCI Medicine in Long Beach VA Medical Center, the first SCI historical library in the world. The articles are in all languages, including English, French, German, Dutch, Italian, and Spanish. Upon my retirement, I started working on updating these subjects.

In order to fully understand the scope of this book, one must first look at what defines a rare disease.

Statistically, there is no single cutoff number has been agreed upon for which a disease is considered rare. A disease may be considered rare in one part of the world, or in a particular group of people, but still be common in another. In the United States, a disease might be considered rare, but common in other parts of the world, which is especially true of genetic diseases and infectious diseases.

The exact definition of rare diseases is not well established and varies widely. Some cases depend on the number of people living with the disease, while others include other factors, such as the existence of adequate treatment or severity of the disease. Globally, in the United States, the Rare Diseases Act of 2002 defines rare disease strictly according to prevalence, specifically "any disease or condition that affects fewer than 200,000 people in the United States," or about 1 in 1,500 people. This definition is essentially like that of the Orphan Drug Act of 1983, a federal law that was written to encourage research into rare diseases and possible cures. In Japan, the legal definition of a rare disease is one that affects fewer than 50,000 patients in Japan, or about 1 in 2,500 people. However, the European Commission on Public Health defines rare diseases as "life-threatening or chronically debilitating diseases which are of such low prevalence that special combined efforts are needed to address them." The term "low-prevalence" is later defined as generally meaning fewer than 1 in 2,000 people.

Diseases that are statistically rare, but not also life threatening, chronically debilitating, or inadequately treated, are excluded from their definition. The European Organization for Rare Diseases (EURORDIS) estimates that as many as 5,000–7,000 distinct rare diseases exist, and as much as 6–8 % of the population of the European Union is affected by one.

Rare diseases are usually genetic and are therefore chronic. EURORDIS estimates that at least 80 % of them have identified genetic origins. Other rare diseases are the result of infections and allergies or due to degenerative and proliferative causes. Symptoms of some rare diseases may appear at birth or in childhood, whereas others only appear once adulthood is reached.

Research publications emphasize rare diseases that are chronic or incurable, although many short-term medical conditions are also rare diseases. The definitions used in the medical literature and by national health plans are similarly divided, with definitions ranging from 1 in 1,000 to 1 in 200,000.

This unique text is presented in a brief synopsis of the collected rare spinal cord cases from the V.A. Long Beach SCI Historical Library. The references collected range from 1930 to present. The information is collected from various languages, including English, French, German, Dutch, Portuguese, Spanish, Italian, and even abstracts in Russian, Japanese, and Chinese. Each case is illustrated with definition, incidence, etiology, pathology, clinical picture, diagnosis, and management. These subjects are divided into congenital (20 %), endocrinal (3 %), iatrogenic (11 %), idiopathic (11 %), infectious (13.5 %), neoplastic (23 %), toxic (2 %), vascular (7 %), and miscellaneous (8 %). This book is presented without illustrations or photos mostly for space and for the reader focus on each case, individually.

References

Aymé S, Schmidtke J. Networking for rare diseases: a necessity for Europe. Bundesgesundheitsblatt Gesundheitsforschung Gesundheitsschutz. 2007;50(12):1477–83.

Solly J, Shyndriayeva G. Managing research advances into a rare disease. Case study of the Myrovlytis Trust. In: Sireau N, editor. Rare diseases, challenges and opportunities for social entrepreneurs. Sheffield: Greenleaf Publications; 2013.

Van de laar FA, Bor H, Van de lisdonk EH. Prevalence of zebras in general practice: data from the Continuous Morbidity Registration Nijmegen. Eur J Gen Pract. 2008;14 Suppl 1:44–6.

Part I

Congenital and Familial Causes of Myelopathy

1 Cervical Myelopathy Due to Exostosis of the Posterior Arch of the Atlas

1.1 Definition

Hereditary multiple exostosis (HME) is also called diaphyseal aclasis, multiple echondromatosis, Ehrenfried disease, hereditary deforming chondrodysplasia, and osteogenic disease. First described by Boyer in 1814, this condition has higher tendency to invade the spine and lead to myelopathy more than solitary osteochondromas, which occur mostly in the appendicular skeleton than the axial one (Mikawa et al. 1997; Palmer and Blum 1980; Schmale et al. 1994).

1.2 Incidence

Incidence of HME is about 0.9 and 2 per 100,000 in Caucasian population, but not quite accurate, some cases do not seek medical advice. Most vertebral exostosis grow from the external parts of the laminae. Only one case was presented arising from the posterior arch (Chooi et al. 2005). Spinal involvment is 7–9 % and usually posterior elements leading to myelopathy.

1.3 Etiology

It is an autosomal dominant disorder, with full penetrance and has an equal gender dominance (Peterson 1989).

Abstracted from Chooi et al. (2005)

I.M. Eltorai, *Rare Diseases and Syndromes of the Spinal Cord*,
DOI 10.1007/978-3-319-45147-3_1

1.4 Pathology

These benign tumors usually arise from the metaphyseal regions of long bones of the legs and occasionally from the ribs. During bone growth in childhood and adolescence the actively growing cartilaginous cap continues to grow. The incidence of malignant transformation is 4–11 % (Decker and Wei 1969). Histiology shows mature trabecular bone with a cartilaginous cap plate. The case described in the posterior arch of the atlas, grew into the spinal cord and compressed the cord at C1.

1.5 Clinical Picture

The symptoms are delayed due t slow growth of the tumor up to 10 years. However, sudden increase in size and pain or neurological changes may suggest malignancy. In the case described by Chooi et al. (2005):

> Progressive numbness and paresis of one arm and both legs over six months, neck pain radiating to the arm, impaired functions of the hand, electrical shock radiating pain, bowel and bladder incontinence, and unsteady gait. Her family history of HME.

1.6 Diagnosis

Diagnosis is based on

1. History of familial HME
2. Slow onset of neurological deficit, sensory-motor.
3. Plain radiography: Increased sclerosis in the region of the posterior arch of the atlas.
4. MRI: exostosis from the right side of the posterior arch anteriorly and compressing the cord at C1.
5. CT Scan: pedunculated bony tumor from the posterior arch anteriorly encroaching on the spinal canal.

1.7 Management

A posterior hemi-laminectomy decompression procedure, the right posterior arch of the atlas removed with a burr. Recovery was uneventful and neurological improvement was noted.

References

Chooi YS, Siow YS, Chong CS. Cervical myelopathy caused by an exostosis of the posterior arch of C1. J Bone Joint Surg [Br]. 2005;87(B):257–9.

Decker R, Wei W. Thoracic cord compression from multiple hereditary exostosis associated with cerebellar astrocytoma: case report. J Neurosurg. 1969;30:310–2.
Mikawa Y, Watanabe R, Nakashima Y, Hayashida T. Cervical spinal cord compression in hereditary multiple exostoses: report of a case and review of the literature. Arch Orthop Trauma Surg. 1997;116:112–7.
Palmer F, Blum P. Osteochondroma with spinal cord compression. J Neurosurg. 1980;52:842–5.
Peterson H. Multiple hereditary osteochondromata. Clin Orthop. 1989;239:222–30.
Schmale GA, Conrad EU, Raskind WH. The natural history of hereditary multiple exostoses. J Bone Joint Surg Am. 1994;76(A):986–92.

2 Myelopathy Due to Congenital Hypoplasia of the Atlas

2.1 Definition

This is a very rare congenital condition, in which there is hypoplasia of the atlantal arch leading to cervical stenosis and subsequent cervical myelopathy.

2.2 Incidence

According to Nishikawa et al. (2001), nine cases of hypoplasia of the posterior atlantal arch, 8 of them developed cervical myelopathy and one case had obstruction of foramen of the Magendie. Only one was female. The symptoms developed between 22 and 82 years of age. Yamashita et al. (1997), recorded one case of 73-year-old female, who had in addition a retrodontoid pseudotumor, treated by laminectomy and occipito-cervical fusion. Okamoto et al., in 1998, reported 77-year-old male with tetraparesis and severe compression myelopathy at C1. Recovery was achieved after resection of the posterior arch of the atlas. Urasaki et al., reported in 2001, 14 year old male with same syndrome treated successfully by laminectomy of the atlas. May et al. (2001), added another case of a 66-year-old male who recovered after posterior decompression.

2.3 Etiology

The embryological ossification of the atlas as follows:

The atlas originates from three ossification centers that arise from the rostal portion of the first sclerotome. The anterior ossification center gives rise to the anterior tubercle and the anterior arch. Complete ossification between the anterior and the

Abstracted from Nishikawa et al. (2001)

I.M. Eltorai, *Rare Diseases and Syndromes of the Spinal Cord*,
DOI 10.1007/978-3-319-45147-3_2

two lateral centers usually occurs between the 6th and 8th year of life. Between the 6th and 7th week of embryogenesis the two lateral centers begin to extend dorsally forming the posterior arch. The chondrification of the posterior arch joins at the middle line during the 4th month of embryogenic life. By birth, the arch is nearly fused. Hypoplasia of the arch could be the result of premature fusion of the posterior ossification centers or insufficient dorsal extension, independent of the time of union. Abnormalities of chondrification is another theory (see Nishikawa et al.)

2.4 Pathology

The normal sagittal spinal canal diameter is 16–25 mm at the level of the atlas. A diameter less than 14 mm at CI level is significant for canal encroachment on the spinal cord. A canal of 10 mm would be symptomatic of cervical myelopathy. The cord shows edema, compression, and later atrophy. Occasionally, hypoplasia of the atlas is associated with retrodontoid pseudotumor, which is associated with osteoarthrosis of the atlantoaxial joint. It is non-neoplastic tumor, mostly a reaction to the hypoplastic atlantal arch.

2.5 Clinical Picture

Although the condition is congenital, the clinical picture shows later in life when the stenosis is aggravated by degenerative changes. Symptoms are:

1. Local or occipital paresthesia
2. Dysthesia of the upper extremities spreading to the lower extremities.
3. Muscle weakness preventing dexterity of the upper limbs and causing ataxic gait
4. Paralysis: tetraparesis and hemiparesis
5. Hypesthesia and hypalgesia

Physical findings are those of etraparesis.

2.6 Diagnosis

Diagnosis is based on the following criteria:

1. X-ray: stenosis of the spinal canal at C1 level, diameter of 10 mm or less, narrow spinal canal 7–8 mm
2. Clinical picture and physical exam.
3. CT scan and MRI: narrow canal, edema of the cord, later atrophy of the cord.

2.7 Management

Atlantal laminectomy

One case of atlanto-axial pseudotumor was treated by occipital cervical fusion. The pseudotumor was removed transorally.

References

May D, Jenny B, Faundez A. Cervical cord compression due to a hypoplastic atlas. Case report. J Neurosurg. 2001;94(1 Suppl):133–6.

Nishikawa K, Ludwig SC, Colon RJ. Cervical myelopathy and congenital stenosis from hypoplasia of the atlas. Spine. 2001;26:E80–6.

Okamoto K, Sumi M, Ikeda M, Sawamura S, Kataoka O. A case of cervical myelopathy with developmental canal stenosis at the level of the atlas. A case report. Kobe J Med Sci. 1998;44(3):135–40.

Urasaki E, Yasukouchi H, Yokota A. Atlas hypoplasia manifesting as myelopathy in a child – case report. Neurol Med Chir (Tokyo). 2001;41(3):160–2.

Yamashita K, Aoki Y, Hiroshima K. Myelopathy due to hypoplasia of the atlas. A case report. Clin Orthop Relat Res. 1997;338:90–3.

Congenital Absence of the Posterior Elements of the Axis

3

3.1 Definition

This is a condition of congenital absence of the pedicles, laminae, and spinous process of the axis associated with its instability and subluxation of C2-C3 leading to compression myelopathy. Occasionally, the defect is only in the spinous processes (spina bifida cervicalis).

3.2 Incidence

Goel et al., reported two cases of their own and quoted only two reports from the literature. Anatomically, defects of the posterior arch of the axis are 1:1,000.

3.3 Etiology

There is a failure either of chondrification or ossification of the right and left primordial cartilages. Thus far no genetic element is quoted.

3.4 Pathology

Complete absence of the posterior arch of the axis leads to instability, subluxation, or dislocation of C2 on C3 with subsequent myelopathy.

A case reported by Goel et al. (1999)

I.M. Eltorai, *Rare Diseases and Syndromes of the Spinal Cord*,
DOI 10.1007/978-3-319-45147-3_3

3.5 Clinical Picture

It may be asymptomatic or mild symptoms as pain in the neck. Neurological picture may develop with minor trauma or magnificent one. Tetraparesis and sensory loss is full blown picture. The symptoms may disappear with cervical traction.

3.6 Diagnosis

Diagnosis is based on the following criteria:

1. Clinical history
2. X-ray: Abscesses of the spinous process and laminae
3. MRI of the spinal cord: the findings are absence of the pedicles, the laminae, and the spinous process of the axis and may show cord indentation.
4. CT scan

3.7 Management

Traction by tongs or halo gives relief of nerological deficits. The final measures are occipito-cervical fusion or anterior decompression by partial corpectomy, hardware fixation with bone grafting.

Reference

Goel A, Gupta S, Laheri V. Congenital absence of posterior elements of axis: a report of two cases. Br J Neurosurg. 1999;13(5):459–61.

Congenital Afibrinogenemia

4

4.1 Definition

This is an ischemic condition of the cervical spinal cord due to vertebral artery dissection (VAD) probably facilitated by congenital afibrinogenemia.

4.2 Incidence

According to Laufs et al. (2004), there was a series of 111 patients with VAD, 2 of them had spinal manifestations. An additional 13 patients, 7 had spinal cord manifestations and 6 had radiculopathy or hemorrhagic complications.

In 1996, Garcia-Mens et al., reported the first case of VAD associated with congenital afibrinogenemia. The same authors stated that until their paper was published, fewer than 200 cases of congenital afibrinogenemia were reported. Lauf et al., reported the second case of VAD associated with congenital afibrinogenemia. Under normal conditions, VAD leads to vertebrabasilar ischemia affecting the posterior circulation. Infarction of the spinal cord is rare and with afibrinogenemia it is more rare.

4.3 Pathology

Arterial dissection occurs when blood enters a vessel wall through an initial tear and a false lumen for blood occurs within the media. According to Laufs et al., involvement of the spinal cord occurs due to:

Abstracted from Laufs et al. (2004)

I.M. Eltorai, *Rare Diseases and Syndromes of the Spinal Cord*,
DOI 10.1007/978-3-319-45147-3_4

- afibrinogenemia and hemiplegia is found in the arterial wall (vertebral) which leads to occlusion of one or multiple feeders of the spinal cord, viz. The radicular branches, which originate from the vertebral second segment (V2). Subcal arteries may be also occluded if the anterior spinal artery (ASA) is involved.
- Possibly embolic occlusion of the descending branch from the intracranial segment of the vertebral artery (V4), which is normally merging with the contralateral to form the ASA. The segments involved are variable; in Garcia-Men's case it involved C2–C4.

The spinal cord ischemia results in infarction of variable size and may be hemispinal size as the case reported by Laufs et al. The dissection may be due to mechanical or trauma.

4.4 Clinical Picture

Women are 2.5 times more likely involved than men. History of trauma may be positive. History of congenital afibrinogenemia may be positive but only very rarely. There may be history of migraine headache, with hemorrhagic tendency. Symptoms may include:

- neck pain radiating to the upper extremities
- facial numbness
- clumsiness and weakness of an upper and lower extremity
- decreased sensation
- ataxic unsteady gait
- Neurological exam
  - cranial nerves within normal
  - Horner's syndrome on one side
  - sensory weakness on one side (pin-prick and proprioception)
  - reflexes are exaggerated

4.5 Diagnosis

Diagnosis is based on

1. History of afibrinogenemia in patient and/or family
2. Neurological exam
3. MRI and MRA of the neck vessels shows VAD from V2 to V3 segments. The infarcted cord shows signal increase on T2-weighted imges. Ultrasonography of the neck arteries may show VAD. The MRI is more diagnostic. Transverse and coronal images localize the extent of the infarct.
4. Laboratory tests: partial thromboplastin time (PTT) and prothrombin time (PT) are prolonged. No clot function. Fibrinogen antigen in plasma is negative.

4.6 Management

According to Laufs et al., Fibrinogen replacement IgM IV to repeat until plasma level >80 mg/dL. Anticoagulation with IV unfractionated heparin. In their case Laufs et al., continued IV heparin for 12 days and was changed to low molecular weight dextran heparin (LMWDH) once daily while reducing fibrinogen therapy. After 3 months LMWDH was discontinued and fibrinogen schedule changed to one a month during the periods of menses. The condition has improved substantially under this regimen. Duplex ultrasound and MRI showed recanalization of the vertebral artery and MRI of the spinal cord showed a small residual lesion.

4.7 Updating

Abstracted from Bas et al. (2009)

Case Presentation

The authors present the third case of afibrinogenemia. A 22-year-old female presented with sudden and severe neck pain and progressive right sided weakness, predominantly with right arm. She had right-sided severe neck pain radiating into the occiput, initiated by neck and head rotation while walking. Pain and numbness ceased for 10 min. After resting for 2 h, right-sided weakness appeared She had congenital afibrinogenemia for 20 years. She had minor hemorrhage around menstruation periods, treated by fibrinogen replacement. No history of hypertension, smoking, or trauma. Right hemiparesis more severe in the arm. CT of the head was normal. She was diagnosed with ischemic stroke and received 300 mg of aspirin.

Blood fibrinogen level was 67 mg/dL (normal range is 144 mg–430 mg/dL). PT and PTT were too high (>150 s). Hemoglobin level was 10.6 g/dL; blood cells and biochemistry were normal. After 12 h from the onset of weakness started on the left side. She was now tetraparetic. Medical Research Council scale 0/5 on the right arm; 1/5 in the right leg; 2/5 in the left arm; and 1/3 in the left leg. Babinski's was negative on both sides. Deep tendon reflexes were absent on the right and significantly diminished on the left. Sensory testing reveled diminished brain sensation below C3 bilaterally. Proprioception was diminished below C4 on the right side. Sense of temperature was unchanged. Horner's syndrome was not noted on the right side. Cranial nerves were intact. MRI of the spine showed spinal cord infarction from upper cervical to mid-thoracic level. T2-weighted images showed hypersensitivity with swelling of the cord predominantly on the right side and less so on the left sided, from C4 to C7 below this level. This appearance was more in the central cord and skipping its periphery. Scattered microhemorrhages were seen in the affected segment in an exaggerated manner on T2 gradient echo sequences (GRE). Fat saturated T1 weighted spin echo images showed hyperintensive mural hematoma in the right vertebral artery, suggestive of dissection with occlusion of the vessel as seen in the pulse sequences. Cranial MRI was normal.

Management

- IV Methylprednisolone 1 g QD/5 days followed by rapid tapering over 12 days.
- Fibrinongen replacement
- thromboprophylaxis
- intensive rehab program

She improved neurologically except some weakness of the right hand and in 4 months she could do daily activities above. There was mild weakness of the left leg. There was patchy sensory loss on the chest and blunting sensation of the left lower limb. MRI at 1 and 6 months later showed severe residual changes from midcervical to lower thoracic segments. The authors did not use heparin since this is a hemorrhagic condition although it was used by the previous authors Lauf et al., and Garcia-Men et al.

Reference
Bas DF, Oguz KK, Yavuz K, Topcuoglu MA. Spinal cord infarction in congenital afibrinogenemia: a case report and review of the literature. J Stroke Cerebrovasc Dis. 2009;18(4):298–303.

Reference

Laufs H, Weidauer S, Heller C, Lorenz M, Neumann-haefelin T. Hemi-spinal cord infarction due to vertebral artery dissection in congenital afibrinogenemia. Neurology. 2004;63(8):1522–3.

Anterior Arch Aplasia with OS Odontoideum

5

5.1 Definition

This is a condition where there is aplasia of anterior arch of atlas with os odontoideum (bipartite atlas). It is usually associated with posterior arch midline defect.

5.2 Incidence

This was described in one case. Currarino et al., reported 11 cases with complete or partial segmentation defect in mid odontoid. Atasoy et al., described a case of bipartite atlas with os odontoideum and posterior arch hypoplasia.

5.3 Etiology

Although os odontoideum may be caused by trauma or vascular disease, this paper will only discuss the congenital form:

In embryogenesis the atlas and the odontoid process develop from the first cervical sclerotome with some contribution from remnants of the proatlas; whereas the body, lateral mass and posterior arch of the axis arise entirely from the second cervical sclerotome. The odontoid process is thought to originate as an addition to or a projection from the anterior part of the atlas. It separates between the 6–7 weeks of gestation, and then moves caudally to join the body of the axis. Ossification of the anterior arch involves one or two ossification centers, which is external and posterolaterally, to fuse with the lateral masses. The os odontoideum may be in the normal posterior position or near the base of the occipital bone in the area of the foramen magnum, where it may be fused to the base of the skull. Failure of the anterior arch to grow is accompanied with the os odontoideum.

A case reported by Garg et al. (2004)

I.M. Eltorai, *Rare Diseases and Syndromes of the Spinal Cord*,
DOI 10.1007/978-3-319-45147-3_5

5.4 Pathology

The presence of the os odontoideum is considered to be a failure of fusion of the ossification of the ossification center within the odontoid process. Aplasia and clefts of the anterior arch are very rare. Anterior midline clefts are usually associated with posterior midline clefts. In the absence of an anterior center of ossification the lateral masses do not fuse anteriorly or no fusion of the two anterior ossification centers. For more details see Garg et al.

5.5 Clinical Picture

Os odontoideum may be clinically silent, may be discovered incidentally by radiography. In cases of instability from os odontoideum, neurological manifestations will be noticed usually in the form of transitory episode of diffused paresis following trauma. Other cases of progressive myelopathy is noted, namely weakness, ataxia, and sensory changes due to the instability. Vascular symptoms may complicate the picture due to vertebral artery compression.

5.6 Diagnosis

Diagnosis is based on the following criteria:

1. Clinical history
2. X-ray
3. MRI: independent ossicle rostral to the axis body in the position of the odontoid process. T2 weighted images show aplasia of the anterior arch of the atlas and os odontoideum. The spinal cord may show hyperintense signal at C2 suggestive of edema of the cord.
4. CT scan: anterior arch aplasia and midline cleft of the posterior arch of the atlas. On flexion of the neck there is ventral displacement of CI over C2 which is reduced on extension.

5.7 Management

Patients with bipartite atlas and os odontoideum have a potentially precarious existence due to spinal cord compression at high cervical level. In symptomatic cases transoral odontoidectomy and posterior fixation of occipit with C2–C3 spinous processes. Asymptomatic cases should be closely observed.

Reference

Garg A, Gaikwad SB, Gupta V, et al. Bipartite atlas with Os odontoideum. Spine. 2004;29:E35–8.

Myelopathy in Pediatric Blau Syndrome

6

6.1 Definition

Blau syndrome is a rare autoinflammatory disorder within the group of pediatric granulomatous diseases. Mutations in nucleotide binding oligomerization domain 2 are responsible for this condition, which has an autosomal dominant pattern of inheritance and variable expressivity.

6.2 Clinical Picture

Clinical picture includes arthritis uveitis, skin rash, and granulomatous inflammation. CNS involvement is seldom reported. Some belated cases of seizures, neurosensorial hearing loss, and cranial nerve palsy.

6.3 Management

The management of Blau syndrome consists of NSAID, corticosteroids, immunosuppressive agents, e.g., antitumor necrosis factor α (TNF-α inhibitor). In refractory cases immunosuppression by methotrexate, azathioprine, mycophenolate mofetil, and interleukin-1 blockers (anakinra). Biological agents, e.g., antitumor necrosis α, such as etanercept, infliximab, and adalimumab.

Entanercept, a soluble recombinant dimmer of human TNF receptor protein fused and bound to human IgG acts competitively to inhibit TNF binding itself to its cell surface receptor. Infliximab and adalimumab are monoclonal antibodies, the first is a murine chimeric and the latter is humanized antibody.

Adverse effects of anti-TNF-α drugs are:

Abstracted from Caraseghi et al. (2011)

I.M. Eltorai, *Rare Diseases and Syndromes of the Spinal Cord*,
DOI 10.1007/978-3-319-45147-3_6

- Local infusion site and systemic reaction
- Opportunistic infections, e.g., fungi and mycobacteria
- Lymphoprolifereative disease
- Systemic lupus erythematousus like syndrome
- Demyelinating diseases, e.g., multiple sclerosis and acute transverse myelitis

6.4 Case Report

A child with Blau syndrome recovering anti-TNF-α, who developed transverse myelitis, which was relieved when the drug was discontinued. A 13-year-old boy presenting with paraparesis, had Blau syndrome at the age of 5 years. His mother had rheumatoid arthritis since childhood. Her genetic study showed a dominant autosomal mutation in the NOD2/CARD15 gene. The child was treated with cortisome and methotrexate from 8 years of age. Then he received etanercept. MRI showed bifocal high intensity white matter lesions on T2-weighted images at C2–C4 and at the conus medullaris L1 enhancing after gadolinium L1. Etanercept was discontinued. Methypredinsolone was given IV 1 g/d for 5 days, followed by oral prednisone 1 mg/kg, which was tapered in 6 weeks. He started to improve progressively so that by the end of the 4 weeks, he was almost fully recovered. After 6 weeks, MRI showed complete resolution. At 3 month follow-up, he was symptom free. He was switched to corticosteroids and methotrexate and TNF-α inhibitor is excluded.

Reference

Caracseghi F, Izquierdo-blasco J, Sanchez-montanez A, Melendo-perez S, Roig-quilis M, Modesto C. Etanercept-induced myelopathy in a pediatric case of Blau syndrome. Case Rep Rheumatol. 2011;2011:134106.

Intradural Extramedullary Bronchgenic Cyst

7

7.1 Definition

According Baumann et al., congenital spinal cysts are of three main classes:

1. Epithelial, endodermal
2. Mesenchymal, including arachnoid cysts
3. Mixed: from multiple layers of the primary germ cell layers

Whereas arachnoid cysts are relatively common, epithelial cysts are rare and include confusing nomenclature: entregenous, foregut cysts, and endodermal cysts. This group is divided into epidermal and ependymal. The epithelial cysts may be gastrointestinal, which is more common and less so are the respiratory. This is the subject of this report.

7.2 Incidence

Neurenteric cysts account for 0.5 % of spinal cord space occupying lesions.

7.3 Etiology

Bronchogenic cysts are developmental abnormalities that may affect the CNS. Their pathogenesis is not fully understood. According to Arnold et al., there are three hypotheses:

Abstracted from Arnold et al. (2009)

I.M. Eltorai, *Rare Diseases and Syndromes of the Spinal Cord*,
DOI 10.1007/978-3-319-45147-3_7

1. The possibility of an ectoendodermal adhesion, which results in incomplete separation of germ cell layers
2. This theory suggest that the cyst originates from ectoderm, which is capable of producing both ectodermal and mesodermal tissues
3. The split notochord syndrome postulated by Bentley and Smith, which describes an incomplete duplication and separation of the notochord that leads to ventral herniation through the notochord, resulting in a fistuala, which runs through the future spinal cord and spine and is eventually closed off as the embryo grows. However, a cystic lesion may remain on the ventral surface. Therefore, the cyst is a remnant of the foregut and this can differentiate into the gut tissues or others of the endoderm

7.4 Pathology

Bronchogenic cysts occur most commonly in the cervical spine, thoracic bronchogenic cysts are extremely rare. Ko et al., reported a case in the sacral region, a thoracolumbar case by Baumann et al. The cysts have been found attached to the sternum, pericardium, skin, diaphragm, in addition to the spinal location. Subdiaphragmatic locations are exceedingly rare. The cyst has a connective tissue base lined with cerebral columnar epithelium. Associated vertebral anomalies may coexist, e.g., spina bifida. The cyst being limited in space grows slowly, and eventually causes compression myelopathy.

7.5 Clinical Picture

The mass of symptoms is slow. Started by pain in the back or neck, depending on the level of cyst:

- Numbness of the lower extremities
- Muscle weakness
- Inability to walk normal, wide based gait
- Loss of sensation of variable degree
- Spasticity of the lower limbs
- Incontinence of urine and/or bowel
- Neurological exam show reduced motor power of lower limbs of variable degree.
- Hypertonicity, Babinski's reflex positive
- Clounus may be initiated
- Some degree of sensory loss
- Spinal bifida or other vertebral anomaly

7.6 Diagnosis

Diagnosis based on:

1. Clinical picture
2. MRI shows the cyst as a an oval or spherical homogeneous swelling in contact with the spinal canal. It is hyperintense on T2 weighted images an hypointense on T1 weighted images. The lesion is shown intradural extramendullary

7.7 Management

Surgery consists of:

1. Through laminectomy, the dura is opened and the mass is dissected by the operative telescope. To facilitate removal aspiration may be done before resection

Reference

Arnold PM, Neff LL, Anderson KK, Reeves AR, Newell KL. Thoracic myelopathy secondary to intradural extramedullary bronchogenic cyst. J Spinal Cord Med. 2009;32(5):595–7.

8 Intramedullary Capillary Hemangioma

8.1 Definition

Capillary hemangiomas are superficial vascular lesions which are not infrequently seen in the subcutaneous tumors such as the scalp, face, neck, oral cavity, and the nasal vault. They may grow internally and may involve the central nervous system.

8.2 Incidence

The first and only case of primary intramedullary hemangioma is described by Hida et al., in 1993, Ianelli et al. (2005), reported a case of an infant with communicating hydrocephalus associated with an intramedullary capillary hemangioma treated by shunting and tumor resection.

8.3 Pathology

The case described by Hida showed angiomatous nests consisting of small capillary-like vessels, telangiectatic vessels, and aggregated venules scattered in the edematous and partially necrotic parenchyma of the spinal cord which is considered to be due to the vascular disturbances in the lesion resulting in parenchymatous damage.

Abstracted from Hida et al. (1993) and Iannelli et al. (2005)

I.M. Eltorai, *Rare Diseases and Syndromes of the Spinal Cord*,
DOI 10.1007/978-3-319-45147-3_8

8.4 Clinical Picture

The patient was 50-year-old male presenting with weakness of the lower extremities, numbness in the right lower extremity, and sphincter dysfunction. The patient's diagnosis was erroneously labeled as syrinx for which syringosubarachnoid shunt was done. The condition neurologically deteriorated to tetraparesis. Reoperation was decided, the shunt was removed, posterior median myelotomy was done and capillary vessels were noted within the cord and were biopsied. Microscopically, they showed telangiectatic veins, engorged arterioles and venules, marked aggregation of the capillaries and vessels. Lymphocytes were perivascularly slight proliferation of astrocytes. Postoperatively slight worsening neurologically occurred, but he went back to the preoperative status shortly afterwards.

8.5 Diagnosis

MRI showed a non-enhanced mass, hypointense in T1-weighted images and hyperintense in T2-weighted images.

8.6 Management

The case described by Ianelli et al., the intramedullary tumor was successfully excised like other intramedullary tumors

References

Hida K, Tada M, Iwasaki Y, Abe H. Intramedullary disseminated capillary hemangioma with localized spinal cord swelling: case report. Neurosurgery. 1993;33(6):1099–101.

Iannelli A, Lupi G, Castagna M, Valleriani A, Becherini F, Bacherini F. Intramedullary capillary hemangioma associated with hydrocephalus in an infant. J Neurosurg. 2005;103(3 Suppl):272–6.

Intradural Extramedullary Capillary Hemangioma

9

9.1 Definition

Capillary hemangiomas are reddish-purple lesions and microscopically by the lobules of capillary-sized channels that are tightly aggregated into nodules nourished by feeding vessels.

9.2 Incidence

Capillary intradural extramedullary hemangiomas are rare. According to Kelleher et al. (2005), fewer than 20 cases have been reported.

9.3 Etiology

The cause is not clear

9.4 Pathology

The feeding vessels come from:

- Nerve roots as cauda equina
- Inner surface of the dura
- Pial vessels

Abstracted from Kelleher et al. (2005)

I.M. Eltorai, *Rare Diseases and Syndromes of the Spinal Cord*,
DOI 10.1007/978-3-319-45147-3_9

The mass is composed of capillary-sized vessels lined by flattened mature endothelial cells. The vessels masses are separated by fibrous septa. The tumor mass acts as a space occupying lesion, which leads to myelopathy or radiculopathy. They are subject to bleeding, which may cause subarachnoid hemorrhage and aggravate the neural deficit.

9.5 Clinical Picture

The tumor may be silent for long, until they reach such a size to cause cord compression. The symptoms are usually pain, sensory and motor changes, depending on the size.

9.6 Diagnosis

It is not easy to predict such a rare tumor and there are external physical signs pointing to it

MRI: The signal intensity of the tumor is isointense on T1-weighted images and hyperintense on T2-weighted images. Details can be seen in papers by Holanda et al. (2004), Choi et al. (2001), and Shin et al. (2000).

Should be differentiated from:

1. Cavernous hemangiomas
2. Arteriovenous malformation (AVM)
3. Hemangioblastoma or angiosarcoma
4. Paraganglioma
5. Metastasis
6. Sarcoidosis
7. Lymphoma
8. Filum terminale ependymoma
9. Neurinoma

Each of these pathologies has characteristic MRI.

9.7 Management

Since the tumor leads to myelopathy and/or radiculopathy it has to be surgically removed. Care is excised for complete hemostatis.

9.8 Updates

Miri et al. (2009)

The authors describe a case of a 20-year-old man complaining of back pain, radiating to both legs and paresthesia of the feet, weakness of the knee flexion and extension, urinary retention, impotence, and retrograde ejaculation. MRI showed an intradural mass, well defined at L3 level isointense at T1-weighted imaging and hyperintense at T2-weighted image with enhancement after gadolinium injection. Laminectomy at L3, after duratomy, a pinkish mass was found attached to one of the rootlets on the cauda equine and was ressected entirely. Histopathology showed capillary hemangioma. Postoperative recovery was attained without evidence of recurrence. The authors state vascular tumors account for 2–7 % of intraspinal tumors. Capillary hemangiomas within the boundries of the dura are extremely rare. They are usually distal in position, i.e., in the conus medullaris or in a root of cauda equine presenting with myelopathy or radiculopathy. As regards to the pathogenesis the capillary hemangioma arises from the vessels of nerve roots or from the subpial vessels. For the pathogenesis there are two hypotheses:

- The lesion may evolve during the early somatic differentiation at the time of angoblastic differentiation (days 21–24 of embryogenesis) due to the impaired movement and differentiation of the primitive mesoderm for the embryonic mesodermal plate.
- It may arise from the vascular structures within the epineurium of the nerve roots during individual during ontogenesis.

As regards to the histopathology the tumor is multilobular with pseudo-capsule. Its structure is made of capillaries lined with flattened endothelium. The lobules are separated by collagen partitions. Mild lymphocytic infiltrations may be found. Histochemical immune tests are positive against neuron-specific enolase and S-100 protein. The tumor cells stain strongly positive for endothelial markers CD31 and CD34, which are compatible with the diagnosis of capillary hemangioma.

Reference

Miri SM, Habibi Z, Hashemi M, Meybodi AT, Tabatabai SA. Capillary hemangioma of cauda equina: a case report. Cases J. 2009;2(1):80.

References

Choi BY, Chang KH, Choe G, et al. Spinal intradural extramedullary capillary hemangioma: MR imaging findings. AJNR Am J Neuroradiol. 2001;22(4):799–802.

Holanda MM, Sarmento SA, Andrade RV, Nóbrega Ede S, Silva JA. Capillary hemangioma of the spinal cord: case report. Arq Neuropsiquiatr. 2004;62(2A):357–9.

Kelleher T, Aquilina K, Keohane C, O'sullivan MG. Intramedullary capillary haemangioma. Br J Neurosurg. 2005;19(4):345–8.

Shin JH, Lee HK, Jeon SR, Park SH. Spinal intradural capillary hemangioma: MR findings. AJNR Am J Neuroradiol. 2000;21(5):954–6.

Spinal Intradural Cerebellar Ectopia 10

10.1 Definition

This is a condition in which cerebellar tissue is found in the spinal canal intradurally. It is independent from the Chiari I malformation, where the cerebellar tonsils are found in the upper cervical canal and from Chiari II, where the vermis is herniated in the spinal canal.

10.2 Incidence

Chung et al., reported the first case of true isolated cerebellar tissue in the lower cervical spine.

10.3 Etiology

The exact cause is not known; however, the authors theorized the development of this anomaly. They think that differentiation of totipotential cells within the dorsal aspect of an endomesenchymal tract lead to the formation of a structure resembling the cerebellar tissue.

10.4 Pathology

The mass was intradural dorsal to the spinal cord. It resembled cerebellar hemisphere with densely packed foliae, the dorsal and lateral wall were covered by thickened arachnoid. Microscopically it showed cerebellar cortex comprised of an outer

Abstracted from Chung et al. (1998)

I.M. Eltorai, *Rare Diseases and Syndromes of the Spinal Cord*,
DOI 10.1007/978-3-319-45147-3_10

and inner molecular granular cells in layers. Deep to the cells were Purkinje cells. An internal medullary layer was also present.

10.5 Clinical Picture

A boy 14 months old came with progressive scoliosis of 6 months duration. When he walked the left foot was everted, mild hyperreflexia of the lower limbs and positive right Babinski sign.

10.6 Diagnosis

Diagnosis is based on the following criteria:

- Radiography: midline segmental anomalies of T1–T3
- MRI: a mass in the spinal canal dorsal to the spinal cord at C6–C7 level. The mass was isointense with spinal cord in both T1 and T2 weighted images but did not enhance with gadolinium injection. Below the mass the spinal canal was wider and a cystic abnormality was seen. T2 showed clefting

10.7 Management

The mass was approached after duratomy and was entirely removed. Twelve months post-operative there was no recurrence and the neurological status was unchanged.

Reference

Chung CJ, Castillo M, Fordham L, Mukherji S, Boydston W, Hudgins R. Spinal intradural cerebellar ectopia. AJNR Am J Neuroradiol. 1998;19(5):897–9.

Cystic Dilatation of the Conus Ventriculus Terminalis

11

11.1 Definition

The ventriculus terminalis (VT) of the conus medullaris referred to as the fifth ventricle is the ependymal-lined space in the middle of the conus. It is present in childhood and its presence in adults is rare as dilatation to form a cyst is also rare. Cystic dilation causes cauda equine syndrome.

11.2 Incidence

Ciappetta et al., reviewed the literature and found 22 cases and added two elderly patients.

11.3 Etiology

The ventriculus terminalis is identifiable in the embryo between 43 and 48 days after conception as part of the caudal neural tube and it regresses after birth although it may be detected by MRI in 2.6 % of children under 5 years of age. For further details of embryology see Ciappetta et al.; for anatomical details see Kernohan et al. The cyst represents failure of regression. Possible etiologies according to Brisman et al.:

1. Failure of fusion of the cranial and caudal neural tube due to congenital disease, trauma, or ischemia
2. Association between spinal dysraphism and tethered cord

Abstracted from Ciappetta et al. (2008)

I.M. Eltorai, *Rare Diseases and Syndromes of the Spinal Cord*,
DOI 10.1007/978-3-319-45147-3_11

3. A type of caudal syrinx or hydromyelia, which is not communicating with the central canal
4. Ciappetta et al., state a possible involvement of the Reissner fiber in the pathogenesis of the VT should not be completely excluded. A Reissner fiber lesion could involve a localized dilatation of the CSF composition and dynamics causing a dilatation of the ependymal canal.

However the exact cause is unknown. Ciappetta et al., based on their study data in surgery and histological characteristic of the lesion stating that the dilatation of the ventriculus termanalis is distinct from other cystic dilatations of the conus medullaris.

11.4 Pathology

The ventriculus terminalis, like a ventricular structure is lined by ciliated ependymal cells and is termed the "fifth ventricle". It is continuous with the central canal of the anterior portion of the spinal cord (Ciappetta et al. 2008). In 11 cases reviewd by Celli et al., one had a sacral lipoma and one had Chiari malformation type I. for detailed histological and ultrastructural characteristics of the VT see Choi et al.

11.5 Clinical Picture

Cystic dilatation of the ventriculus terminalis (CDVT) may be asymptomatic and may be discovered by an MRI done for other purposes. When symptoms develop they may be mild or severe and in between. The course may be acute or chronic. The symptoms are pain in the lower back, lumbar-sacral, sciatica-like. When the cauda and the conus are involved the patient develops shooting pains in the legs, muscle weakness, gait trouble, sphincter dysfunction, especially incontinence urinary and rectal. Sensory impairment may be detected. The distal tendon reflexes are reduced. The clinical picture is that of conus compression and/or the cauda equine.

11.6 Diagnosis

Diagonsis is based on:

1. History
2. Neurological signs
3. MRI: The cyst is well outlined and ahs signal intensity identical to the CSF on both T1 and T2 weighted images. Usually there is no contrast enhancement. The surrounding tissue is thinned out to about 2 mm.
4. Ultrasonography: can be done as preliminary test

11.7 Management

1. Asymptomatic cysts and these incidentally discovered should be treated conservatively, with a follow up clinically and by MRI.
2. Symptomatic cases with neurological deficit should be operated upon to avoid further disabilities (cauda equine syndrome). Surgery is done through a laminectomy, a midline myelotomy and cyst drainage may be enough.
3. Others use marsupialization or cystosubarachnoid tube drainage or cyst fenestration. (see Brisman et al. 2006, for further details)

The results of surgery are satisfactory with reversal of most neurological deficits, although not all of them. Post-operative follow up is important to rule out recurrence and to monitor the result of surgery.

References

Brisman JL, Li M, Hamilton D, Mayberg MR, Newell DW. Cystic dilation of the conus ventriculus terminalis presenting as an acute cauda equina syndrome relieved by decompression and cyst drainage: case report. Neurosurgery. 2006;58(3):E585; discussion E585.

Ciappetta P, D'urso PI, Luzzi S, Ingravallo G, Cimmino A, Resta L. Cystic dilation of the ventriculus terminalis in adults. J Neurosurg Spine. 2008;8(1):92–9.

Syringomyelia in Association with Dandy-Walker Syndrome

12

12.1 Definition

Dandy-Walker complex (DWC) is a condition in which there is atresia of foramena of Magendie and Luschka causing congenital hydrocephalus. There is partial or complete absence of the cerebellar vermis, posterior fossa cyst formation, continuous with the fourth ventricle. The cyst expands in the middle line causing the occipital bone to bulge and to dislodge the tentorium and torcula upward. There is an obstruction of the foramen magnum with alteration of the CSF flow dynamics resulting in cervicothoracic syrinx.

12.2 Incidence

Hammond et al., reviewed the literature and tabulated 17 cases and added their own adult case of herniation of the DW cyst which blocked the foramen magnum resulting in cervicothoracic syrinx, which was reduced in size after cystoperitoneal shunting. In 2008, Kasliwal et al. (2008), reported a pediatric case of Dandy-Walker malformation associated with syringomyelia.

12.3 Etiology

The cause of DWC formation is atresia or occlusion of foramen of Magendie or foramen of Luschka, resulting in congenital hydrocephalus with dilatation of the fourth ventricle, the aqueduct, the third and lateral ventricles. A cystic structer representing the dilated fourth ventricle expands the midline and eventually herniated; blocking the foramen magnum and the end result is a syrinx.

Abstracted from Hammond et al. (2002)

I.M. Eltorai, *Rare Diseases and Syndromes of the Spinal Cord*,
DOI 10.1007/978-3-319-45147-3_12

12.4 Clinical Picture

The condition may be observed in neonates, some of whom may not survive due to other abnormalities. They will show hydrocephalus, possible papilledema, and occasional cranial palsy.

12.5 Diagnosis

Diagnosis is based on:

1. Clinical picture
2. X-ray and MRI: will show syrinx and DWC

12.6 Management

Cystoperitoneal shunting, sometimes ventriculopertioneal shunting in addition or posterior fossa decompression.

References

Hammond CJ, Chitnavis B, Penny CC, Strong AJ. Dandy-Walker complex and syringomyelia in an adult: case report and discussion. Neurosurgery. 2002;50(1):191–4.

Kasliwal MK, Suri A, Sharma BS. Dandy Walker malformation associated with syringomyelia. Clin Neurol Neurosurg. 2008;110(3):317–9.

13 Myelopathy Due to Duplication of the Laminae

13.1 Definition

This is a congenital condition in which the laminae are duplicated causing a mass effect resulting in cord compression

13.2 Incidence

Two cases have been reported by Cushman.

13.3 Etiology

This is a congenital abnormality of which the cause is not clear

13.4 Pathology

There is a duplication of the laminae encroaching on the spinal canal causing stenosis and cord compression. The embryology of the laminae can be consulted in textbooks of embryology.

13.5 Clinical Picture

The condition is asymptomatic in childhood and teenage years. With development of the bone and perhaps a minor trauma, symptoms appear. In the case reported a 23-year-old man developed weakness of the lower extremities and became

Abstracted from Cushman (1988)

I.M. Eltorai, *Rare Diseases and Syndromes of the Spinal Cord*,
DOI 10.1007/978-3-319-45147-3_13

paraplegic in a few months with sphincteric dysfunctions and parasthesias of the lower extremities. The reflexes were exaggerated with ankle clonus and positive Babinski.

13.6 Diagnosis

Diagnosis is based on the following criteria:

1. Radiography of the spine: sharply marginated osseous density inside the posterior elements
2. CT scan: severe spinal stenosis with cord compression due to a posterior wall marginated osseous density representing the duplication of the laminae.
3. Myelography: complete block at T10–T11

No electrophysiological studies were performed.

13.7 Management

Cord compression was diagnosed and surgical decompression was done. After exposure of the posterior elements, the laminae were removed. Incomplete recovery was attained postoperatively.

Reference

Cushman JD. Duplication of cord laminae resulting in cord compression. AJNR Am J Neuroradiol. 1988;9(2):408–9.

14 Compression Myelopathy Due to an Intramedullary Cyst Containing Ectopic Choroidal Plexus Tissue

14.1 Definition

This is a unique condition where there is ectopic choroid tissue in the spinal cord causing pressure myelopathy.

14.2 Incidence

This is a single case reported, whereas intracranial cysts containing ectopic choroid plexus or choroid-like tissue has been rare rarely reported (five cases).

14.3 Etiology

The choroid plexus develops from the tela choroidea and projects into the lateral ventricle on its medial aspect, roof of the third ventricles and roof of the fourth ventricle. Such tissue or tissue like it has been found in the epithelial linked non-communicating cysts intracranially. The exact causative factor is still unknown. It is considered as a developmental abbreviation with a theory that the same origin and that the ectopic choroid is formed by metaplasia of the ependymal rest.

14.4 Pathology

The histopathology and the immunohistochemical exam showed a normal choroid plexus consisting of a single layer of choroid epithelium arranged in microvillar pattern with a microvascular core. Immunohistochemical staining showed with glia

Abstracted and reported by Dwarakanath et al. (2005)

I.M. Eltorai, *Rare Diseases and Syndromes of the Spinal Cord*,
DOI 10.1007/978-3-319-45147-3_14

fibrillary acid protein and epithelial membrane architecture suggestive of a normal choroid plexus confirming the ectopic choroid plexus nature.

14.5 Case Report

A 30-year-old man complained of progressive descending weakness from the upper to the lower limbs giving the neurological picture of tetraparesis.

14.6 Diagnosis

Diagnosis is based on the following criteria:

1. MRI of the spine: Expansion of the spinal canal; C6–T2 intramedullary cystic lesion: hypointense on T1 weighted images and hyperintense on T2 weighted images. More details show holocord syrinx.

14.7 Management

Since the patient had compression myelopathy microsurgery was through laminectomy C6–T2, the dura was expanded, opened, the cord distended, paper thin myelotomy and syringostomy through the cyst, which was dissected and removed with its choroid content. Laminoplasty with miniplates and screws was done with uneventful post-operative course.

Reference

Dwarakanath S, Suri A, Mahapatra AK, Mehta VS, Sharma MC. Intramedullary ectopic choroid plexus: report of a rare case. Neurosurgery. 2005;56:869.

Chiari 1 Malformation and Holocord Syringomyelia in Hunter Syndrome

15

15.1 Definition

Hunter syndrome, mucopolysaccharidosis type II, MPS-II, or iduronate-2-sulphatase deficiency is cause by deficiency of enzyme L-iduronate-2-sulphate. Hunter syndrome has two clinical subtypes. It shows X-linked recessive inheritance and is the only one of mucopolysacchariodosis in which the mother alone can pass the defective gene to the son.

Chiari malformation I (CM1) is a congenital cerebellar tonsil downward ectopically causing holocord syringomyelia.

15.2 Incidence

Hunter syndrome develops in 1:100,000 to 150,000 male births. Chiari malformation 1 (CM1) appears in 1:100 of pediatric population.

15.3 Etiology

MPS-II is an X-linked recessive lysosomal storage disorder caused by iduronate-2-sulphatase (IDS) deficiency. The resulting lysosomal accumulation of upstream metabolites affects a variety of organ systems, including visceral organs, skeleton, connective tissue, and the CNS.

Abstracted from Manara et al. (2014)

I.M. Eltorai, *Rare Diseases and Syndromes of the Spinal Cord*,
DOI 10.1007/978-3-319-45147-3_15

15.4 Pathology

Skeletal changes glycosaminoglycans (GAG) accumulation in the growing cartilage results in the dens dysplasia and atlantoaxial instability. Subsequent periodontoid fibrocartilaginous tissue deposition with upper cervical stenosis results in compression myelopathy and holocord syringomyelia.

Other skeletal abnormalities scoliosis, kyphosis, joint stiffness

Cranial abnormalities CM1 as described in the case report

Chiari malformation Chiari malformation I is due to the underdevelopment of mesenchymal structures forming the clivus and posterior cranial fossa bones. In 90 % of cases holocord syringomyelia there is also CM1. In CM1 there are congenital impingements of the cerebellar tonsils due to discrepancy between the size of the posterior cranial fossa and the volume of the cerebellar structures. The abnormal postion of the cerebellar tonsils interferes with cerebrospinal fluid dynamics at the foramen magnum is possibly the cause of spinal cord damage, leading to holocord syringomyelia, which may involve the medulla oblongata.

Soft connective and mesenchymal tissues are affected by MPS-II leading to abnormalities of bone growth e.g., dysostosis multiplex and possibly CM1.

15.5 Clinical Picture

Primary mesenchymal involvement of the cranio-occipital region, the coexistence of CM1 and MPS-II might not be unexpected and complicate further the disease in these patients. Strict monitoring a prompt treatment might be of foremost importance for preventing major neurological complications. At birth the child appears normal; gradually, the child develops morphologic changes: recurrent respiratory infections, joint stiffness and organomegaly. About 10 % of MPS-II patients with severe upper spinal canal stenosis causing compression myelopathy, this may require decompression surgery. The signs and symptoms may overlap with those of other systems involved. Diagnosis and monitoring will depend on MRI findings in the craniocervical region particularly for spinal stenosis and CM1. In the cranium underdevelopment of mesenchymal structures forming the clivus and the cranial fossa are to be observed. The onset is insidious and slowly progresses. In CM1 there is headache, neck pain and brain stem dysfunction and syringomyelia e.g., motor and disassociate sensory impairments and scoliosis.

15.6 Diagnosis

Diagnosis is based on the following criteria:

1. Clinical examination
2. Biochemical examination
    - Urinary glycosaminoglycans are high
    - L-iduronate-2-sulphatase activity of leukocytes is low
    - Genetic studies reveals c.589-592 del CCTG of IDS gene
3. MRI reveals shows the J-shaped pituitary sella, enlargement of the perivascular (Virchow-Robin) spaces in the corpus callosum and semiovale bilaterally. Moderate ventricular enlargement. Ectopic cerebellar tonsils 6 mm below the foramen magnum, evidence of CM1. MRI of the craniocervical region shows dens hypoplasia with periodontoid cap leading to stenosis of the cervical spinal canal. MRI of the brain shows cerebral atrophy. MRI of the spine shows syringomyelia and compression of the cord, a holocord syrinx from the cervico-medullary junction to the conus medullaris.

15.7 Management

- Enzyme replacement therapy: idursulfase (Elaprase (R)) at a dose of 0.5 mg/kg per week
- Surgical therapy:
  - Decompressive suboccipital craniectomy
  - C1 laminectomy
  - duraplasty

The result was clinical and neurological improvement and relief from neurological symptoms and bladder and bowel incontinence and complete disappearance of the syrinx.

In conclusion this case highlights that a cerebellar tonsils impingement in MPS-II patients does not strictly depend on the size of the posterior cranial fossa and that a low position of the tonsils should be noted even in the presence of an enlarged cisterna manga. The cerebellar tonsil impingement in MPS-II patients may require very close monitoring with MPS-II myelomalacia and multi-organ involvement. The MPS-II related instability of the atlanto-axial junction leads to spinal canal stenosis and consequent syringomyelia. The roll of surgery is important in MPS-II patients with syringomyelia to improve the neurological impairment.

Reference

Manara R, Concolino D, Rampazzo A, et al. Chiari 1 malformation and holocord syringomyelia in hunter syndrome. JIMD Rep. 2014;12:31–5.

Myelopathy in Infantile Myofibromatosis

16

16.1 Definition

Infantile myofibromatosis (IMF) is a congenital disease characterized by formation of benign tumors either single or multiple, arising form cells supporting and binding the tissues of the body as well as smooth muscle tissues. The potentially massive tumors arise from the skin, subcutaneous tissues, muscles, bones, and viscera.

16.2 Incidence

According to Tamburrini et al., it is the commonest fibrous disorder of infancy and childhood. According to Wada et al., in 1998, six cases of spinal canal involvement were reported and added a case of their own. Tamburrini et al., reported the first solitary case of spinal canal IMF.

16.3 Etiology

The condition is congenital. Extensive search did not show the genetics of this tumor.

16.4 Pathology

The tumor is benign, but it tends to be massive and has a tendency to regress with age. It is either solitary or multicenteric. It involves many tissues e.g., skin, subcutaneous tissues, muscles, bones, central nervous system (CNS) and viscera. It is

Abstracted from Tamburrini et al. (2003)

I.M. Eltorai, *Rare Diseases and Syndromes of the Spinal Cord*,
DOI 10.1007/978-3-319-45147-3_16

encapsulated. Histologically it consists of spindle shaped cells without mitosis, lymphocytic infiltration, collagen bundles, and a prominent vascular pattern simulating hemangipericytoma in the central pattern. According to Wada et al. (1998), immunohistochemistry shows immuo-reactivity for vimentin but desmin, neurofilament, neuron-specific enolase and leukocyte common antigen are negative. They report gross necrosis hemorrhage and dystrophic calcification. The paravertebral tumor in the authors' case extended into the spinal canal through the intervetebral foramen. The pelvic tumor compressed the ureter leading to hydronephrosis. There was bone involvement. They referred to nine intracanal involvement cases usually epidural calvarial masses causing compression. Adickes et al., reported a case of multicenteric tumors on the spinal epidural surface and within the parenchyma of the spinal cord.

16.5 Clinical Picture

IMF may be detected after birth (congenital) or within the first few weeks during which the tumor is becoming hypertrophic or it may initially appear within the first 2 years of life. Small non-visceral tumors may be asymptomatic. Generally there is a period of rapid growth, then stabilization and then regression. Small or residual tumors may eventually regress completely. Multicenteric progressive visceral tumors are life threatening due to complications. The spinal cord may be involved by compression in the presence of a paravertebral tumor or the tumor may intramedullary as in the case reported by Tamburrini et al. In either case there is paralysis of the lower extremities and bladder dysfunction. It may be associated with cerebral symptoms due to intracranial involvement peripheral nerves or viscera. Intrapelvic tumors give rise to pressure on ureter resulting in hyperureter and hydronephrosis. Osseous lesions give rise to pathological fractures. Diminick reported a case with cervical myofibromatosis leading to tetraparesis, at the same patient had a parietal mass. Adickes et al., reported a case of spinal and cerebral involvement.

16.6 Diagnosis

Diagnosis is base on:

1. Clinical history from patients
2. Neurological assessment
3. The presence of mass especially paravertebral
4. X-ray: shows extremity fractures
5. CT scan: showed paravertebral tumor invading the spinal canal
6. MRI: showed involvement of the spinal canal and rarely intraperichymatous involvement of the spinal cord.
7. Brain studies: show epidural mass

8. Histopathology: CT guided needle biopsy will show the pathology as mentioned aboved.

It should be differentiated from disseminated neuroblastoma, soft tissue sarcoma, histiocytosis X, lymphangiomatosis and neurofibromatosis.

16.7 Management

- Small non-visceral asymptomatic masses may be left alone with frequent monitoring, since spontaneous regression is possible.
- Involvement of the spinal cord: in the presence of paralysis mass reduction is indicated, the residual mass will usually regress.
- Intrapelvic mass may be resected if causing visceral pressure such as hydronephrosis.
- Chemotherapy and/or radio therapy have been tried in children with unresectable or rapidly progressive disease.

References

Wada H, Akiyama H, Seki H, Ichihara T, Ueno K, Miyawaki T, Koizumi S. Spinal canal involvement in infantile myofibromatosis: case report and review of the literature. J Pediatr Hematol Oncol. 1998;20(4):353–6.

Tamburrini G, Gessi M, Colosimo Jr C, Lauriola L, Giangaspero F, Di Rocco C. Infantile myofibromatosis of the central nervous system. Childs Nerv Syst. 2003;19(9):650–4. Epub 2003 Apr 29.

Tetraparesis in Laurence-Moon-Biedl-Bardet Syndrome

17

17.1 Definition

Laurence-Moon-Biedl-Bardet (LMBB) syndrome is manifested by:

- Polydactyly
- Obesity
- Hypogonadism
- Retinitis pigmentosa
- Mental retardation

To diagnose the syndrome at least four of the above features must be present. There are seven heredity syndromes related to LMBBS deafness, ataxia, diabetes mellitus, renal involvement, quadriparesis, or paraplegia.

17.2 Incidence

The authors refer to a few cases previously reported.

17.3 Pathology

No data available. Their case had spinal stenosis causing myelopathy, which was the first case.

Nyska et al. (1991)

I.M. Eltorai, *Rare Diseases and Syndromes of the Spinal Cord*,
DOI 10.1007/978-3-319-45147-3_17

17.4 Clinical Picture

A 36-year-old male presented with postataxial polydactyly, retinitis pigmentosa, obesity, hypogonadism and borderline mental retardation. He suffered inability to walk with micturition dysfunctions.

Neurological exam showed lead-pipe quadriplegia. Spasticity was more marked in the lower than the upper limbs and the right side more than then left. Patellar and ankle reflexes were brisk, with patellar and ankle clonus and had bilateral Babinki sign. Sensory damage was bilateral hypoesthesia from C2 downwards. Hip joint movements were limited. According to JOA score to be one point. Urodynamics showed spastic sphincter, necessitating a sphincterotomy.

Radiography and CT scan showed cervical and lumbar stenosis. The narrowness interpedicular distance of the cervical spine was 15 and 14 mm in the lumbar vertebrae. The smallest anteroposterior distance was 3 mm at C3 and 10 mm at L3 vetebra. There was also platyspondyly and Schmorl nodes of almost all thoracic vertebral bodies. MRI showed almost complete block of the cervical cord with almost complete block of the cervical canal with atrophy of the cord at C3–C4 and C6. Similar changes were seen in the lumbar spine.

17.5 Management

Laminoplasty C3–C6. Three months post-op, the cervical cord was wide; 6 months the patient could only stand with help but still with spastic tetraparesis.

Reference

Nyska M, Mozes G, Howard C, Bar-ziv J, Dekel S. Quadriparesis in the Laurence-Moon-Biedl-Bardet syndrome: case report. Paraplegia. 1991;29(5):350–4.

18 Lymphangiomatosis

18.1 Definition

Lymphangiomatosis is a disease of childhood, although was described in adults or elderly. It is characterized by abnormal lymph tissue in different sits of the body, except the neural tissue. There is skeletal and visceral involvement, the former leads to bone lysis, resulting in deformity, instability, and compression myelopathy.

18.2 Incidence

The disease is rare. The authors report 2 cases both are children.

18.3 Etiology

The disease is considered a congenital anomaly, although the neoplastic nature is still considered. Familial cases have been described.

18.4 Pathology

The disease is multifocal collections of endothelial lined tissues containing eosinophilic stained material or lymph, this is contrast with hemangiomas in which red blood cells are found in endothelial lined spaces and both types may be combined to hemangiolymphogioma. Extraskeletal involvement is common 75 % in the liver, spleen, and lungs. Skeletal involvement is up to 67 % and affects skull, ribs,

Watkins et al. (2003)

I.M. Eltorai, *Rare Diseases and Syndromes of the Spinal Cord*,
DOI 10.1007/978-3-319-45147-3_18

shoulder, girdle, spine, and pelvis. Other nomenclature given to the disease depending on its pathological picture:

- Generalized lympangiectosis
- Cystic lymphangiotosis
- Diffused skeletal angiomatose
- Massive osteolysis
- Gorham's disease or disappearing bone disease is different being unifocal and not accompanied by extraskeletal changes.

18.5 Clinical Picture

Usually children are subjects of lyphangiomatosis, 65 % but older adults and even elderly presented the disease. There is usually a swelling in the neck, there is pain, spinal deformity. Different sites are involved, especially the ribs, skull, and the spine. Cord compression is manifested by weakness, inability to walk, and sensory changes. Chylothorax and/or chylophericardium may be seen.

18.6 Diagnosis

Diagnosis based on:

1. Clinical history, which may date to infancy
2. Physical exam: swelling
3. Deformities of the cervical and thoracic spine, possible pathological fracture
4. Neurological assessment
5. Evoked potentials
6. Radiological

18.7 Management

Surgery is indicated when lymphangiomatosis causes neural compression and instability of the spine. Surgical outcome is strongly influenced by extraskeletal involvement.

Reference

Watkins RG, Reynolds RA, Mccomb JG, Tolo VT. Lymphangiomatosis of the spine: two cases requiring surgical intervention. Spine. 2003;28(3):E45–50.

Ischemic Myelopathy Due to Marfan's Syndrome

19

19.1 Definition

Marfan's syndrome (MFS) is an inherited disorder that affects the connective tissue as an autosomal dominant disorder with muscoskeletal, ocular, and cardiovascular manifestations. Patients usually have unusual height, large hands and feet and involvement of the lungs.

19.2 Incidence

It affects about 1 in 5,000–10,000 individuals. There are sporadic cases of spinal involvement, exact incidence is not known. Spinal cord infarcts are rare. Wityk et al., in a study of 513 patients 18 patients had neurovascular diagnosis (3.5 %). Two cases had spinal cord ischemia (0.38 %), one was an infarct and one with spinal cord subarachnoid hemorrhage.

19.3 Etiology

Clinical expression of the genetic defects however, can be variable both within and between families. It is one of the most common genetic disorders of connective tissue. Approximately 75 % of patients inherited the disease through family members, and 25 % are sporadic.

Abstracted from Wityk et al. (2002)

I.M. Eltorai, *Rare Diseases and Syndromes of the Spinal Cord*,
DOI 10.1007/978-3-319-45147-3_19

19.4 Pathology

In two genes FBN1 (causing MFS1) and TGFBR2 (MFS2) have been associated with MFS. Wityk et al. have studied the neurovascular complications of MFS, which is the principal source of this paper. We will forgo the cerebral complications and focus on the spinal cord. In medium and large sized arteries defects in fibrillation are associated with disruption of the elastic fibers predisposing to arterial aneurysms and arterial dissection, which cause brain and spinal cord ischemia (10–20 %) of patients with MFS. The possible causes of ischemia are:

- Arterial dissection reading the spinal arteries
- Hemorrhage due to anticoagulants
- Embolism from prosthetic valves and arterial fribrillation.

19.5 Clinical Picture

Infarction or compression of the cord results in paraplegia with sensory-motor deficits and sphincteric dysfunction. The patient has typical MFS and most probably family history (75 %).

19.6 Diagnosis

Diagnosis is based on the following criteria:

1. Family history
2. Clinical picture
3. Paresis and sensory deficit
4. Cardiovascular abnormalities

Angiography should be performed if safe

19.7 Management

- Vascular management e.g., grafting for dissecting aneurysm
- Anticoagulation for embolism or thrombosis
- Spinal cord infarct is not reversible
- Compression by hematoma may need decompression

Reference

Wityk RJ, Zanferrari C, Oppenheimer S. Neurovascular complications of marfan syndrome: a retrospective, hospital-based study. Stroke. 2002;33(3):680–4.

Myelopathy in Neurocutatneous Melanosis

20

20.1 Definition

The neural crest is the common embryonic origin of both the melanotic cells of the skin and the leptomeninges. According to these authors neurocutaneous melanosis (NCM) is a congenital syndrome characterized by the development of congenital melanocytic naevi and benign or malignant melanotic tumors of the CNS. NCM is considered a rare complication of giant congenital meano-cytic-naevus (GCMN).

20.2 Incidence

The risk of developing benign or malignant melanotic tumors in carries of GCMN is unknown; just over 100 cases were reported (2001). Involvement of the brain will not be discussed. Myelopathy is the subject of this presentation.

20.3 Etiology

NCM is thought to be due to an error in the embryogenesis of the embryological neuroectoderm.

20.4 Pathology

There is melanotic pigmentation of the spinal arachnoid and adjacent leptomeninges. Cord compression is usually due to development of melanotic arachnoid cyst or to direct infiltration or syringomyelia. The chance of malignant progression and

Abstracted from Holmes et al. (2001)

I.M. Eltorai, *Rare Diseases and Syndromes of the Spinal Cord*,
DOI 10.1007/978-3-319-45147-3_20

prognosis are unknown. Twenty percent of cases show or display widespread pigmentation and thickening of the full length of the spinal cord meninges. Malignant transformation in the CNS is estimated to be up to 50 %.

20.5 Clinical Picture

Patients with GCMN on the extremities never develop NCM. Posterior axial nevi are more subject to NCM. CNS involvement excluding intracranial lesions may be asymptomatic. Cord compression or infiltration will give the picture of myelopathy. Radicular syndrome is also common.

20.6 Diagnosis

Diagnosis is based on:

1. Congenital nevi
2. Neurological findings
3. MRI: for symptomatic patients and all asymptomatic patients with large multiple lesions of the head and neck or lesions of the posterior midline.

20.7 Management

Close observation of these lesions regularly by the dermatologist. There is no therapy for leptomeningial melanotic changes. Space occupying lesions may be approached neurosurgically.

Reference

Holmes G, Wines N, Ryman W. Giant congential melanocytic naevus and symptomatic thoracic arachnoid cyst. Australas J Dermatol. 2001;42(2):124–8.

21 Myelopathy in Osteogenesis Imperfecta

21.1 Definition

Osteogenesis imperfecta (OI) is heterogeneous group of congenital disorders of collagen synthesis, characterized by generalized osteoporosis and multiple fractures. It is caused by a genetic mutation in abnormal production of type-I collagen. The major clinical characteristics of OI:

- osteopenia
- bone fragility (fragilitas ossium)
- blue sclera
- dentinogenesis imperfecta
- short stature
- loss of hearing

There are seven major types of OI. The classification is based on disease severity and progression. However, the disease is presented as a continuum and it is hard to put any patient in a certain category. Also patients of the same category may have different histological pictures. Of the seven types of OI, types V, VI, and VII are not associated with type-I collagen defects. More details about genetics can be seen in the article by Roughley, Rauch, and Glorieux.

21.2 Incidence

OI may affect more than 1:10,000 individuals

Abstracted from Daivajna et al. (2005)

I.M. Eltorai, *Rare Diseases and Syndromes of the Spinal Cord*,
DOI 10.1007/978-3-319-45147-3_21

21.3 Etiology

The hereditary trait is usually transmitted as an autosomal dominant with variable expressivity. As to the cause of the deformity, poor bone mass, fractures, laxity of ligaments, microfractures of the growth plate will result in a congenital hemi-vertebrae.

21.4 Pathology

Microscopically the cortical is thin to the point of porosity. As to the cancellous trabeculæ, they are slender, delicate, widely separated, and few in number. Few osteoblasts can be seen; osteocytes are crowded together by virtue of a lake of intervening matrix. The collagen fibers of the bone are thinner than normal and the collagen bundles have different dimensions. Wedged vertebra may be associated with disordered growth of the compressed vertebra.

21.5 Clinical Picture

Intrauterine death may occur due to fractures and hemorrhage or shortly thereafter. Survivors have a slower rate of growth and are libel to fractures in different sites. The picture of the patient has characteristics mentioned above; in addition, the neck is short and the skull is deformed. The skull may be so incomplete that it is a mere membranous bag or few boney plates; further ossification may present a large number of Wormian bones. There may be hydrocephalus. Deformities of the spine are usually are thoracolumbar kyphosis, scoliosis, cervical spondyloptosis, and rarely cervical kyphosis or loss of the cervical lordosis. As a result of the deformities craniocervical regions deformities develop as complications, namely, basilar impression (vertebral basilar invagination), atlantoaxial dislocation, and syringomyelia caused by obstruction of cerebral spinal fluid (CSF) outflow caused by basilar impression. The basilar impression may be caused by brainstem compression. In some cases atlantoaxial dislocation may lead to compression myelopathy upper motor tetraparesis. These deficits are exaggerated by myelopathy.

21.6 Diagnosis

In some cases, an ultrasound can identify bone abnormalities at 14–18 weeks. Cells obtained through chorionic villus sampling or amniocentesis can also be analyzed for a genetic mutation. Diagnosing OI is primarily a clinical process. It is often difficult or inconclusive without a physician familiar with the disorder.

21.7 Management

Currently, as a consequence of improved understanding of the molecular mechanisms of OI, medical treatments aimed at increasing bone mass and strength are gaining popularity, and surgery is reserved for functional improvement. Surgery remains a pillar of treatment for patients with OI, but it should be performed only if it is likely to improve function and only if the treatment goals are clear. Surgical interventions include intramedullary rod placement, surgery to manage basilar impression, and correction of scoliosis.

Reference

Daivajna S, Jones A, Hossein Mehdian SM. Surgical management of severe cervical kyphosis with myelopathy in osteogenesis imperfecta: a case report. Spine. 2005;30(7):E191–4.

22 Prader-Willi Syndrome

22.1 Definition

Prader-Willi syndrome (PWS) is a congenital condition due to loss of part or all of chromosome 15; specifically, the chromosome 15 from the father. It is characterized by hypotonia, hypogonadism, hypomentia, and obesity for which the acronym HHHO is given. It is usually associated with scoliosis, rarely kyphosis and spinal stenosis.

22.2 Incidence

Myelopathy due to PWS is very rare. Kyphosis has been described in 1991.

22.3 Etiology

PWS is a congenital condition due to partial or total loss of chromosome-15 from the father.

22.4 Pathology

Spinal cord compression is due to kyphosis, developmental stenosis, and dynamic factors (hypotonia or atonia) may include the etiological factors for myelopathy. Kyphosis itself is probably due to cervical muscles hypotonic and heaviness of the head. Hypotonia, mental retardation, and obesity may account for minor trauma, which may trigger the myelopathy to be manifested clinically.

Abstracted and reported by Tsuji et al. (1991)

I.M. Eltorai, *Rare Diseases and Syndromes of the Spinal Cord*,
DOI 10.1007/978-3-319-45147-3_22

22.5 Clinical Picture

The patient has typical picture of PWS with history of hypotonia, hypogonadism, mental retardation, slow development, hyperphagia or even bulimia and obesity. After minor trauma the picture of compression myelopathy is due to cervical kyphosis. It starts with weakness of the extremities, it progresses to tetraparesis, inability to walk or stand. Urinary dysfunction is also noted. The reflexes are exaggerated, and sensation may be preserved.

22.6 Diagnosis

Diagnosis is based on the following criteria:

1. X-ray findings reveal kyphosis with spondylitic changes, narrow spinal canal, may show some osteophytes.
2. MRI of the spinal cord shows cord compression.

22.7 Management

Initially Hal-Vest traction to correct the kyphosis and provide stability may improve the symptoms. According to Tsuji et al., surgery was done later by anterior cervical releasing followed 1 week later by anterior interbody fusion and halo-vest application for cervical spine stability and correction of the kyphosis, although the latter was not achieved.

Reference

Tsuji M, Kurihara A, Uratsuji M, Shoda E. Cervical myelopathy with Prader-Willi syndrome in a 13-year-old boy. A case report. Spine. 1991;16(11):1342–4.

Compression Myelopathy in Proteus Syndrome

23

23.1 Definition

Proteus syndrome is manifested by a disturbance of cell growth including benign tumors under the skin, overgrowth of the body, more on one side (hemihypertrophy), overgrowth of the fingers (macrodactyly) and spinal deformaties.

23.2 Incidence

The syndrome was first identified by Choen in 1973. The name coined by Widerman in 1983, after the Greek God Proteus, presumably due to various manifestations in the first unrelated boys first described. Since then 120 cases were reported, but not all are typical of the syndrome. In 1991, Ring and Snyder reported a case with compression myelopathy. Skovby et al., described two cases of spinal stenosis with cord compression.

23.3 Etiology

Spinal stenosis occurs as a result of:

- Ventral anomalies, e.g., high or irregular shaped vertebrae and pedicles, dystrophia and intervertebral discs, spondylomegaly, megaspondylodysplasia. These anomalies may account for elongation of the neck and or the trunk
- Scoliosis or kyphoscoliosis, which vary from mild to severe
- Cord compression may occur due to thoracic lipomatosis or angiolipoma that infiltrate the spinal canal and cause compression of the cord.

Abstracted from Skovby et al. (1993)

I.M. Eltorai, *Rare Diseases and Syndromes of the Spinal Cord*,
DOI 10.1007/978-3-319-45147-3_23

23.4 Pathology

This cord compression is due to spinal stenosis, vertebral deformities, anomalies of the vertebrae and soft tissue tumor infiltration through the intervertebral formena into the spinal canal. Takabayashi et al., discussed scoliosis in detail.

23.5 Clinical Picture

Proteus syndrome has characteristic pleomorphic manifestation. There are seven clinical manifestations at least four of them are associated with Proteus syndrome. These are included in the syndrome described by Samlaska et al., macrocephaly, eye abnormality, hemihypertrophy, macrodactyly, exostosis, epidermal nevi, cerebriform mass of the palmar and plantar surfaces, scoliosis, and metal deficiency. Other manifestations are loss of subcutaneous fat, hamartomas e.g., lipomas and hemangiolipomas or lymphangiomas, or lyphangiolipomas. Spinal stenosis, vertebral deformities, hamartomas lead to spinal cord compression. It is manifested by sensory and motor changes, as well as sphincteric disturbances.

23.6 Diagnosis

Diagnosis based on:

1. The morphology of the abnormalities of the Proteus syndrome: see clinical picture.
2. Neurolgical findings: mental status may or may not be deficient
3. Radiological findings: spinal deformaties, anomalies of the vertebrae, digital exostosis, macrocephaly.
4. CT scan may show spinal stenosis. Compression of the cord by myelography. Intrathoracic neoplasm: lipoma or hemangiolipoma with cord compression.
5. MRI shows cord compression

23.7 Management

Patients with Proteus syndrome are usually high risk in surgery, because they have thrombocytopenia and may develop pulmonary embolism. Intrathoracic tumors may be hemangiolipomas, which are vascular and risk of massive bleeding even after embolization. Decompressive laminectomy may be performed. For kyphoscoliosis, two-stage spondylodesis is the appropriate procedure. For irremovable tumors attempt steroids and interferon-alpha. For recurrent angiolipomas Cytoxan may be attempted.

Updates

Abstract from Yamamoto et al. (2012)

Proteus syndrome is a rare, sporadic, hamartomatous disorder manifesting with multifocal overgrowth of tissue. The features seem to develop most often during childhood. Vertebral overgrowth with severe spinal canal stenosis is unusual, although scoliosis with abnormal vertebral bodies is one of the typical features of Proteus syndrome. We report a case of Proteus syndrome with severe spinal canal stenosis, scoliosis, cervical kyphosis, and thoracic deformity with airway obstruction because of asymmetrical overgrowth of vertebrae and ribs associated with a tethered cord, lipomas, strawberry hemangioma, flat nasal bridge, and bilateral hypoplasty of the first metatarsal bones with hyperplasty of soft tissue.

Reference

Yamamoto A, Kikuchi Y, Yuzurihara M, Kubota M, O'uchi T. A case of Proteus syndrome with severe spinal canal stenosis, scoliosis, and thoracic deformity associated with tethered cord. Jpn J Radiol. 2012;30(4):336–9.

Reference

Skovby F, Graham JM, Sonne-holm S, Cohen MM. Compromise of the spinal canal in Proteus syndrome. Am J Med Genet. 1993;5:656–9.

Segmental Spinal Dysgenesis

24

24.1 Definition

Segmental spinal dysgenesis (SSD) is a rare congenital condition in which a segment of the spine and spinal cord fails to develop properly.

24.2 Incidence

The disease is rare, no world literature is available. Tortori-Donati et al., in their report in 1999, collected ten cases form two institutions in Italy and France from 1975 to 1998. In 2006 Bristol et al., reported four cases of SSD, in the same article in their review of the literature SSD have involved the lumbar or thoracic spine. Their case at C7–T1 shows the highest level of involvement.

24.3 Etiology

From Desai et al.:

> The embryogenesis of SSD is unclear. The probable cause is segmental maldevelopment of the neural tube. Programmed cell death, i.e. apoptosis, is a process of cell elimination that occurs in the course of normal development and represents a crucial phenomenon during various steps of embryogenesis. These apoptotic events occur at the time of axial identity and segmentation in the mesenchyme and neuroepithelium; wrongly specified cells in terms of their reostrocaudal position are eliminated (positional apoptosis). During human gastrulation, the prospective chorda-mesodermal cells migrating through the primitive pit and into the ectoderm-endoderm interface have a genetically determined destination along the longitudinal embryonic axis. An error in this positional imprinting could activate apoptotic events so that wrongly specified cells are eliminated and, eventually, fewer cells or even no

Abstracted from Tortori-Donati et al. (1999) and Desai et al. (2003)

I.M. Eltorai, *Rare Diseases and Syndromes of the Spinal Cord*,
DOI 10.1007/978-3-319-45147-3_24

cells at all form the chordo-mesoderm at a given abnormal segmental level. The consequences of such segmental chorda-mesodermal paucity are manifold and affect the development of the spinal column, spinal cord and nerve roots. These embryologic events manifest as a spectrum of spinal cord, nerves and vertebral column abnormalities described as SSD.

The real cause is still unknown.
Theories to the etiology

- Failure of caudal notocord
- Arrest of development of the caudal cell mass
- Trauma
- Vascular insult
- Maternal diabetes
- Toxins
- Medication: teratogenic drugs
- Vitamin A deficiency

Experimental details can be seen in the article by Desai et al.

24.4 Pathology

There is localized agenesis or dysgenesis of the lumbar, thoracolumbar, or rarely the lumbosacral spine. There is kyphosis and kyphoscoliosis and focal abnormalities of the spinal cord and its roots. The spinal cord is thinned or even discernible. Distally there may be a bulky, low lying segment of the cord caudal to the defect. Desai et al., reported a case of thoracic amyelia associated with SSD. Dysphasia may involve cord above and below the defect. Other associated anomalies may be present: closed spinal dysraphism including diastatomyelia, dermal sinus, lipoma, thickened filum terminale, and spina bifida. More details can be found in an article by Tortori-Donati et al., other abnormalities may be encountered in the spine, kidney, bladder, heart, ribs, feet, dysraphism, and amyelia.

24.5 Clinical Picture

Various pictures are encountered depending on the level and degree of the anomaly and associated anomalies. The consistent sign is an irregular kyphosis. Associated anomalies such as dysraphism, meningoma, lipomas, anomalies of the other organs, and deformities of the lower extremities can be seen in SSD. There is paraplegia, spastic or flaccid sensory loss and neurogenic bladder, the result of which is urinary tract infection, sepsis and vesico-ureteral reflux. Other spinal anomalies are sometimes encountered sacrococcygeal agenesis, butterfly vertebra, etc.

24.6 Diagnosis

Diagnosis is based on the following criteria:

1. Clinical findings include: gibbus, unstable spine, paraparesis or paraplegia, associated anomalies, and deformities of the lower extremities
2. Neuro-radiography: varies according to the extent and level of the dysgenesis.
   - Kyphosis or kyphoscoliosis,
   - defect of the missing vertebrae,
   - various anomalies including: aplastic, hypoplastic, or incompletely segmented vertebra,
   - narrow spinal canal, which may be absent at the apex of the gibbus.
3. MRI: The spinal cord above the defect is normal, in the defect is thinned or discernible no roots. The distal cord is bulky. There may be no distal cord due to hypoplasia. Amyelia has been described once (Desai et al.)

For neurological studies see Tortori-Donati et al.

24.7 Management

The common procedures are decompression and arthrodesis. Other procedures performed as indicated, e.g., release of tight filum terminale, disconnecting a neurenteric cyst and corrective surgeries on deformities of the lower limbs. Since the series of Tortori-Donati et al., is one of the largest I'll quote the procedures they had in their series followed up to 23 years. In their series of 100 spinal surgery was done in seven children; three patients had arthrodesis of the spine.

1 had posterior arthrodesis at age 1 year
1 had 2 posterior arthrodesis at age of 1 and 2.5 years
1 had posterior arthrodesis at age of 5 years, anterior arthrodesis at age of 5.2 and another posterior arthrodesis at age of 5.5
4 patients had surgical decompression anterior or posterior.

According to Desai et al.,

> There is considerable debate regarding optimal treatment of children with SSD. The role of spinal decompression is unclear because neurological deficits are related to the congenital hypoplasia in absence of an entire segment of the spinal cord and are irreversible. Detethering may be considered in cases where additional evidence of a closed dysraphism. Surgery is indicated in patients with relatively preserved neurological functions below the level of the anomaly and when significant compression of the cord is demonstrated on radiological examination. Decompression and spinal stabilization are needed as kyphosclerosis can cause neurological worsening.

On the other hand Bristol et al., states

> …incomplete ossification of the vertebral bodies and poor results of allografts materials restricts fusion option. Neurological deficits prevent ambulation and decrease the axial loading forces that enhance fusion. We allow spinal mobilization for 12–18 months before spinal fusion preferably rib or fibular allograft.

Bristol et al., do not allow instrumentation in infants except when the second graft is not enough by itself.

References

Desai K, Nadkarni T, Bhayani R, Goel A. Congenital thoracic cord segmental amyelia: a rare manifestation of segmental spinal dysgenesis. Pediatr Neurosurg. 2003;38:102–6.

Tortori-Donati P, Fondelli MP, Rossi A, Raybaud CA, Cama A, Capra V. Segmental spinal dysgenesis: neuroradiologic findings with clinical and embryologic correlation. AJNR Am J Neuroradiol. 1999;20:445–56.

Ischemic Myelopathy Due to Sickle Cell Trait

25

25.1 Definition

Sickle cell anemia or sickle hemoglobin (Hb S) disease is due to the characteristic phenomena of Hb S, which under conditions of low oxygen tension is crystallizes and this leads to sickling of the erythrocytes, which become trapped in the terminal arterioles and capillaries resulting in more hypoxia and consequently more sickling which results in thrombosis and ischemic infarction. Tissues that have blood at low oxygen tension e.g., the pulmonary arterioles and the renal parenchyma are more liable to sickling although tissues that have relatively oxygenated blood, e.g., the brain or spinal cord are not exempt. The sickle cells are rigid and less flexible and more fragile so they hemolyze. The possible complications of sickle cell anemia fall into five categories:

- painful crisis especially in the bone
- infection
- fat embolism: due to sickle cells accumulation in the bone marrow capillaries leading to fat necrosis, see Loupy et al. 2008
- vascular disease
- loss of vision

The focus of this paper will be on the last three and specifically the spinal cord.

25.2 Incidence

Stroke due to sickle cell anemia is common in childhood and accounts for high mortality. The overall prevalence of stroke in sickle cell patients is 20 %. Spinal cord infarct on the other hand is very rare. Few cases have been reported by Wolman and Hardy (1970) and Rothman and Nelson (1980).

Abstracted from Wolman and Hardy (1970)

I.M. Eltorai, *Rare Diseases and Syndromes of the Spinal Cord*,
DOI 10.1007/978-3-319-45147-3_25

25.3 Etiology

The genetic aspects of sickle cell anemia are beyond the presentation of this paper and can be consulted in hematology references. The etiology of the infarct in vascular occlusion is not clear it is proposed that:

- Hypodynamic circulation leads to endothelial damage by the sickle cell leading to thrombosis. Also leucocyte-endothelial adhesion.
- An opposite view that chronic stasis leads to thrombosis.
- The sickle cells occlude the vasa vasara of large vessels producing ischemia of the vessel wall, which leads to thrombosis.

More detailed studies can be seen in the works of Kaul et al., and Mohandes and Evans. Quoting from Kaul et al.:

In the oxy-condition, initiation of sickle cell vaso-oclusion may involve:

- Microvascular topographical characteristics, perfusion pressure changes, arterio-venous wall shear rate gradient, and the loss of vascular adjustments.
- Continuation of specific density classes in the adhesion and obstruction.
- The inverse correlation of sickle cell adhesion with the vascular diamteres in accordance with the wall shear rate profiles in the microcirculation.
- Random trapping of intravascular sickle cells at the arteriolar-capillary bifurcation points and selective secondary trapping of the densest cells in the post-capillary venules, where sickle cells have preferentially adhered.

25.4 Pathology

Postmortem cases show multiple infarcts of the spinal cord with necrosis evidenced by vascular occlusions. Cerebral infarcts are also detected.

25.5 Clinical Picture

The disease has a racial predisposition usually African descent. Other manifestations of sickle cell disease may be manifested: anemia, bone pain, cerebral ischemia, fat embolism etc. Neurological manifestations are usually vague initially and may be misdiagnosed. From the case described by Wolman and Hardy, there was pain, loss of sensation, muscle weakness, and eventually paraparesis or tetraparesis.

25.6 Diagnosis

Diagnosis is based on the following criteria:

1. Ethnicity
2. Symptoms of anemia
3. History of other manifestation of sickle cell anemia e.g. acute attacks, fat embolism
4. Body pains, parathesia, anesthesia, muscle weakness, paresis, sphincter dysfunction
5. Change in mental status
6. High lesions may lead to respiratory distress or even arrest
7. Blood picture: sickle cell erythrocytes, evidence of anemia, hemolysis. ESR is elevated.
8. CSF: high protein content and presences of red blood cells
9. MRI, MRA, and CT scan to rule out any hemorrhage and epidural abscess

25.7 Management

- hydration
- blood transfusion
- antibiotics: penicillin
- Tissue plasma activator (TPA) if bleeding is ruled out by MRI
- possibly exchange transfusion to reduce vascular occlusions
- antiplatelet drugs
- rehab therapy
- Hyperbaric oxygen (HBO) is being used in some centers especially in Europe for treatment of stroke. It may be thought of in spinal cord infarct since there is no evidence of its use.

Updating

Márquez et al. (2012)

Spinal cord ischemia due to sickle cell disease is extremely rare. To the best of their knowledge only one case has been reported.

The patient was initially diagnosed by diffusion weighted images (DWI); follow-up MRI confirmed the diagnosis.

Case Report

A 19-year-old male African American developed acute flaccid tetraplegia with bladder dysfunction. He was diagnosed with sickle cell disease at the age of 5. He had multiple admissions for chest syndromes and pain crises; the last of which was

1 month prior to the present condition. He was diagnosed 6 years ago as having a silent cerebral infarct. On admission, MRI of the spine was normal; however, DWI showed a high signal in the spinal cord from C2–C7 with compounding restricted diffusion on the attenuation diffusion coefficient (ADC) map suggesting infarction. Three days later another MRI showed enlargement of the spinal cord at the same levels. There was low intensity signal in T1-weighted images and high signal intensity on T2-weighted images. Another DWI showed restricted diffusion.

Management
Exchange transfusion keeping his hemoglobin A at a higher level than 70 % to prevent further ischemia.

Outcome
The patient improved with rehabilitation and was able to walk, although the left upper extremity remained paralyzed.

Reference
Márquez JC, Granados AM, Castillo M. MRI of cervical spinal cord infarction in a patient with sickle cell disease. Clin Imaging. 2012;36(5):595–8.

References

Loupy A, Laissy JP, Klein I, et al. Fat emboli unleashed: an exceptional etiology of encephalitis in sickle cell disease. Ann Hematol. 2008;87(11):939–41.

Rothman SM, Nelson JS. Spinal cord infarction in a patient with sickle cell anemia. Neurology. 1980;30(10):1072–6.

Wolman L, Hardy AG. Spinal cord infarction associated with the sickle cell trait. Paraplegia. 1970;7(4):282–91.

26 Sotos Syndrome as a Cause of Compression Myelopathy

26.1 Definition

Sotos syndrome (cerebral gigantism) is a rare overgrowth syndrome, characterized by distinct facies, above average birth weight and length, joint laxity, pes planus, acromegaly, excessive growth rate, advanced bone age, and developmental delay. Very rarely are the spine or vertebra involved.

26.2 Incidence

Sotos syndrome only has slightly more than 300 cases reported in the English literature to date. Prior cases report only spinal or vertebral involvement with an increased rate of scoliosis. However in 2004, Carlo and Dormans (2004) reported a patient with Sotos syndrome and an incidental finding of cervical instability, causing C3–C4 anterolisthesis with pinching of the spinal cord.

26.3 Etiology

The disease is congenital in origin, and the genetic code has not been reported.

26.4 Clinical Picture

In Sotos syndrome the child has a head circumference and height above normal. The palms and feet length are at the 97th percentile. Generalize ligamentous laxity will be noticed. In Carlo and Dormans' case There is scoliosis and in the cervical spine

Abstracted from Carlo and Dormans (2004)

I.M. Eltorai, *Rare Diseases and Syndromes of the Spinal Cord*,
DOI 10.1007/978-3-319-45147-3_26

there was 50 % anterolisthesis at C3–C4, which was incompletely reducible on extension of the neck. There was impingement on the spinal cord for which the patient had surgery manifested by hyperreflexia in the lower extremities. In general, children have higher rates of cervical laxity than adults because of the disproportionally large heads, horizontal orientation of cervical facet joints, and greater neck weakness.

26.5 Diagnosis

The syndrome has some similarity to Downs except for the anterolisthesis at the cervical region. Radiography reveals the anterolisthesis at C3–C4 in the case described; magnetic resonance imaging (MRI) shows anterolisthesis causing mild spinal canal stenosis with evidence of chronic compression and mild atrophy of the spinal cord.

26.6 Management

Because of the cervical anterolisthesis and spinal cord compression surgery is indicated. Surgery was done by posterior approach and posterior spinal wire and fusion of C3–C4 by wiring with titanium sublaminar cables and iliac crest autograft. The postoperative was somewhat stormy but 10 weeks after surgery there was radiologic evidence of stable reduction and arthrodesis of the fused segment. Carlo and Dormans recommend awareness of the syndrome for early diagnosis and management before neurological injury.

Reference

Carlo W, Dormans JP. Cervical instability in Sotos syndrome: a case report. Spine. 2004;29(7):E153–6.

Atlantoaxial Instability in Spondyloepiphyseal Dysplasia Congenita

27

27.1 Definition

Spondyloepiphyseal dysplasia congenita (SEDC) is a rare systemic skeletal disease characterized by congenital dwarfism, a short trunk, and epiphyseal dysplasia of the long bones and vertebral bodies and frequently suffers from atlantoaxial instability associated with os odontoideum, leading to spinal cord compression and occasionally to sudden death.

27.2 Incidence

It is a rare disease. Eleven cases of SEDC were reviewed by Sawaizumi and Kitamura and added a case of their own. The ages ranged from 5 to 56; the male to female ratio is even.

27.3 Etiology

Congenital anomaly genetically not yet known.

27.4 Pathology

- Atlantoaxial instability
- Os odontoideum
- Spinal stenosis
- Scoliosis

Abstracted and reported by Gembun et al. (2001)

I.M. Eltorai, *Rare Diseases and Syndromes of the Spinal Cord*,
DOI 10.1007/978-3-319-45147-3_27

27.5 Clinical Picture

Neurological symptoms may occur without trauma. Trauma may cause much damage to the spinal cord which may not recover after decompression.

27.6 Diagnosis

Diagnosis is based on the following criteria:

1. Radiography will reveal:
   (a) Atlantoaxial instability
   (b) Flexion extension views
   (c) Os odontoideum
   (d) Spinal stenosis
   (e) Scoliosis
   (f) Flat vertebrae
   (g) Epiphyseal dysplasia of the long bones
2. Urine glucosamnogly level is normal to differentiate from Morquio's disease
3. MRI: high signal lesion in T2 weighted images.

27.7 Management

Laminectomy of C1. Occipitocervical fusion using SS rod and bone iliac graft

Reference

Gembun Y, Nakayama Y, Shirai Y, Miyamoto M, Sawaizumi T, Kitamura S. A case report of spondyloepiphyseal dysplasia congenita. J Nippon Med Sch. 2001;68(2):186–9.

Brown Séquard Syndrome Associated with Sprengel's Deformity

28

28.1 Definition

Sprengel's deformity (SD) is a congenital condition in which there is failure of the scapular descent during intra-uterine growth. The neurological syndrome was due to spina bifida of C4–6 and defect of posterior arch of the fifth cervical vertebra and the presence of an ectopic bone on the left side of the spina bifida. There was an omovertebral bridge attached to cervical spine. The congenital anomalies lead to Brown Séquard syndrome in the case described by Hauman et al.

28.2 Incidence

Sprengel's deformity (SD) occurs in 1–2 per 3,000 births. The condition is usually sporadic, but may be inherited as an autosomal dominant trait. Brown-Séquard syndrome (BSS) was only once reported and our search brought no other cases reported since 1986

28.3 Etiology

SD is congenital and rare familial (Carno Disease). BSS was found to be due to cervical spina bifida, absence of hemi-arch of C5 and small mass of bone causing compression of the cord on the left side.

Abstracted from Hauman et al. (1986)

I.M. Eltorai, *Rare Diseases and Syndromes of the Spinal Cord*,
DOI 10.1007/978-3-319-45147-3_28

28.4 Pathology

There was cord compression which when relieved a neurological recovery was attained. The deformity may be associated with syringomyelia, Klippel-Feil syndrome, or a cervical rib, hemivertebra, diastematomyelia, aortic cortication, hyperplasia of the shoulder muscles, pectoris major, serratus anticus, trapezius, and latissus dorsi.

28.5 Clinical Picture

The patient recorded was 13 year old with inherited SD through his mother. He developed right hemithermoanalgesia and pyramidal syndrome on the left. He was diagnosed with BSS with C6 sensory level.

28.6 Diagnosis

Diagnosis is based on the following criteria:

1. right congenital elevated scapula
2. left pyrmadial hemiparesis
3. Radiography shows the following:
   - Elevated right scapula
   - Omovertebral bridge with upper angle of the scapula linked to the cervical spine and is imbedded in the right half of the a large posterior arch defect of C5
   - Spina bifida of C4 and C6
   - To the left of the midline there is a boney fragment included in the spina bifida
4. Myelogram: showed a block at C4
5. CT scan showed:
   - aplasia of the medial part of the left posterior arch and deficit of C5
   - aberrant boney fragment embedded spina bifida
   - compression of postrolateral aspect of the cervical dura
   - spinal cord compression by the small left fragment at C4
   - MRI was not performed

28.7 Management

Surgery consisted of:

- Removal of the boney fragment responsible for the compression from the cleft in the posterior arch of C4
- Vertebral omo connection was not removed

The result of the surgery was regression of the spinal cord compression. The authors recommend surgery to be done between 3 and 7 years of age; in older children there is an increased risk to the brachial plexus from stretching or compression by the clavicle.

Reference

Hauman H, Wilms G, Roussel JM, Van den bergh R. Congenital elevation of the scapula and Brown-Sequard syndrome. Clin Neurol Neurosurg. 1986;88(4):289–92.

Synovial Chondromatosis 29

29.1 Definition

This is a condition of cartilaginous proliferation with synovium and may be calcified or ossified. It may be extruded from the synovium, forming a loose body.

29.2 Incidence

The condition occurs in large joints most commonly in the knees. In the spine, only nine cases have been reported. Median age is 39 years. There is a male to female ratio of 5:4.

29.3 Etiology

There is no definite causative factor; however, the condition may be primary arising in healthy joints or secondary in pathologic joints: osteoarthritic, rheumatoid and neuropathic joints, osteonecrosis, tuberculosis, and osteochondral fractures. Whether spinal cord is metaplastic or neoplasic the former is more rare.

29.4 Pathology

The tumor is well defined proliferating within the subsynovial space. The synovium is preserve, but may be attenuated. The chondrocytes have small round nuclei, as seen in benign chondromas. Some chondrocytes may have larger irregular nuclei. Incomplete ablation results in recurrence (15 %). Gallia et al. (2004) reported two

---

Abstracted from Abdelwahab et al. (2008).

I.M. Eltorai, *Rare Diseases and Syndromes of the Spinal Cord*,
DOI 10.1007/978-3-319-45147-3_29

cervical cases, the first transformed into a low-grade chondrosarcoma, which is a common change in nonspinal chondromas. Secondary changes may occur, viz. calcification of osteochondral changes. Atypical cells may be seen, chondroblasts. The synovial cells may proliferate on top. Most reported cases arose from the facet joint synovia, Kyriakos et al. (2000) Out of the nine reported cases, four were cervical, two were thoracic, two were lumbar, and one was costotransverse joint. Compression myelopathy results as the mass grows more towards the spinal cord.

29.5 Diagnosis

Diagnosis is based on the following criteria:

1. Pain is the most common complaint 89 %.
2. Neurological deficit in 77 %: sensory deficits, sphincteric dysfunction, weakness, paresis, paralysis.
3. Localized tenderness at the tumor site.
4. MRI of the spinal cord: (in the case presented) a lobular mass, which had an isointense signal on T1-weighted images and a hyperintense signal on T2-weighted images. These MRI findings are highly suggestive of a cartilaginous mass or a cyst e.g. discal cyst, perineural cyst, extradural arachnoid cyst, synovial cyst from the facet joint.

Other cartilogenous tumors of the spine that should be differentiated from chondromatosis are chondromas, enchondromas, osteochondromas, chondroblastomas, and chondromyxoid fibromas, which may cause cord compression.

29.6 Management

Surgical removal of the tumor is necessary through hemilaminectomy with microsurgery. Close followup is required both neurologically and by imaging.

References

Abdelwahab IF, Contractor D, Bianchi S, Hermann G, Hoch B. Synovial chondromatosis of the lumbar spine with compressive myelopathy: a case report with review of the literature. Skeletal Radiol. 2008;37(9):863–7.

Gallia GL, Weiss N, Campbell JN, Mccarthy EF, Tufaro AP, Gokaslan ZL. Vertebral synovial chondromatosis. Report of two cases and review of the literature. J Neurosurg Spine. 2004;1(2):211–8.

Kyriakos M, Totty WG, Riew KD. Synovial chondromatosis in a facet joint of a cervical vertebra. Spine. 2000;25(5):635–40.

30 Myelopathy Due to Tourette's Syndrome

30.1 Definition

According to Lin et al., Tourette's syndrome is manifested in a broad spectrum of motor, vocal and behavioral disturbances. Movement disorders, such as tics, may contribute to the development of cervical myelopathy owning to the effects of involuntary movements on the neck. According to the dictionary of medical syndromes: "it is a psychological disorder characterized by chorea, coprolalia, echolalia, and tic." It affects children usually boys between 5 and 10 years of age. It is manifested by tics of the hands, arms, or face and then it spreads to the rest of the body. Eventually, combined movements with variable frequencies. The tics are sometimes accompanied by uncontrollable noises and utterances, as well as features of attention deficit hyperactivity disorder (ADHD), obsessive compulsive disorder (OCD), poor impulse control, and other misbehaviors. Common motor tics include eye blinking, head jerking, eye movements, and different facial expressions, such as grimacing and noise twitching, grunting and hiccupping may become more frequent.

30.2 Incidence

Cervical myelopathy has been reported by Lin et al., Dobbs and Berger, Brill et al., Krauss and Jankovic, Muroi et al., and Nomura et al. The disease occurs most frequently in Ashkenazy Jews and people of Mediterranean descent, rarely in blacks. Transmission as an autosomal dominant trait is suspected.

Abstracted from Dobbs and Berger (2003) and Lin et al. (2007)

I.M. Eltorai, *Rare Diseases and Syndromes of the Spinal Cord*,
DOI 10.1007/978-3-319-45147-3_30

30.3 Pathology of the Cervical Cord

The cause of myelopathy is believed to be due to repetitive stretching and compression of the spinal cord; also ischemia and venous congestion during the frequent forceful tics. The forceful tics may cause herniation of the nucleus pulposus and with chronicity there may be some degree of spondylosis. Children with spinal stenosis are more liable to the myelopathy; however, the forceful frequent extension, flexion, and thrusting movements of the neck are believed to be the direct cause of the myelopathy.

30.4 Pathology

There is no autopsy report found of the syndrome. MRI shows disc prolapse and compression myelopathy. Brain MRI was normal (Lin et al.)

30.5 Clinical Picture

In childhood the patient gets typical Gilles de al Tourette's syndrome (see definition) and usually the myelopathy is manifested in adults by tetraparesis with upper motor neuron clinical picture.

30.6 Diagnosis

Diagnosis is based on:

1. History and clinical picture
2. MRI shows:
   - Disc herniation and cord compression
   - Non-enhancing focus of T2 signal rostral to the area of compression
3. Laboratory tests to rule out MS and SCD
4. Electrophysiologic studies confirm compression: visual and brain stem evoked potentials. EMG for denervation

30.7 Management

- Medical treatment of the tics according to Lin et al. (2007):
  - Olanzapine
  - Selegiline
  - Flunazine
  - Trihexyphenidyl
  - Haloperidol

- Decompression laminectomy and cervical discectomy: according to Lin et al., the result is variable, since there are variable causes of the myelopathy viz. the disc, the stenosis, or the spondylosis
- Rehabilitation program
- Botox neck muscle block. This may prove to be valuable in preventing cervical myelopathy in this syndrome. According to Lin et al., perioperative BTX followed by halo vest may improve the outcome after surgery. However, due to surgical risk and postoperative lack of control of the tics conservative treatment is an alternative.

References

Dobbs M, Berger JR. Cervical myelopathy secondary to violent tics of Tourette's syndrome. Neurology. 2003;60(11):1862–3.

Lin JJ, Wang HS, Wong MC, Wu CT, Lin KL. Tourette's syndrome with cervical disc herniation. Brain Dev. 2007;29(2):61–3.

Part II

Endocrine Causes of Myelopathy

31 Adrenomyeloneuropathy Causing Spastic Paresis

31.1 Definition

Adrenomyeloneuropathy (AMN) is a variant of adrenoleukodystrophy (ALD), both of which are rare inherited disorders of perixosomes characterized by the accumulation of very long chain fatty acids in plasma, the central and peripheral nervous systems, adrenal glands, and testes, which leads to dysfunction of these organs and systems.

Historical Note (according to Moser et al.)

> X-linked ALD (X-ALD) was first described in Germany, by Siemerling and Creutzfeldt in 1923. They named it "Bronzekrankheit und Sklerosierende Encephalitis" because of the unique combination of primary adrenal insufficiency with an inflammatory demyelinating process that affects the cerebral hemispheres. In Vienna, Paul Schilder provided a detailed description of the neuropathology, which led to its designation as "Schilder's disease." X-linkage was proposed in 1963 on the basis of pedigree analysis. The name "adrenoleukodystrophy" was introduced 1970 by Michael Blaw and is now generally used.

31.2 Incidence

The overall frequency of X-ALD is estimated to be 1:17000. All ethnic groups are affected with no apparent differences in frequency. From Moser et al., laboratories they identified 1441 kindreds with 3831 affected males and 3356 women who are heterozygous for X-ALD. Markedly different phenotypes often co-occur within a family.

Abstracted from Moser et al. (2005)

I.M. Eltorai, *Rare Diseases and Syndromes of the Spinal Cord*,
DOI 10.1007/978-3-319-45147-3_31

31.3 Etiology

According to Spurek et al. (2004), the causes of primary adrenal insuffiency are:

Autoimmune disorder	70 %
Tuberculosis	20 %

The other 10 % of causes include:

Fungal Infection
Adrenal hemorrhage
AID
Metastases
ALD or AMD
Congenital adrenal hypoplasia
Drug us (ketoconazole, mitotane, metyrapone, aminoglutethemid)

According to Fatemi et al.,

> AMN was first recognized in 1976 as the non-inflammatory adult variant of X-ALD, a genetic disorder characterized by accumulation of very long chain fatty acids (VLCFA) in the central nervous system, adrenal glands, and testes. The gene deficient in X-ALD, *ABCD1*, codes for a peroxisomal membrane protein that is a member of the adeosine triphosphate binding cassette transporter superfamily. Forty percent of the men with the genetic defect of X-ALD present with the childhood cerebral from, while 45 % present initially with AMN.

According to Moser et al., and Kemp:

> X-ALD is an X-linked disorder, i.e. it affects only males, and is transmitted by a female carrier. In men with one X-chromosome it is not protected and the disease can be manifested in males, whereas in females there are two X's, the second is protective. Approximately half of the women heterozygous for X-ALD develop an AMN-like syndrome in later years.

31.4 Pathology

Pathologic changes in AMN as well as in heterozygotes are mainly confined to the spinal cord, where there is distal axonapathy involving most severely the ascending tracts of the dorsal column in the cervical region and the corticospinal tracts in the lower thoracic and lumbosacral regions. Brain changes occur in 20 % of adult patients with AMN. Those that have no brain changes are designated as pure AMN. Adrenal insufficiency is common. Spinal cord atrophy was noticed.

31.5 Clinical Picture

AMN appears usually in the late 20s as a spastic paraparesis with loss of the vibratory sensation and dysthesia and bowel and bladder dysfunction. The disease is slowly progressive. In few cases, cerebral manifestations are noticed. Addison's disease may occur without neurological manifestations.

31.6 Diagnosis

Diagnosis is based on:

1. Family history
2. Neurological findings
3. Laboratory tests:
   - Very long chain fatty acids in blood
   - DNA-based blood test
   - Genetic analysis: ALD gene
   - Adrenal functions
   - CSF: $C_{26:0}/C_{22:0}$ ratio and $C_{24:0}/C_{22:0}$ ratio were both elevated
   - Electrophysiology
4. Imaging
   - MRI of the spinal cord and brain
   - Magnetization transfer-weighted MRI (see Fatemi et al. (2005))

31.7 Management

- Intensive rehabilitation program
- Adrenal replacement: this is required for patients with Addison's manifestations. It improves patient's general condition and well-being, but has no effect on the paralysis.
- Lorenzo's oil therapy (diet)
  - This consists of 4:1 ratio of:
    - Glyceryl trioleate
    - Glyceryl trierucate
    - It normalizes plasma very long chain fatty acid levels in X-ALD within 4 weeks. It does not stop cerebral lesions progress, but it may be prophylactic. It is generally used for X-ALD in young boys.
- The following experimental treatments:
  - Hematopoietic stem cell transplant for cerebral X-ALD
  - Bone marrow transplant for X-ALD
  - Pharmacotherapy: levostatin and phenylbutyrate
  - Investigation of gene therapy

References

Fatemi A, Smith SA, Dubey P, et al. Magnetization transfer MRI demonstrates spinal cord abnormalities in adrenomyeloneuropathy. Neurology. 2005;64(10):1739–45.

Moser HW, Raymond GV, Dubey P. Adrenoleukodystrophy: new approaches to a neurodegenerative disease. JAMA. 2005;294(24):3131–4.

Spurek M, Taylor-gjevre R, Van Uum S, Khandwala HM. Adrenomyeloneuropathy as a cause of primary adrenal insufficiency and spastic paraparesis. CMAJ. 2004;171(9):1073–7.

Copper Deficiency

32

32.1 Definition

Copper deficiency is a condition which results in a clinical picture similar to subacute combined degeneration. It is manifested by prominent gait difficulty, sensory ataxia due to dorsal column dysfunction and lower limb spasticity.

32.2 Incidence

Copper deficiency myelopathy is not common disease subsequently, there are no national statistics; although, in a brief English literature search it was found about 20 cases with neurological manifestations in association with copper deficiency.

32.3 Etiology

Copper deficiency myelopathy may be congenital in humans, Menkes disease. The gene responsible for Menkes disease (ATP7A) encodes a P-type adenosine triphosphatase that has multiple copper-binding motifs near its amino terminus. Copper deficiency manifested in childhood is that of neurological disorder due to inherited copper malabsorption. In adults the causes copper deficiency are:

- in patients with malabsorption syndrome
- nephrotic syndrome
- prolonged parenteral nutrition
- as a complication of zinc, penicillamine
- self-administered high dose of zinc gluconate over long periods of time
- possible excess iron intake
- chemotherapy regimens using tetrathiomolybdate

Abstracted from Kumar et al. (2004)

I.M. Eltorai, *Rare Diseases and Syndromes of the Spinal Cord*,
DOI 10.1007/978-3-319-45147-3_32

Copper deficiency is known to cause an ataxic myelopathy in ruminants called swayback.

32.4 Pathophysiology

The site of copper absorption in humans remains unclear; however, Mason stated that it appears to take place in the stomach and proximal duodenum. Copper is a key component of various metalloenzymes and proteins, which have a vital role in mitochondrial metabolism and structure and function of the nervous system. It is a constituent of cytochrome oxidase (oxidase phosphorylation), superoxide dismutase (antioxidant defense), ceruloplasmin (iron metabolism), tyrosinase (melanin synthesis, and dopamine β-monooxyygenase (catecholamine synthesis). The pathology is that of demyelination and axonal degeneration of the spinal cord especially in the posterior column. There is also neuropathy as evidenced by demyelination of the peripheral nerves and occasionally the optic nerve. The picture simulates subacute combined degeneration.

32.5 Clinical Picture

The picture is that of progressive myeloneuropathy in association with copper deficiency. It is primarily in the lower limbs and rarely in the upper. The gait is ataxic, with mild stiffness of the lower extremities. The sensory deficit is in the proprioception. The vibration sense is severely affected. Perception of pinprick and touch are variably reduced in a stocking distribution (peripheral neuropathy). No sensory levels are identified over the trunk. The knee jerks are mostly increased, but they may be normal, or may be decreased. The ankle jerks are mostly decrease, but may be increased. Babinski sign and Romberg sign may be positive; clonus is usually negative. The upper limbs may be spared or only mildly affected. Optic neuritis may rarely be manifested.

Continuing with Kumar, et al., findings: the blood picture of copper deficiency shows anemia and leukopenia. Cerebral spinal fluid (CSF) examination is usually normal with the exception of occasional mild elevation of the proteins. Magnetic resonance imaging (MRI) of the spinal cord may show T2 signal in the paramedian dorsal cervical cord and may extend from the upper cervical and/or thoracic. The brain MRI showed nonspecific findings including lancunes, mild atrophy, and nonspecific foci of increased T2 signal. Other changes in the brain may be detected but are nonspecific. Electromyelography (EMG) and nerve conduction studies will show varying degree of axonal neuropath, mostly mild, sensory and motor are of variable degrees. Occasionally myelopathic potentials may be detected. Somatosensory evoked potentials show impairment of central conduction. Nerve biopsy may show axonal degeneration; whereas muscle biopsy may be normal or may show vacuolar changes. Small intestinal biopsies are performed in suspicious cases of coeliac disease. Vitamin B12 levels may be reduced as they were in patients who had gastrectomy or gastric bypass, or terminal bowel resection for Crohn's disease.

32.6 Prognosis

Once the diagnosis is made, copper supplementation improves the condition and prevents deterioration of spinal cord. The degree of improvement is variable especially in the position and vibration perception. Somatosensory evoked potentials show variable degree of central conduction improvement. Nerve conduction studies may show improvement or may be unchanged. The chemical studies, especially copper and zinc levels show improvement.

32.7 Management

The medical treatment for copper deficiency is intravenous (IV) 2 mg cupric sulfate; if there is no improvement another course of IV 2 mg/dL ceruloplasmin. Vitamin B12 may be added if the serum level is low. Clinically, the impairment of parathesia, perception of touch and pinprick sense of position, ataxia and gait, all seem to improve in physical therapy and rehabilitation.

Reference

Kumar N, Crum B, Petersen RC, Vernino SA, Ahlskog JE. Copper deficiency myelopathy. Arch Neurol. 2004;61(5):762–6.

33 Diabetic Myelopathy

33.1 Definition

Diabetic myelopathy is a condition, which pathological changes occur in the spinal cord as a result as a result of diabetes mellitus.

33.2 Incidence

Major long-term complications of diabetes mellitus include neuropathy, retinopathy, nephropathy, and angiopathy. Peripheral neuropathy is the commonest chronic complication. In the CNS there is a two to sixfold incidence of cerebrovascular disease in diabetes than non-diabetes. Stroke related morbidity and mortality are increasing in the diabetic population. Diabetic myelopathy has not been assessed clinically in diabetic patients.

33.3 Etiology and Pathology

The pathogenesis of peripheral neuropathy (PNP) remains poorly understood. It is suggested to be due to metabolic changes, such as hyperglycemia and vascular changes (micro-angiopathy). Most of the clinical research has concentrated on the structural and functional aspects of the peripheral nerves. However, potentially important area of research is the spinal cord. There is some evidence from autopsy studies and neurophysiological studies that the peripheral nerves and the spinal cord may be affected by the pathogenic factors from the generalized disease e.g. diabetes mellitus. A common observation is that electric stimulation of the spinal cord does not control the neuropathy. This may suggest involvement of the cord.

Collateral evidence comes from two works:

1. Autopsy studies by Slager showed: Posterior column demyelination in 27 % of cases. She considered these changes are due to a common metabolic or toxic effect to both the peripheral nerves and to the spinal cord. Spinal cord infarcts

Abstracted from multiple sources

I.M. Eltorai, *Rare Diseases and Syndromes of the Spinal Cord*,
DOI 10.1007/978-3-319-45147-3_33

were found in 19 % secondary to arteriopathy of the intrinsic vessels of the spinal cord. These changes had a predilection to white matter and are commoner in diabetics that non-diabetics and unrelated to age. The author found diabetic myelopathy in 42 % of 37 autopsies.

2. MRI findings: Eaton et al., have measured cross sectional area of these regions of the spinal cord including the cervical and lumbar enlargements. In patients with distal symmetrical polyneuropathy (DSP) the spinal cord cross sectional area was significantly reduced in 2 of the 3 regions compared with the controls. From this pilot study the data were consistent with contributory spinal cord pathology in DSP. The authors stated significant differences in mean cord area found at the levels of C4–5 and T3–4. Whether spinal cord involvement is primary or secondary event in DSP is unclear. One possibility is that damage to the peripheral nerves causes the cord to die back. The other possibility is that the primary damage starts in the spinal cord. However, the necropsy findings show microangiopathy in both the spinal cord as well as the peripheral nerves indicating a common pathogenic mechanism.

33.4 Clinical Picture

There is no typical picture of diabetic myelopathy since the predominant picture is that of peripheral neuropathy, especially distal symmetrical polyneuropathy.

33.5 Diagnosis

Diagnosis is based on the following criteria:

1. History
2. Clinical picture: sensory loss of different modalities, trophic changes in the skin, motor weakness, muscle atrophy, osteoporosis and diabetic arthropathy, and vascular insufficiency
3. Laboratory tests: nerve induction studies, general metabolic assessment (GMA) evoked potentials, ultrasonography, peripheral nerve biopsy
4. MRI of the spinal cord: rule out myelopathy

33.6 Management

- Medical management of diabetes
- No specific treatment yet available for disseminated peripheral neuropathy.

Management can be found in textbooks on diabetes and endocrinology

Suggested Reading

Meiners T. Sequelae of diabetes mellitus in the vertebral column and spinal cord. Orthopade. 2003;32(3):236–40.

Prick JJ, Prevo RL, Hoogenraad TU. Transient myelopathy of the cervical posterior columns in a young man with recently diagnosed diabetes mellitus. Clin Neurol Neurosurg. 2001;103(4):234–7.

Selvarajah D, Wilkinson ID, Emery CJ, et al. Early involvement of the spinal cord in diabetic peripheral neuropathy. Diabetes Care. 2006;29(12):2664–9.

Seo JH, Park SH. Diabetic cervical radiculopathy with adhesive capsulitis of the shoulder. Yonsei Med J. 2003;44(6):1114–8.

Cervical Myelomalacia in Laron Syndrome

34

34.1 Definition

Laron Syndrome (LS) is characterized by inability to respond normally to growth hormone of endogenous or exogenous origin (Laron et al. 1993). Most growth hormone effects are mediated by insulin-like growth factor 1 (IGF-1), which is the anabolic effector hormone of the pituitary growth hormone. In LS a deficit occurs in the growth hormone receptor gene or the post-receptor pathways, resulting in defects in growth hormone signal transmission and thereby in a failure to generate IGF-1 (Laron et al. 1993). Patients have therefore high serum growth hormone but undetectable IFG-1.

34.2 Incidence

LS was first described in 1966 and in 1968 in a group of Oriental Jewish patients. Since then 100 of patients have been reported worldwide, mostly of Mid-Eastern origin (Kornreich et al. 2002, 2008). These authors in a study of 11 patients found cervical focal myelomalacia at C1 in two patients, an incidence less than 20 %.

34.3 Etiology

LS is an autosomal recessive disease caused by deletions or mutations in the growth hormone receptor gene or the post-receptor pathways resulting in defects in growth hormone signal transmission and, thereby inability to generate IGF-1, which is effector hormone of the pituitary growth hormone. The patients will fail to respond to growth hormone of endogenous or exogenous source.

34.4 Pathology

The disease is due to pathophysiology, based on genetic delinquency.

Abstracted and reported by Kornreich et al. (2002, 2008).

I.M. Eltorai, *Rare Diseases and Syndromes of the Spinal Cord*,
DOI 10.1007/978-3-319-45147-3_34

34.5 Clinical Picture

- There is a progressive dwarfism with final stature from 3′6″ to 4′5″ in women and 3′10″ to 4′8″ in men.
- Acromicria and organomicria
- Small genitalia and gonads
- Craniofacial abnormalties:
  - Subnormal head circumference
  - Underdevelopment of facial bones
  - High pitched voice in children and many adults
  - Adults become obese and have hypercholesteremia and insulin resistance
  - Although sexual maturity is retarded they eventually have reproductive ability
  - The mediolateral diameter of the oropharynx is much smaller than the normal and patients frequently have sleep apnea

34.6 Diagnosis

Diagnosis is based on the following criteria:

1. Morphology of the patient
2. Radiography: Cervical spine shows significant narrowing of the spinal canal associated with abnormalities of the dens, degenerative changes of the atlanto-odontoid joint. It shows smaller dimensions of the oropharynx. Spinal stenosis is common finding in the cervical spine due to retarded bone mutation, due to growth hormone insensitivity. This syndrome places the patient at greater risk of neurological deficit at the occurrence of degenerative disk disease and spondylitic changes (Kornreich et al. 2002, 2008) in one of their patients a disk bulge with compression of the thecal sac was evident at the age of 36.
3. MRI of the spinal cord: Sagittal T2-weighted images show spinal stenosis of the cervical spine. Multiple bulging disks may show compression of the thecal sac. Anomalies of the dens may be seen and may be compatible with os odontoideum. The atlanto-axial joint may show osteoarthritis.
4. Biochemical assay: There is a high serum level of growth factor and undetectable serum IGF-1.

34.7 Management

IGF-1 replacement therapy at the early age before skeletal changes and possibly cord compression. Subsequent changes are to be treated accordingly, e.g. orthopedic treatment.

References

Kornreich L, Konen O, Schwarz M, et al. Abnormalities of the axial and proximal appendicular skeleton in adults with Laron syndrome (growth hormone insensitivity). Skeletal Radiol. 2008;37(2):153–60.

Kornreich L, Horev G, Schwarz M, Karmazyn B, Laron Z. Laron syndrome abnormalities: spinal stenosis, os odontoideum, degenerative changes of the atlanto-odontoid joint, and small oropharynx. AJNR Am J Neuroradiol. 2002;23(4):625–31.

Laron Z, Klinger B, Eshet R, Kaneti H, Karasik A, Silbergeld A. Laron syndrome due to a post-receptor defect: response to IGF-I treatment. Isr J Med Sci. 1993;29(12):757–63.

35 Compression Myelopathy due to Tophaceous Gout

35.1 Definition

This is a condition of compression myelopathy secondary to gouty tophus, usually associated with hyperuricemia, which is uncontrolled for a long time leading super-saturation of tissue fluids.

35.2 Incidence

The first case of compression myelopathy due to gouty tophus was recorded in 1953 by Koskoff et al. Occasional similar cases have been reported since then. According to Saketkoo et al., 125 cases have been reported.

35.3 Etiology

Although gouty polyarticular disease is not uncommon gouty spondylitis is rare and it may be associated with intraspinal tophi. These consist of monosodium urate crystals in chronic cases of gout with poor control of uricaemia.

35.4 Pathology

The intraspinal thophi may be extradural and rarely intradural. The crystals form a foreign body granuloma, consisting of multinucleated (giant cells) histiocyts, and fibroblasts surrounding an amorphous acellular material uric acid level greater than 70 mgm/L results in deposition of urate especially in cooler avascular tissues such as tendons. With chronic hyperuricemia internal organs, especially the kidneys leading to decreased clearance, especially with chronic renal failure, leukemia, lymphoma, hemolytic uremia and high dietary purines, alcohol intake. Such conditions may be kept in mind if a compression myelopathy is detected. Any level of the

Abstracted from Saketkoo et al. (2009)

I.M. Eltorai, *Rare Diseases and Syndromes of the Spinal Cord*,
DOI 10.1007/978-3-319-45147-3_35

spinal cord may be affected, the cervical, thoracic, lumbar, including the cauda equina and the filum terminale.

35.5 Clinical Picture

The patient has history of gouty arthritis either peripheral or spinal. The onset may be fever. Back pain in the form of radiculopathy; neurological symptoms attributable to mass lesions may appear (parasethesias, anesthesia, motor weakness, paresis, paralysis, and sphincter disturbances). Peripheral arthritic thophi may be detected (big toe, elbow, ear, etc). Occasionally, neurogenic claudication is the main symptom.

35.6 Diagnosis

Diagnosis based on:

1. Clinical picture
2. Neurological exam
3. Laboratory studies: hyperuricemia, high ESR, elevated CRP, metabolic changes, BUN
4. Aspiration of tophus for urate crystal CT guided
5. Gadolinium MRI amy show extradural or occasionally a calcified shadow on T2 weighted images can show an enhancing lesion

Plain x-ray may be negative. Should be differentiated from other space occupying lesions, epidural abscess, hematoma, neoplasia, diskitis, osteomyelitis

35.7 Management

Surgery consists of:

1. Laminectomy with or without stabilization. However, suppression of serum urate with allupurinal.

May arrest the pathological deposition of uric acid with possible regression of the tophi and possible successful non-surgical treatment, but this should be not too long to avoid further cord deficit.

Reference

Saketkoo LA, Robertson HJ, Dyer HR, Virk ZU, Ferreyro HR, Espinoza LR. Axial gouty arthropathy. Am J Med Sci. 2009;338(2):140–6.

Part III

Iatrogenic

36 Myelopathy due to Acupuncture

36.1 Definition

Acupuncture is an ancient oriental modality of healing, which stood the test of time in the orient and that contributed to its survival. In the last several decades it has been introduced to the West and like other modalities of treatment it has been scrutinized scientifically and technologically. Like all therapeutic measures it is not free from complications.

36.2 Incidence and Etiology

Ernest and White (1997) published the adverse reaction after acupuncture after thorough review. These are summarized as follows:

36.2.1 Infection

Infection due to lack of sterility and the reuse of the needles. Transmitted diseases reported include: hepatitis B or C, H.I.V., subacute bacterial endocarditis. Hepatitis was seen more in endemic areas or in asymptomatic patients or carriers especially after tattooing or blood transfusion. Bacterial infections resolved and were asymptomatic. Septicemias due to staphylococous aureus infection were also reported and resolved. Local infections, as a complication of acupuncture included cellulitis, and abscesses. Distant infection, e.g. in bilateral lumbar paraspinal acupuncture, bilateral psoas abscesses developed. Epidural infection will be discussed in detail.

Abstracted from numerous sources please see references

I.M. Eltorai, *Rare Diseases and Syndromes of the Spinal Cord*,
DOI 10.1007/978-3-319-45147-3_36

36.2.2 Trauma

1. local tissue injury
2. pneumothorax unilateral or bilateral
3. puncture of the heart through a formen in the sternum (10 % in males and 4 % in females leading to fatal cardiac tamponade
4. abdominal injuries were reported to the kidney, intestine, and urinary bladder
5. peripheral nerve injuries e.g. the median in the carpal tunnel and the lateral popliteal (fibula) behind the knee
6. vascular injuries e.g. arterial puncture leads to thromobosis or false aneurysm, injuries to the vein leads to iatrogenic venous thrombosis
7. injuries to the spinal cord will be discussed separately

36.2.3 Spinal Cord Injuries Due to Acupuncture

According to Perker et al., 10 cases of injuries to the spinal cord or the spinal nerve roots. In four cases migration of the needle fragments were responsible for the lesions and six were caused by direct injury. The level of injury C1-C2 in four cases, C6 in one case, L4-L5 in two cases, S1 in one case. Focal neurological signs up to paraplegia were reported. Spinal epidural hematoma and subarachnoid hemorrhage was reported (Keane et al. 1993). Spinal epidural hematoma leading to paraplegia (Chen et al. 2006). Needle migration to the cord or even the medulla.

36.2.4 Spinal Cord Infection Due to Acupuncture

A long needle may penetrate into the spinal canal and may carry bacteria from the skin especially staphylococcus aureus. In some cases the needle penetrated the colon and rectum, resulting in bacteremia and septicemia especially in those with low immunity, e.g. diabetics. In the lumbar region paravertebral acupuncture may lead to iliopsoas abscess and vertebral osteomyelitis, diskitis (Bang and Lim 2006). Epidural abscess may also develop leading to paraplegia or tetraplegia (Yazawa et al. 1998). Abdominal symptoms may be the source of spinal infection (Studd et al.) or retroperitoneal suppuration may be the source (Cho et al.).

36.3 Pathology

The spinal cord may be injured in different ways, just as seen in the *myelopathy due to cervical manipulation* entry

1. Injury causing contusion, edema, or hematoma, partial Brown Séquard syndrome or subtotal injury
2. Epidural abscess

Epidural abscess causes cord compression and if not treated early enough ischemia will cause permanent pathological changes.

36.4 Clinical Picture

In cases of epidural hematoma will lead to cord compression immediate or late. In subarachnoid, hemorrhage the picture is that of headache, painful neck stiffness, nausea, and vomiting (Keane et al. 1993). In infection, epidural abscess starts by back pains. If the epidural abscess is lumbar, neck pain and stiffness; if it is in the cervicothoracic region fever may be low or high grade, chills may be present, and stiffness of the neck in high abscesses. If left untreated weakness of the extremities inability to walk, then paraplegia; in cervical cases tetraplegia. In high lesions there may be shortness of breath, which may require ventilator assistance. Septicemia may lead to septic shock and paresis may be late in diagnosis.

36.5 Diagnosis

Diagnosis is based on:

1. History of acupuncture
2. Physical examination for needle puncture sites especially with signs of infection, spinal stiffness, tenderness, edema in paraspinal soft tissue
3. Neurological signs: sensory, motor deficits, increased reflexes, loss of temperature sensation, proproception, touch
4. Lumbar puncture: granulocyte pelocytosis and increased proteins in infective cases. Culture may be positive for cocci and/or bacilli. In hemorrhagic cases anthochromatisis, high number of red cells, and also white cells.
5. Radiography: may show osteomyelitic changes
6. CT scan: may show a block to the cord
7. MRI: in abscess an epidural mass with an increased high intensity on T2-weighted images and the periphery of the mass is low intensity on T1-weighted images. The spinal cord may be swollen or displaced and may be delineated by peripheral enhancement with gadolinium. In epidural hematoma, MRI shows hyperintensive mass in the epidural space with compression and/or displacement of the cord

36.6 Management

Epidural infection should be treated very early by triple antibiotics and may abort the infection. In rare cases may reverse neurological deficit. Short course of intravenous methylprednisolone sodium will help resolve the inflammatory edema. MRI follow up is important. If the cord remains compressed surgical drainage is indicated.

For subarachnoid hemorrhage conservative treatment is adopted. For the epidural hematoma compression of the cord leading to paraplegia intravenous methylprednisolone sodium with large bolus 30 mg/kg body weight followed by 1 mg/kg/h (Chen et al. (Chen et al. 2006)). Decompressive laminectomy and evacuation of the hematoma with thorough hemostasis may help neurological recovery.

36.7 Prophylactic Management

Licensure of acupuncturists should be based on good anatomical knowledge, thorough theoretical education and application of the bylaws of the medical boards to acupuncturists whether physicians or technicians. Strict asepsis is required. Publication and education of complications however minor they may be. This is essential as almost all complications are avoidable.

References

Anderson DW, Datta M. The self-pith. AJNR Am J Neuroradiol. 2007;28(4):714–5.

Bang MS, Lim SH. Paraplegia caused by spinal infection after acupuncture. Spinal Cord. 2006;44(4):258–9.

Chen JC, Chen Y, Lin SM, Yang HJ, Su CF, Tseng SH. Acute spinal epidural hematoma after acupuncture. J Trauma. 2006;60(2):414–6.

Ernst E, White A. Life-threatening adverse reactions after acupuncture? A systematic review. Pain. 1997;71(2):123–6.

Filshie J. Safety aspects of acupuncture in palliative care. Acupunct Med. 2001;19(2):117–22.

Keane JR, Ahmadi J, Gruen P. Spinal epidural hematoma with subarachnoid hemorrhage caused by acupuncture. AJNR Am J Neuroradiol. 1993;14(2):365–6.

Yazawa S, Ohi T, Sugimoto S, Satoh S, Matsukura S. Cervical spinal epidural abscess following acupuncture: successful treatment with antibiotics. Intern Med. 1998;37(2):161–5.

Bronchial Artery Embolization (BAE) for Severe Hemoptysis 37

37.1 Definition

This is an acute paraplegia due to infarction of the spinal cord due to embolization of the anterior spinal artery (ASA) during embolization of the bronchial artery for severe recurrent hemoptysis.

37.2 Incidence

The complication of BAE occurs in 1.4–6.5 % of various reports.

37.3 Etiology

- Inadvertent embolization of the artery of Adamkiewicz
- Abnormal migration of the gel foam used for embolization
- Stagnation of spinal artery circulation
- Prolonged hypotension
- Contributory factors are
  - Atherosclerosis
  - Polycythemia
  - Severe kyphoscoliosis, which changes the anatomical course of the vessels
  - Arteriovenous malformation (AVM)
  - Hypercoagulability with malignancy Hypercoagulability
  - The presence of an epidural hematoma
  - Bronchopulmonary dilatation or Rasmussen's aneurysm

Abstracted and reported by Lekhra and Dosi (2013).

I.M. Eltorai, *Rare Diseases and Syndromes of the Spinal Cord*,
DOI 10.1007/978-3-319-45147-3_37

37.4 Pathology

Inadvertent embolization of the ASA will lead to acute ischemia of the spinal cord with consequent infarction, resulting in paraplegia (ASA syndrome) i.e. loss of motor functions below the level of injury with intact or partially impaired sensory functions. The substances used for embolization are:

- Gel foam
- PVA (polyvinyl alcohol)
- Tris-acryl gelatin microspheres
- thrombin

BAE is approached through the descending aorta via the femoral or subclavian artery through angiography.

37.5 Case Report

A 56-year-old man presenting with expectorant streaked with blood for 5 months. He received medical treatment, viz. styptics, antibiotics for tuberculosis, anti-inflammatory drugs, and hematinics. Six months later he developed severe hemoptysis. CT scan showed right upper lobe fibrocavitory with a possible Rasmussen's aneurysm. The bronchial tree was normal on bronchoscopy. Microbiology showed methicillin sensitive streptococcus pneumonia for which he received antibiotics. The bronchial artery leading to the cavity was embolized. A few hours post-op he developed numbness and weakness of the lower extremities. Twenty-four hour hours later he developed full paraplegia, 50% sensory loss, deep tendon reflex (DTR) absent. Differential diagnosis included: epidural hematoma, epidural abscess, and spinal cord infarction. MRI revealed ASA syndrome. He was put on full rehabilitation program. Three months later he recovered reasonably well and hemoptysis did not recur.

Reference

Lekhra OP, Dosi R. Bronchial artery embolization – an unusual cause of paraplegia and review of literature. IOSR J Dent Med Sci (IOSR-JDMS). 2013;6(5):11–4.

Spinal Cord Infarction Following Central Line Insertion

38

38.1 Definition

This is a condition of spinal cord infarction resulting in tetraplegia after central line insertion in acute dialysis patient.

38.2 Incidence

Unique case by Williams et al.

38.3 Etiology

Central line insertion for dialysis is liable to complications presented by the authors:

> The internal jugular vein is the first choice for catheter insertion in acute dialysis setting. There is 6.2 % rate of complications in this setting.

Some of the complications are pneumothorax, hemothorax, brachial plexus injury, thoracic duct damage, air embolism, laryngeal hematoma, cardiac tamponade, ruptured superior thyroid artery; and the authors added spinal cord infarction.

38.4 Pathology

The patient reported, was on peritoneal dialysis complicated by peritonitis. Acute hemodialysis was planned by insertion of double lumen dialysis catheter in the left internal jugular vein. He developed a hemothorax, which was aspirated and a

A unique case reported by Williams et al. (2003)

I.M. Eltorai, *Rare Diseases and Syndromes of the Spinal Cord*,
DOI 10.1007/978-3-319-45147-3_38

femoral hemodialysis was conducted. Recurrence of the left hemothorax took place with marked hypotension, which is common in dialysis patients. The mediastinal shift and the hypotension lead to spinal cord infarction in the distribution to the anterior spinal artery.

38.5 Clinical Picture

With the extensive left hemothorax resulting from the internal subclavian perforators and mediastinal shift and the severe hypotension, the patient developed tetraplegia with a sensory level at T4. Thoracotomy was done to evacuate the blood and to repair the leaking left subclavian vein.

38.6 Diagnosis

Diagnosis is based on the following criteria:

1. X-rays: massive left hemothorax and shift of the mediastinum
2. MRI: below T4 there was increased signal within the cord ill-defined on T2-weighted images. The lower cord was swollen and occupied almost all of the spinal canal

38.7 Management

Dialysis was continued, but the paralysis was permanent.

Reference

Williams A, Little M, Gibbs J, Warwicker P, Farrington K. Spinal cord infarction following central-line insertion. Ren Fail. 2003;25(2):327–9.

39 Chemical Myelopathy due to Cervical Myelography

39.1 Definition

This is an iatrogenic condition secondary to intramedullary injection of a contrast material during cervical myelography.

39.2 Incidence

Simon et al., collected 26 cases from the literature and added a case of their own.

39.3 Etiology

Cervical myelography is now replaced by MRI; however, there are a few cases in which it may be indicated:

- Patients who are unable to undergo MRI
- Those whose pathology is inadequately demonstrated as to explain the patient's symptoms.

  The procedure is risky due to the possible injection of contrast into the cord.

Abstracted from Simon et al. (2002)

I.M. Eltorai, *Rare Diseases and Syndromes of the Spinal Cord*,
DOI 10.1007/978-3-319-45147-3_39

39.4 Pathology

There is spinal cord damage due to:

- Kinetic element depending on the injected amount and its pressure
- Neurotoxicity of the contrast

The injection of contrast, lohexol, through a lateral approach between C1-2 gives an adequate dye load with a minimum contrast dose and it reduces the need to reposition of the patient during the procedure for contrast dispersion throughout the subarachnoid space. But sill intramedullary injection is a risk leading to cord injury although it may be reversed by methylpredinisolone.

39.5 Clinical Picture

During the procedure there is intense neck pain, which may radiate to the ipsilateral side of the face, arm, or leg. Neurologic deficit appears soon after the injection and usually do not progress due to the discontinuing the injection instantly. With the use of high does of predisolone there is resolution of neural deficit, but these may persist even after a small dose of contrast. It also depends on the type of contrast and the location of the injection in the cord parenchyma. More persistent neural deficit follows melizemide injection.

39.6 Diagnosis

Diagnosis is based on the following criteria:

1. History of cervical myelography with instant pain.
2. Neurological deficit: sensory and motor with hyperreflexia, Babinski's sign, Hoffman's reflex etc.
3. Post myelography CT scan and MRI show: intraparenchymal contrast and edema of the spinal cord.

39.7 Management

High dose of methylpredinsolone IV or bolus of 30 mg/kg followed by 5.4 mgm/kg IV per hour for 48 h. Neurological resolution may occur to a greater or lesser degree. Some deficits may persist as well as some physical signs. Oral prednisone may continue for weeks with tapering. Rehabilitation is recommended for permanent disability. MRI follow-up is recommended.

Reference

Simon SL, Abrahams JM, Grady S, LeRoux PD, Rushton SA. Intramedullary injection of contrast into the cervical spinal cord during cervical myelography. Spine. 2002;27:E274–7.

40 Myelopathy due to Cervical Spinal Manipulation

40.1 Definition

Neck pain is one of the very common orthopedic problems. A popular modality of treatment is manipulation therapy, which is a part of manual medicine as a mechanicotheraputic procedure. Chiropractors, physicians, therapists, osteopaths, and bonesetters, especially in the Orient, generally practice it. The procedure is not totally risk free. Myelopathy is one of its serious complications apart from others, e.g. vertebral artery dissection leading to stroke, skeletal injury and disc prolapse, soft tissue, and nerve injuries

40.2 Incidence

Patjin showed a complication rate in one in 518,886 manipulations. According to a survey by 117 California neurologists over 2 years (Lee et al.) there were 16 myelopathy, 30 radiculopathies, and 55 strokes, following chiropractic manipulations. They found persistent neurological deficit in 86 % of patients and 97 % of patients with radiculopathy when examined 3 months after the onset of the complication.

Abstracted from Lee et al. (1995)

I.M. Eltorai, *Rare Diseases and Syndromes of the Spinal Cord*,
DOI 10.1007/978-3-319-45147-3_40

40.3 Etiology

Predisposing causes:

- Ankylosing spondylosis
- Osteoporosis
- Spinal stenosis (Pavlov's ratio less that .8, spinal canal diameter less than 9–11 mm as measured by CAT scan) (Torg et al. 1986)
- Hypermobility of the spine
- Pathological lesions are actually contraindications
  - Vertebral bony abnormalities
  - Hypermobility syndrome
  - Infections
  - Severe diabetes
  - Anticoagulation therapy
  - Rheumatoid arthritis
  - Spurs
  - Inflammatory and malignant conditions
  - Preexisting myelopathy
  - Trauma to the spine
  - Preexisting space occupying lesions
- Rotational manipulations and high velocity chiropractic manipulations are particularly dangerous.

40.4 Pathology

The spinal cord may be injured in different ways:

- Spinal injury causing contusion, edema, partial Brown Séquard syndrome or subtotal injury
- Ischemia due to vascular injury
- Hemorrhage causing hematoma that leads to compression myelopathy

Partial or incomplete resolution of the trauma site may occur especially with emergency case with high steroid therapy. Delayed pathological changes include syrinx and myelomalacia.

40.5 Clinical Picture

There is a history of chiropractic manipulation followed soon by pain in the back of the neck, which may be radiating to the upper extremities. Parathesia, anesthesia, analgesia, to the upper and may be the lower extremities, motor weakness and paralysis in the form of tetraparesis. Sphincteric dysfunction may occur. The paresis may be isolated to one side of the body (Brown-Sèquard Syndrome). Cerebrovascular complications (stroke) may be another complication.

40.6 Diagnosis

Diagnosis is based on:

1. History of cervical manipulation
2. Clinical symptoms
3. Neurological signs: sensory, motor deficits, increased reflexes, Brown-Sèquard syndrome, loss of temperature sensation, proproception, touch and transient tetraplegia has been reported in patients with spinal stenosis
4. MRI of spinal cord: showed a collection anterior to the spinal cord from C1-T5 and post-epidural collection from T3-T5 and another collection form T11-L3.
5. Radiography: showed bone and joint abnormalities
6. CT scan: show hematoma and cord displacement or compression
7. MRI: edema of the cord will show increased signal intensity in sagittal and axial T2 weighted images. In Brown-Sèquard syndrome there will be enlargement on one side of the cord. Ligamentous and soft tissue injuries may be seen as well as other pathological conditions i.e. multiple sclerosis, space-occupying lesions, etc. In cases of epidural hematoma gives a bright signal on T1-weighted images with cord compression or displacement. Centrally the hematoma has a low signal with a peripheral rim of bright signal on T2-weighted images.

40.7 Management

As soon as the diagnosis is established, steroid therapy should be instituted if the MRI shows cord edema. If decompressive laminectomy is indicated, it may be on multiple levels. Steroids seem to be helpful for neuronal recovery (Chung 2002). For the hematoma evacuation is indicated. Minor injuries may resolve with conservative therapy. Preventative treatment is important by avoiding manipulation on patients predisposed to cord injury and by experience and knowledge. Turning to hand medicine only after medical treatment fails.

References

Chung OM. MRI confirmed cervical cord injury caused by spinal manipulation in a Chinese patient. Spinal Cord. 2002;40(4):196–9.

Lee KP, Carlini WG, Mccormick GF, Albers GW. Neurologic complications following chiropractic manipulation: a survey of California neurologists. Neurology. 1995;45(6):1213–5.

Torg JS, Pavlov H, Genuario SE, et al. Neurapraxia of the cervical spinal cord with transient quadriplegia. J Bone Joint Surg Am. 1986;68(9):1354–70.

Paraplegia Following Chemonucleolysis 41

41.1 Definition

This is an iatrogenic paraplegia following inadvertently injecting chemolytic agent into the lumbar theca for degenerative disc disease.

41.2 Incidence

This complication is rare, a case was reported by Smith in 1967 and a case reported by Eguro; and the case of reference is that reported by Dyck. One case of transverse myelitis is reported by Haag et al.

41.3 Etiology

Chymopapain is a disclytic agent and is used for treatment of disc degenerative disease. Injection into the subarachnoid space leads to hemorrhage and neurotoxicity resulting usually in cauda equine lesion or as Eguro reported transverse myelitis.

41.4 Pathology

Chymopapain is a neurotoxic and causes subarachnoid hemorrhage both leading to paresis. Other side effects are mentioned by Haag et al.

Abstracted from Dyck (1985)

I.M. Eltorai, *Rare Diseases and Syndromes of the Spinal Cord*,
DOI 10.1007/978-3-319-45147-3_41

41.5 Clinical Picture

Back pain, radiating to the lower limbs, weakness of the legs ending in paraplegia with sensory and motor changes and sphincteric dysfunction.

41.6 Diagnosis

Diagnosis is based on the following criteria:

1. history
2. neurological examination
3. CT scan
4. MRI
5. CSF exam

41.7 Management

- Prevention of intrathecal injection of the chymopapain very careful handling into the disc after laminectomy and lavage of the clots out. Steroids may help a little.
- If it happens CSF barbotage is recommended. In case of paresis due to subarachnoid clot formation evacuation of the clot is recommended.

Reference

Dyck P. Paraplegia following chemonucleolysis. A case report and discussion of neurotoxicity. Spine. 1985;10(4):359–62.

Spinal Cord Injury After Chest Compressions

42

42.1 Description

The authors report the first case of an infant who had asystole and ventricular fibrillation needing resuscitation. There have been sporadic reports spinal cord injury after chest compressions, including a case by Azuma et al. in 1986 and the case presented, by Samson et al. in 2012.

42.2 Case Report

A male infant born with a complete aterioventricular septal defect with a hypoplastic left ventricle. At 3 days of age he underwent the first stage of Damus-Kaye-Stansel and Sano procedures (for further details on the procedures see article by Tomasian et al. 2009). He developed progressive and refractory low cardiac output because of tricuspid regurgitation, at 3 months postoperatively he had a transient attack of reduced cardiac output requiring inotropic support with milrinone infusions and diuretics with many other pediatric medications.

Three weeks postoperative he had routine cardiac catheterization and biopsy to rule out rejection. The child was in the ICU on mechanical ventilation but was awake with movements in the extremities. The procedure was done through the right femoral vein under fluoroscopy. The procedure took 45 min uncomplicated. He developed brief period of asystole and ventricular fibrillation. CPR was done by chest compression for 10 min. He needed 3 defibrillations (2 J/kg). He was given adrenalin, sodium bicarbonate, calcium and a single dose of amiodarone. He was deeply sedated for 5 days in the ICU on a ventilator. When sedation was discontinued, he had little movement in the upper extremities and none in the lower extremities. He had flaccid paraplegia.

Abstracted from Samson et al. (2012).

I.M. Eltorai, *Rare Diseases and Syndromes of the Spinal Cord*,
DOI 10.1007/978-3-319-45147-3_42

42.3 MRI

MRI showed 5 mm subdural hematoma (SSH) and hemorrahagic contusion of the cord from T4 to T10 with subarachnoid hemorrhage extending from T10 to S2. Brain MRI showed severe extraventricular hydrocephalus and intraventricular hemorrhage and ischemic areas. There was no evidence of coagulopathy international normalized ratio (INR) of 1.13, a prothormbin of 14.8 s. Because of the poor prognosis and ischemic lesions, life support was discontinued. Autopsy confirmed the above findings.

42.4 Pathogenesis

The pathogenesis of chest compression complications include:

- Compression fractures of the chest wall and vertebrae
- SSH is due to increased intravascular pressure due to compression and to the low subdural pressure leading to bleeding.

The cerebral spinal fluid (CSF) pressure does not increase to neutralize the intravascular pressure because of the shielding effect of the spinal column. The great disparity of pressure between vessels and CSF in the subdural spaces causes the SSH.

The bleeding in SSH is very slow and may take days to manifest itsclf especially its origin is mostly venous. The intramedullary hemorrhage is explained on the same factors. The authors elaborate more on theories of bleeding. The elasticity of the infantile spine also predisposes to cord contusions.

References

Azuma SS, Mashiyama ET, Goldsmith CI, Abbasi AS. Chest compression-induced vertebral fractures. Chest. 1986;89(1):154–5.

Samson MÈ, Willems A, Lapierre C, Jouvet P. Spinal cord injury and hemorrhage after chest compressions: a case report. J Pediatr Neuroradiol. 2012;1(1):55–7.

Tomasian A, Malik S, Shamsa K, Krishnam MS. Congenital heart diseases: post-operative appearance on multi-detector CT-a pictorial essay. Eur Radiol. 2009;19(12):2941–9.

43 Cervical Myelopathy Contrast Injection

43.1 Definition

This is a condition of cervical myelopathy developing after accidental injection contrast into the spinal cord.

43.2 Incidence

Simon et al. reported one case and reviewed eight papers from the literature between 1983 and 2001, which included 26 patients.

43.3 Etiology

The cord drainage is due to:

- Mechanical effects of the contrast material i.e. physical compression.
- Toxic effect of the contrast material. Iohexol is less toxic than Metrizamide.

The amount injected varied between 1.1 and 15 ml of either Iohexol or Metrizamide.

Abstracted from Simon et al. (2002)

I.M. Eltorai, *Rare Diseases and Syndromes of the Spinal Cord*,
DOI 10.1007/978-3-319-45147-3_43

43.4 Pathology

Parenchymal reactions to pressure of the injection and chemical toxicity. The greater the volume injected, the more injury and more profound the neurologic deficit. More damage was seen with Metrizamide even with small doses of contrast medium.

43.5 Clinical Picture

Cervical myelopathy through C1–C2 lateral approach is rarely indicated as long as MRI can be done. It is indicated it's the patient is unfit for MRI those whose pathology could not be adequately demonstrated by MRI. When there is intramedullary contrast injection the patient generally feels pain in the neck, site of the face, and arm. Numbness of the upper and lower extremity, weakness, paresis and anesthesia. Most of these are reversible, especially after giving high doses of Methylpredinsolone although sensory and motor weakness may persist. Two patients died amongst the 26 cases and these were before the Methylpredinsolone intensive therapy era.

43.6 Diagnosis

Diagnosis is based on

1. Onset of sudden pain, numbness, weakness of one or more extremities during myelography
2. Neurologic signs
3. Radiography shows a longitudinal contrast stripe in the spinal cord, which gains more length and breadth with more contrast injection

43.7 Management

Intravenous Methylpredinsolone bolus 30 mgm/kg body weight, followed by a 5.4 mgm/kg body weight per hour for 48 h followed by tapering doses of oral methylpredisolone. In the case if ordered by Simon et al. patient almost totally recovered.

Reference

Simon SL, Abrahams JM, Sean Grady M, Leroux PD, Rushton SA. Intramedullary injection of contrast into the cervical spinal cord during cervical myelography: a case report. Spine. 2002;27(10):E274–7.

44 Acute Transverse Myelitis in an Infant After Dtap Vaccination

44.1 Definition

This is a condition of edema of the spinal cord developing after vaccination with diphtheria-tetanus-acellular pertussis (DTaP) vaccination as evidenced by neurological exam and MRI imaging.

44.2 Incidence

The case report by Riel-Romero seems to be the only one developing acute transverse myelitis after DTap 17 days earlier, although the child had two previous vaccinations (DTaP) without reaction. Kulenkampff et al. described a case of an infant, 6-month-old, who developed flaccid quadraparesis with respiratory compromise 17 days after DTaP vaccination (1974). Other cases of acute transverse myelitis (ATM) in childhood were reported due to hepatitis B vaccination (Fonseca et al. 2003; Iniguez et al. 2000). A case of Japanese B encephalitis vaccine was followed by transverse myelitis (Matsui et al. 2002). Whittle and Robertson reported a case of a 7-month-old infant who developed flaccid paraplegia after receiving DT inoculation and oral polio vaccine (1977). Zanoni et al. in 2002, reported a 15-month-old girl who developed ATM 21 days after receiving measles-mumps-rubella vaccination; similarly, Lim et al. 2004 with a 9-year-old girl who developed ATM 16 days post measles and rubella vaccination.

Abstracted from Riel-Romero (2006)

I.M. Eltorai, *Rare Diseases and Syndromes of the Spinal Cord*,
DOI 10.1007/978-3-319-45147-3_44

44.3 Etiology

The cause of developing ATM after DTaP vaccination is not quite clear:

- Riel-Romero's hypothesis is that the infant had acute respiratory infection 2 weeks before the onset of the myelitis, suggesting a viral agent. In an analysis of 33 patients of ATM post vaccination the author found, including adults, that 45 % had a preceding infection, most of them were respiratory with 73 %, gastrointestinal infection was 13 and 13 % had flu-like symptoms (Jeffery et al. 1993).
- The offending agent triggers an autoimmune reaction to the myelin sheath of the central nervous system (CNS), mainly to the spinal cord (Kerr and Ayetey 2002). The risk of ATM as an autoimmune response may depend on genetically predisposed child.
- Myelitis may have developed as an incidental condition.

44.4 Pathology

There is no pathological data in these cases; however, in hepatitis B vaccination it shows the inflammatory reaction, edema, and demyelination (Sindern et al. 2001). The disease seems to be self and time limited illness and is generally monophasic. Improvement occurs in 2–12 weeks after maximal development, but the faster the development the worse the prognosis is. Resolution occurs especially after steroid therapy; however, a scar is formed and motor recovery is minimal.

44.5 Clinical Picture

(From Riel-Romero 2006) An infant 7-months-old was admitted for leg weakness 17 days after DTaP vaccination. He received two injections without problems. He developed priapism and dribbling of urine. He had constipation previously, which was resolved with fleet enema. His past history was negative except for acute upper respiratory infection before admission. Examination of his systems was unremarkable. The neurological exam showed flaccid paraplegia. Noxious stimuli of the legs gave triple flexion response (no anesthesia). The lower limbs tendon reflexes were +1.

44.6 Diagnosis

Diagnosis is based on:

1. Clinical picture
2. Laboratory tests

(a) Blood count shows leucocytosis 16,000 and poly 67 %
(b) CSF showed 2 RBC/uL and 7 WBC/uL, 4 lyphocytes, and 3 monocytes
(c) Myelin basic protein was increased at 4.9 mg/dL (normal: 0–2.3)
(d) Other tests were within normal including IgG, and tests for viruses and bacteria were negative.

3. MRI: brain was negative. Spine showed diffused edema of the spinal cord with increased T2 signal within the spinal cord from C3 to T6, dorsal and ventral veins were normal and no evidence of AVM. After gadolinium injection there was a faint and patchy encroachment of the spinal cord.

The diagnosis was, from the clinical and imaging pictures, ATM 17 days after DTaP vaccination.

44.7 Management

Riel-Romero gave the following treatment:

- IV methylpredinsolone: 1.5 mgm/kg/day for 7 days followed by
- Oral predinsolone tapering at 1 mg/kg/day for 2 weeks
- Acyclovir pending on the result of CSF, HSV-DNA PCR.
- Bowel and bladder care
- Rehabilitation program

Within a week priapism resolved and the lower extremities gained tone and there was a clonus. At three weeks the constipation resolved and urine stream was established but signs of pyramidal involvement persisted. Three months later MRI showed resolution of the cord edema and its signals but showed reduction of the cord caliber. Ten months after the onset spastic paraplegia persisted.

References

Fonseca LF, Noce TR, Teixeira ML, Teixeira AL, Lana-peixoto MA. Early-onset acute transverse myelitis following hepatitis B vaccination and respiratory infection: case report. Arq Neuropsiquiatr. 2003;61(2A):265–8.

Iñiguez C, Mauri JA, Larrodé P, López del val J, Jericó I, Morales F. [Acute transverse myelitis secondary to hepatitis B vaccination]. Rev Neurol. 2000;31(5):430–2.

Jeffery DR, Mandler RN, Davis LE. Transverse myelitis. Retrospective analysis of 33 cases, with differentiation of cases associated with multiple sclerosis and parainfectious events. Arch Neurol. 1993;50(5):532–5.

Kerr DA, Ayetey H. Immunopathogenesis of acute transverse myelitis. Curr Opin Neurol. 2002a;15(3):339–47.

Lim S, Park SM, Choi HS, et al. Transverse myelitis after measles and rubella vaccination. J Paediatr Child Health. 2004;40(9–10):583–4.

Matsui M, Kawano H, Matsukura M, Otani Y, Miike T. Acute transverse myelitis after Japanese B encephalitis vaccination in a 4-year-old girl. Brain Dev. 2002;24(3):187–9.

Riel-Romero RM. Acute transverse myelitis in a 7-month-old boy after diphtheria-tetanus-pertussis immunization. Spinal Cord. 2006;44(11):688–91. Epub 29 Nov 2005.
Sindern E, Schröder JM, Krismann M, Malin JP. Inflammatory polyradiculoneuropathy with spinal cord involvement and lethal [correction of letal] outcome after hepatitis B vaccination. J Neurol Sci. 2001;186(1–2):81–5.
Whittle E, Robertson NR. Transverse myelitis after diphtheria, tetanus, and polio immunisation. Br Med J. 1977;1(6074):1450.
Zanoni G, Nguyen TM, Destefani E, Masala L, Nardelli E, Tridente G. Transverse myelitis after vaccination. Eur J Neurol. 2002;9(6):696–7.

45 Paraplegia After Endovascular Repair of Abdominal Aortic Aneurysm

45.1 Definition

This is an ischemic condition of the spinal cord resulting in paraplegia 3 weeks after endovascular repair of an abdominal aortic aneurysm (AAA)

45.2 Incidence

This is the first case after endovascular repair of AAA. After open surgical technique the incidence of spinal cord ischemia is 0.25 %. According to the Eurostar database, the incidence of cord ischemia is 0.21 %. Smaller arterial endovascular procedures do not lead to spinal cord ischemia.

45.3 Etiology

Spinal cord ischemia after AAA repair is due to the following:

- interruption of the cord circulation due to clamping
- atheromatous embolization
- hypoperfusion due to hypotension
- interruption of the artery of Adamkiewicz
- reperfusion edema leading to cord hypoperfusion and ischemia

CSF drainage can increase spinal cord perfusion, acting against the upper mechanisms.

Abstracted from Godstein et al. (2010)

I.M. Eltorai, *Rare Diseases and Syndromes of the Spinal Cord*,
DOI 10.1007/978-3-319-45147-3_45

45.4 Pathology

There is ischemia, edema of the cord, leading to demyelination and apoptosis, resulting in permanent myelopathy.

45.5 Clinical Picture

The case presented is a 75-year-old man: diabetic, chronic renal failure, coronary heart disease, aortic valve replacement, and an asymptomatic 5.5 cm infrarenal AAA, and concomitant 3.5 cm right common iliac artery aneurysm

45.6 Diagnosis

CT scan showed a fusiform aneurysm 3 cm below the right renal artery.

45.7 Management

Endovascular repair by aorticuniiliac (AUI) graft and femoral-femoral bypass. The patient developed several pressure ulcers postoperatively, which got septic. Twenty-one days post-op he was found paraplegic. MRI showed diffuse edema of the cord, due to ischemia. He needed feeding gastrotomy tube and left iliac colostomy and tracheostomy. There was no further report.

Reference

Goldstein LJ, Rezayat C, Shrikhande GV, Bush HL. Delayed permanent paraplegia after endovascular repair of abdominal aortic aneurysm. J Vasc Surg. 2010;51(3):725–8.

46 Spinal Cord Infarction After Endoscopic Esophageal Varix Ligation

46.1 Definition

According to Stedman's medical dictionary "an infarct is an onset of necrosis, resulting from a sudden insufficiency of arterial or venous blood supply."

46.2 Incidence

These cases are rare. Tofuku et al. reported a case in 2007. Debette et al. reported a case in 2003. In 1996, Heller et al. reported on case. The number of cases is very small.

46.3 Etiology

The causes of spinal cord venous infarction are:

- congenital arteriovenous malformation (AVM)
- epidural hematoma
- tumors
- iatrogenic: ligation of esophageal varices; sclerotherapy of esophageal varices
- decompression sickness

Because of the rarity of cases the etiology is not quite clear.

Abstracted from Tofuku et al. (2008)

I.M. Eltorai, *Rare Diseases and Syndromes of the Spinal Cord*,
DOI 10.1007/978-3-319-45147-3_46

46.4 Pathology

The ligation or injection of the esophageal varices leads to hemodynamic changes in venous circulation of the cord resulting in congestion and thrombosis, which ultimately leads to tissue ischemia and necrosis.

46.5 Clinical Picture

Following varices interruption by 1–3 days, a sense of numbness of the extremities, followed by weakness and paralysis with sphincter dysfunction.

46.6 Diagnosis

Neurological exam will detect motor and sensory loss and usually hyporeflexia.

MRI with and without gadolinium. Lab tests include INR, platelet count, liver function tests.

46.7 Management

Conservative treatment of paraplegia. Tofuku et al. used hyperbaric oxygen therapy (HBO2) at 2 ATA wit 15 min descent and 15 min ascent for 1 h daily for 20 days, with good outcome. Experience with HBO2, treatment in decompression sickness DCS justified its use in the particular case.

Reference

Tofuku K, Koga H, Yamamoto T, Yone K, Komiya S. Spinal cord infarction following endoscopic variceal ligation. Spinal Cord. 2008;46(3):241–2.

Subacute Combined Degeneration Provoked by Nitrous Oxide Anethesia Patients with Cobalamin Deficiency

47

47.1 Definition

Vitamin B_{12} deficiency leads to neuropathological changes in humans, principally subacute combined degeneration (SCD) of the spinal cord and polyneuropathy. Less commonly it causes encephalopathy leading to degeneration and optic neuropathy. Myelopathy may develop after nitrous oxide anesthesia in asymptomatic patients or those with borderline vitamin B_{12} deficiency or overlooked cases. It can result from chronic recreational use of N_2O or industrial exposure. This presentation will focus on myelopathy and SCD.

47.2 Incidence

SCD is a manifestation of vitamin B_{12} deficiency in one-third of the patients. Following nitrous oxide anesthesia cases of SCD are rare. In our English literature search we came across 11 reported cases, which means extreme rarity.

47.3 Etiology and Pathology

Kando et al. showed that nitrous oxide causes multiple defects in Cb1 metabolism. N_2O is a patent oxidant that disrupts the methonine synthetase reaction by causing oxidation of Co^{++} to Co^{+++}, which blocks regeneration of the cobalamine coenzyme methylcobalamin producing a condition simulating Cbl deficiency, inhibits methylation of myelin phospholipids, and alters incorporation of fatty acids into myelin sheaths. In patients with normal Cbl stores, a sufficient quantity of unoxidized Cbl

Abstracted from Ahn and Brown 2005

I.M. Eltorai, *Rare Diseases and Syndromes of the Spinal Cord*,
DOI 10.1007/978-3-319-45147-3_47

may be available to maintain enzyme function; in patiens with borderline Cbl stores, even short exsposures to N_2O may be suffienct to precipitate Cbl deficiency syndrome. The mature cobalamine is excreted so that exposure to N_2O will deplete the Cbl store.

47.4 Clinical Picture

The duration of anesthesia varies from 2 to 8 h; the onset is usually after 2–6 weeks. SCD is manifested by:

- Parathesia, numbness, weakness of the extremities, optic changes, loss of muscle tone, loss of position sense, gait instability, ataxia, and eventual spastic paraplegia.

The picture is modified in the presence of peripheral neuropathy. Bladder and bowel dysfunctions may be observed.

47.5 Diagnosis

Clinical picture confirmed by neurological exam, electromyography EMG, nerve conduction studies, Cbl serum level, Schilling test, evoked potential.

MRI will show High intensity signals in the post-lateral column.

47.6 Management

A short course of IV hydroxoocabalamin 5000 µg/day followd by IM cyanocobalamin 1000 µg/day × 5 days followed by 5000 µg QOD and then weekly and then monthy until recovery. This may take months since N_2O irreversibly oxidizes the cobalt ion of cobalamin.

Updates

2009

Chaugny et al.

Nitrous oxide is widely used in anesthesia. It is usually safe but may be associated with severe side effects when it is used repeatedly or on a prolonged time. Here, we report a case of drug-induced subacute combined spinal cord degeneration related to cobalamin deficiency.

Case Report

A 20-year-old man with sickle-cell disease (SS) who was followed for severe recurrent vaso-occlusive crisis with repeated hospital admissions presented with ascending motor and sensitive neurological deficits that were later associated with bladder dysfunction. He was first considered to develop Guillain-Barre syndrome. However, persisting neurological signs despite adequate treatment lately led to diagnose subacute combined medullar degeneration due to abnormal cobalamin (vitamin B12) metabolism induced by repeated use of nitrous oxide during painful episodes of sickle-cell disease. Inhaled nitric oxide is widely used in the treatment of vaso-occlusive crisis. Clinicians should be aware of possible severe neurologic side effects.

Reference

Chaugny C, Simon J, Collin-masson H, et al. Vitamin B12 deficiency due to nitrous oxide use: unrecognized cause of combined spinal cord degeneration. Rev Med Interne. 2014;35(5):328–32.

2015

Pugliese et al.

Recreational Use of Nitrous Oxide

A case of subacute combined degeneration (SCD) of the spinal cord manifesting as severe ataxia and urinary retention in a patient with a history of heavy nitrous oxide abuse and self-supplementation with cyanocobalamin is reported.

Case Report

A 27-year-old woman was treated in the emergency department for complaints of abdominal pain and inability to urinate for about 12 h. The patient also complained of worsening lower-extremity weakness for 10 days and a "pins and needles" sensation in the lower extremities for approximately 1 year. She reported nitrous oxide abuse over 3 years (an average of 100–200 "whippit" cartridges daily on 3 or 4 days per week), as well as long-term self-medication with oral and i.m. cyanocobalamin for the purpose of preventing nitrous oxide-induced neurologic symptoms. Results of magnetic resonance imaging (MRI) were highly suggestive of SCD, which is typically seen in primary vitamin B12 deficiency but has been reported in the context of chronic nitrous oxide exposure. Treatment was initiated with cyanocobalamin 1000 μg i.m. daily, to be continued for 5 days and followed by a four-week regimen of 1000 μg i.m. weekly. The patient was discharged after 3 days, despite continued symptoms, with instructions to obtain ongoing care but was lost to follow-up.

Reference

Pugliese RS, Slagle EJ, Oettinger GR, Neuburger KJ, Ambrose TM. Subacute combined degeneration of the spinal cord in a patient abusing nitrous oxide and self-medicating with cyanocobalamin. Am J Health Syst Pharm. 2015;72(11):952–7.

Reference

Ahn SC, Brown AW. Cobalamin deficiency and subacute combined degeneration after nitrous oxide anesthesia: a case report. Arch Phys Med Rehabil. 2005;86(1):150–3.

48 Myelopathy due to Cervical Spine Flexion for Pediatric Tracheal Resection

48.1 Definition

This is a paraplegic condition resulting from cervical spine flexion after tracheal resection for tracheal stenosis.

48.2 Incidence

After Silver, who made a literature review of paraplegia due to cervical spine flexion found 4 case reports.

48.3 Etiology

The cause is not fully understood:

- in children there is undue hypermobility of the cervical spine, which may result in cord damage without bony injury
- the presence of Schuerman's disease may cause stretching the cord across kyphotic spine
- in the elderly with spondylotic cervical spine acute flexion may cause transient dislocation, which results in tetraplegia. In the elderly, also vascular damage may cause cord infarction with resultant ischemic myelopathy. However, this does not apply to children.

Abstracted from Silver (2007)

I.M. Eltorai, *Rare Diseases and Syndromes of the Spinal Cord*,
DOI 10.1007/978-3-319-45147-3_48

48.4 Pathology

According to Vaget et al:

According to the distinctive anatomical and physiologic features of children and adolescents along with growth and development are responsible for the unique manifestations and complications of SCI in the pediatric population.

SCI without radiologic abnormalities (SCIWORA) and the delayed onset of neurologic deficits are relatively unique to that population. The unique anatomic and biomechanical characteristics of the youthful spine are responsible for the higher incidence of SCIWORA. These characteristics include:

- increased elasticity of the spine
- less flexibility of the spinal cord
- shallow and horizontally oriented facet joints
- anterior wedging of the vertebral body
- vulnerability of the growth zone of the vertebral end plates
- poorly developed uncinate processes

Pathology of spinal cord:

- minor hemorrhage
- traumatic edema
- severe hemorrhage
- incomplete cord injury
- traction on the cord and extremities

48.5 Clinical Picture

Silver's case was a child born with tracheal stenosis and had repeated resections until he was 17-years-old when the stenosis recurred causing shortness of breath and tracheal resection was done and his neck was flexed and his chin was sutured to his chest, to avoid tension on the tracheoplasty and was kept under light anesthesia for 48 h. When anesthesia was discontinued, he woke up with weakness of the left upper limb and complete paraplegia with sensory level at T8. MRI showed small annular disc herniation at C6-C7. Gadolinium showed no enhancement. Upper extremity weakness improved, but paraplegia persisted.

48.6 Management

Prevention of prolonged flexion and resorting to some other procedures of tracheoplasty.

In the early phase, steroid therapy may be useful.
In persistent deficit full rehab program is needed

Reference

Silver JR. Paraplegia as a result of tracheal resection in a 17-year-old male. Spinal Cord. 2007;45(8):576–8.

49 Spinal Cord Stimulator Scar Tissue

49.1 Definition

This is an iatrogenic complication resulting and compression myelopathy due to a foreign body reaction to spinal cord stimulation for chronic refractory pain.

49.2 Incidence

This is the first case of this nature.

49.3 Etiology

For the last 30 years spinal cord stimulation (SCS) has been used for:

- Failed spinal surgery syndrome
- Radicular pain syndrome
- Epidural fibrosis
- Arachnoiditis
- Complex regional pain syndrome
- Reflex sympathetic dystrophy

Abstracted from Guzzi et al. (2015)

I.M. Eltorai, *Rare Diseases and Syndromes of the Spinal Cord*,
DOI 10.1007/978-3-319-45147-3_49

SCS is used after all conservative measures have been tried. The complications SCS are:

- Pre- and post- OP complications viz.: puncture of the dura, CSF leak, injury of the cord, hematoma, and in the spinal cord.
- Delayed complications: malfunction, fibrosis and the equipment and manipulation of the spinal cord electrode. A foreign body giant – cell granuloma.

Foreign body reaction to this cord stimulator forming a mass as in the case presented, which has not been reported previously.

49.4 Pathology

A foreign body mass as a reaction to this stimulator occurs with giant cells and macrophage as a chronic inflammation response due to invasive procedure and chronic inflammatory response with poorly absorbed substance in the tissue.

49.5 Case Report

Fifty nine year old woman with history of back and all extremities pain and was placed on SCS says the painless refractory to standard measures. The stimulator was replaced due to fracture of the electrode wire. The system was fully exploited do to its fracture it was replaced by a simulator to C3 – C5 and can (see details in the article). There was a staph wound infection necessitating removal of the electrode. Recurrence of pain was worse than before. She also had loss of balance, she had upper extremity weakness 4/5. She had numbness and tingling and the stocking and glove distribution and exaggerated deep tendon reflexes. MRI: severe cervical stenosis secondary to intraspinal mass compressing of the cord at the site of the previous stimulator.

49.6 Management

Decompression laminectomy and removal of the mass, which gave her recovery. Pathology of the mass showed fibrous tissue with giant cell reaction to foreign body.

Reference

Guzzi G, Volpentesta G, Chirchiglia D, Della torre A, Lavano F, Lavano A. Cervical spinal cord compression from delayed epidural scar tissue formation around plate lead for SCS. Case report and literature review. J Neurosurg Sci. 2015 (in Pubmed: 26430719).

Neonatal Paraplegia Through Umbilical Catheterization

50

50.1 Definition

This is a condition of spinal cord infarction through umbilical artery catheterization (UAC) for therapeutic purposes.

50.2 Introduction

A brief abstract of the fetal circulation is presented from Gray's Anatomy

The fetal blood is returned to the fetus from the placenta (with nutrition) through the umbilical vein, which passes under the liver at the edge of the falciform ligament, gives off 2 or 3 branches, the larger one goes into the left lobe of the liver and the other two to the quadrate and caudate lobes.

At the porta hepatis it divides into two branches, the larger is joined by the portal vein to enter the right lobe, the smaller continues upwards to join the inferior vena cava (and is called the ductus venosus). The blood reaching the inferior vena cava (IVC) through the hepatic veins and the ductus venosus is admixed with the blood returning from the liver extremities and the abdominal wall. All IVC blood reaches the right atrium and is directed by IVC valve into the foramen ovale to the left atrium where it mixes with a small amount returning from the lungs. Then it is distributed after passing through the left ventricle and the ascending aorta to head and neck and upper extremities, a small portion goes to the lower extremities.

From the head and neck and upper limbs blood is returned via the superior vena cava to the right atrium, it goes into the right ventricle and from there to the pulmonary artery to the lungs, it returns to the left atrium, the greater part passes through the ductus arterious into the aorta where it is mixed with a small portion

Abstracted from Brown and Phibbs (1988)

I.M. Eltorai, *Rare Diseases and Syndromes of the Spinal Cord*,
DOI 10.1007/978-3-319-45147-3_50

coming from the left ventricle. Part of the aortic blood is distributed to the abdominal and pelvic viscera and lower limbs; the greater part is conveyed through the umbilical arteries to the placenta.

50.3 Incidence

In 1988, Brown and Phibbs reported two cases of spinal cord infarction through catheterization. The collected and reviewed the previous six cases. In our extensive literature search 2 additional cases were found: Munoz et al in 1993 and in 1996, Lemke et al., reported a case of UAC after switch operation for great vessels transposition.

50.4 Etiology

Catheterization is used for infusion of blood and sometimes hypertrophic solutions. The cause of the infarct is either the tip of the catheter reaching the arterial blood supply of the spinal cord, principally the artery of Adamkiewicz leading to thrombosis. Also could be due to embolism (see entry under embolism). Catheters are also used for blood samples, administration of fluids or medications. Another causative factor is vasospasm. These newborns are very sick usually in shock, which together with the use of hypertonic solutions are predisposed for thrombosis. There is a possibility that blood transfusion may be causative. High insertion of the tip of the catheter may impinge on the opening of the artery of Adamkiewicz.

Etiology of neonatal paraplegia after UAC, according to Aziz et al., the complications of UAC are thrombosis in 95 % of infants, embolism, vascular perforation, vasospasm, damage from hypertonic solutions, hemorrhage, infection, and cardiac arrhythmias. As a result of vascular complications an infarct develops in the spinal cord especially in the lower thoracic region, the territory of the artery of Adamkiewicz.

50.5 Pathology

The autopsy of the case reported by Brown and Phibbs showed gliosis of the anterior part of the spinal cord demyelination with focal necrosis of the anterior segment due to infarction. A picture of anterior spinal artery occlusion (Spiller's syndrome) spinal infarct has been demonstrated by MRI (Lemke et al.) which demonstrated hemorrhagic infarct, possibly due to trauma by the catheter tip.

50.6 Clinical Picture

The cases recorded were infants less than 1 week of age and half of them were preterm. They were sick, needing emergency care including UAC e.g. hyperbilirubinemia secondary to ABO, hemolytic disease, respiratory failure due to hyaline membrane disease, respiratory failure due to cardiac arrest shortly after birth, Rh hemolytic disease, and congenital heart disease.

Emergency intensive care is required and UAC is life saving, especially for transfusions or exchange transfusions, medications injected and lab tests. Cord infarction is manifested by motor and sensory and sometimes mottling of the lower extremities without vascular occlusion as in the case of Brown and Phibbs. MRI shows cord swelling in the thoracic region and increased signal intensity indicating infarction. Later atrophy of the cord is manifested on MRI.

50.7 Diagnosis

Diagnosis is based on:

- Neurological findings: flaccid paralysis of the lower extremities, loss of sensation especially to pain, mottling of the skin.
- MRI: shows swollen edematous spinal cord usually in lower thoracic and lumbar regions (the zone of artery of Adamkiewicz).

50.8 Management

Survivors are followed up in pediatric rehabilitation. The infant who lived and followed by Brown and Phibbs paraplegia was permanent but sensation was intact.

50.9 Preventative Management

Brown and Phibbs favor having the catheter tip either low i.e. at or below the third lumbar vertebra or higher above the tenth thoracic vertebra confirmed radiologically. Transfusions and hypertonic solutions should be limited to necessity. Transfusions should be carefully administered, diluted with normal saline, slow and careful infusion with port-filters. According to Aziz et al., it is better to direct the tip of the catheter towards the aortic bifurcation far below the artery of Adamkiewicz.

Reference

Brown MS, Phibbs RH. Spinal cord injury in newborns from use of umbilical artery catheters: report of two cases and a review of the literature. J Perinatol. 1988;8(2):105–10.

Malfunction of a Ventriculo-Peritoneal Shunt

51

51.1 Definition

This is a condition of paraparesis secondary to a malfunction of ventriculo-peritoneal shunt for hydrocephalus resulting in acute expansion of cervical syrinx.

51.2 Incidence

According to Lee et al., a retrospective study showed 4 cases of weakness of the lower extremities amongst 70 cases of ventriculoperitoneal shunt malfunctioning.

51.3 Etiology

A ventriculoperitoneal malfunction or obstruction force reopening of the central canal and propagates increasing pressure in it and causing expansion of the syrinx, especially when the fourth ventricle foramina are blocked by previous meningitis. This increased syrinx pressure causing mechanical pressure on the neural tracts as well as vascular compromise resulting in paraparesis.

51.4 Clinical Picture

From the case described by Beswick et al.:

> The 16-year-old female patient had the vetriculoperitoneal shunt for post-meningitis hydrocephalus. She had repeated malfunctions, which were corrected by reinsertion. She developed paraparesis associated with head, neck, and shoulder pains. She underwent posterior

Abstracted from Beswick et al. (2005)

I.M. Eltorai, *Rare Diseases and Syndromes of the Spinal Cord*,
DOI 10.1007/978-3-319-45147-3_51

fossa decompression for Chiari I. Reinsertion of the shunt gave temporary relief. She developed spastic paraparesis. CT scan showed enlarged ventricles and MRI showed an extensive syrinx from C1-T10. The syrinx acts as a fifth ventricle for the obstructed shunt.

51.5 Management

Revision of the malfunctioning shunt as early as possible especially in the presence of a syrinx. Although it has been suggested that prompt revision may result in good outcome this does not appear to be universally so.

Reference

Beswick E, St George EJ, Solanki GA. Paraparesis secondary to expansion of cervical syrinx: an unusual presentation of ventriculo-peritoneal shunt malfunction. Pediatr Neurosurg. 2005;41(6):334–6.

52 Viper Antivenin Induced Brown-Séquard Syndrome

Description This is a unique case of myelopathy induced by antivenin injection. Guillian-Barré Syndrome, which follows a viral infection or immunization, and is an acute inflammatory demyelinating neuropathy of acute onset affecting the peripheral and cranial nerves, there is no similar affection of the spinal cord.

The case presented was a 40-year-old woman who received antivenin (polyvalent enzyme-refined globulin). She developed an immunological inflammation. The snake was a green pit viper and the antivenin was prepared in India. She manifested Brown-Séquard syndrome, confirmed by computerized tomography. It was manifested by right hemiplegia and absence of pain and temperature sensation on the left half of her body below the 4th rib. There was loss of vibration sense and joint position sense on the right side of the body. The neurological examination indicated a deficit at the level of C6. The follow up of the patient showed recovery after 2 years.

Although, the pathology of the lesion was not determined this complication from the antivenin may be important since there are many areas in the United States where snakebites are not uncommon. There will be a possibility of such a complication of the antivenin serum; although, rarely. The venin itself may cause myelopathy. There is no definite Pathophysiology of the Brown Séquard syndrome; it might be an immune reaction to the serum with an inflammatory manifestation in the spinal cord itself. Since Guillian-Barré syndrome has developed as a reaction to immunization (flu vaccine) this might be a weak supportive cause.

Abstracted from Biswas et al. (2004)

I.M. Eltorai, *Rare Diseases and Syndromes of the Spinal Cord*,
DOI 10.1007/978-3-319-45147-3_52

Reference

Biswas R, et al. Anti-venom-induced myelopathy in semipoisonous snakebite. Int J Clin Pract. 2004;58(6):645–6.

Part IV

Idiopathic

Baastrup's Disease Causing Neurogenic Claudication

53

53.1 Definition

This is a condition where the adjacent spinous processes (kissing spines) come in close contact due to hyperextension and increasing lumbar lordosis and when continued it leads to neoarthosis and osteoarthritis with synovial lining. Also called Lumbar Interspinous Bursitis

53.2 Incidence

Bywaters and Evans conducted an autopsy study on 152 lumbar spines to find out the prevalence of Baastrup's disease (BD). They noted pseudojoints, chondroid metaplasia, endochondral ossification and gross osteoarthritic bone erosion with eburnation. They defined a "bursal index" to identify spines at risk of developing this disease. The range was from 6.2 to 22.1 %. The spines with lower index were more predisposed to the disease. Hagner suggested that there is higher prevalence in professional divers mostly at L3-L4, L4-L5.

53.3 Etiology

Kissing spines occur in chronic hyperextension of the spine as in professional divers adopting that position. It also develops in people with increasing lordosis. Associated instable disc segments may contribute to the development of the disease. Diffused fatty degeneration of the paraspinal muscles may predispose the disease due to accompanying lordosis, obesity, and chronic limitations of hip flexion.

Abstracted from Rajasekaran et al. (2003)

I.M. Eltorai, *Rare Diseases and Syndromes of the Spinal Cord*,
DOI 10.1007/978-3-319-45147-3_53

53.4 Pathology

As mentioned above there are kissing spines processes with chondrification, ossification, degeneration, and bursa formation, associated lumbar degenerative conditions.

53.5 Clinical Picture

Only one case of jumbo-bursa developed and penetrated in ligmentum flavum epidurally and caused cauda equina symptoms as reported by Rajasekaran et al., and is the main source for this subject and from which the clinical picture is summarized:

A 50-year-old female presenting with chronic lower back pain increasing with activity and becoming progressive to neurologic claudication pain. Physical exam showed palpable steps at L3-L4 and L4-L5, which were tender. Paraspinal muscles were spastic on flexion.

Radiography showed Grade I anterolisthesis of L3 over L4 and Grade II L4 over L5.

MRI T2-weighted images: neoarthrosis between the spinous processes with interspinous bursitis, indicating Baastrup's disease. A cyst was seen in posterior epidural space at the same level with resultant spinal canal compromise mass. Minor disc degeneration was seen; no pressure was noted.

53.6 Management

Surgery was indicated to resolve the spinous process artherosis, pain and to the intraspinal cyst. At surgery neoarthrosis was confirmed. The adjacent surfaces of the spinous processes were facetted with well-formed pseudoarthotic cavity, of which was formed by a thick fibrous wall and was found to have an hourglass communication intraspinally through midline cleft of the ligamentum flavum. The intraspinal cyst, thin walled, filled with fluid and tense was causing epidural compression. The spinous processes were removed, the cyst excised and vertebral stabilization done by posterior Moss-Miami fixation along with intertransverse fusion.

The result was relief of spinal pain and neuroclaudication. In other cases there may be a failure due to associated degenerative diseases, such as disc prolapse, osteoarthritis, spina bifida occulta, spinal stenosis, etc.

Gato et al., reported a case of cervical myelopathy caused by osteophytic lipping and pseudoarthosis between the posterior tubercle of C1 and the spinous process of C2

Updates

Abstracted from Signla et al. 2014

Case Report

A 67-year-old male presented with a gradually progressive low back pain of 2 years duration. The patient had no history of trauma, radiation of pain, or any suggestion of claudication, nor was there any comorbidity. The pain was aggravated by extension and relieved by flexion. Swelling and neurological deficit were not present; however, muscle spasm was Radiographs of the spine revealed degenerative changes in the lumbosacral spine, along with articulation of spinous processes at lumbar spine at all levels, suggestive of Baastrup's disease, commonly know as kissing spine. The patient chose a conservative course, with week's course of analgesics and muscle relaxants and then started spinal flexion exercises. At 6 month follow up he had significant improvement.

Reference

Singla A, Shankar V, Mittal S, Agarwal A, Garg B. Baastrup's disease: the kissing spine. World J Clin Cases. 2014;2(2):45–7.

Reference

Rajasekaran S, Pithwa YK. Baastrup's disease as a cause of neurogenic claudication: a case report. Spine. 2003;28(14):E273–5.

Castleman's Disease

54

54.1 Definition

Castleman's disease (CD) is a rare lymphoproliterative disorder of unknown causes, which involves the lymph nodes and less commonly the extranodal tissues.

Synonyms: angiofollicular hyperplasia, nodal hyperplasia, giant lymph node hyperplasia, angiomatous lymphoid hamartoma, follicular lymphoreticuloma.

54.2 Incidence

CD is rare and its involvement of the central nervous system (CNS) is rarer. In the spinal canal, only four cases have been reported: by Alper et al. (1996), from C6 to T2; by Eisenstat et al. (2002), from T8 to T11 by Kachur et al. (2002), from T3 to T5; and by Lee et al. (2002), from T2 to T3.

54.3 Etiology

The disease has no definite etiology. It is theorized to be:

- inflammatory origin
- bacterial: although, no bacteria have been isolated
- hamartomatous process
- a response to an unknown stimulus with defective immunoregulation

I.M. Eltorai, *Rare Diseases and Syndromes of the Spinal Cord*,
DOI 10.1007/978-3-319-45147-3_54

54.4 Pathology

The sites affected by Castleman's disease are:

- The nodal sites of CD involves most commonly the mediastinum, cervical, axillary, less commonly it involves the mesenteric, retroperitoneal, and pelvic glands.
- The extranodal sites have been described in the larynx, thymus, lung, pericardium, and vulva.
- In the CNS it presents as leptomeningeal mass, which may be well circumscribed and may cause compression.

Microscopic findings of CD are that it is a distinct lymphoproliferative disorder characterized by lymphoid hyperplasia, with blood vessel proliferation. CD is divided into two types: hyaline-vascular and plasma cell. The former is more common and is characterized by lymphoid follicles penetrating vessels and interfollicular vascular proliferation. This kind is usually asymptomatic. The plasma cell form however, is associated with systemic symptoms. Large hyperplastic follicles with intervening sheets of plasma cells create the plasma cell form of CD.

54.5 Clinical Picture

Although the disease is benign and frequently asymptomatic, the multicentric forms may be aggressive; it is most commonly mediastinal. However, this presentation focuses on compression myelopathy by CD. Involvement of the brain is far more common than that the spinal cord. Four cases have been reported, which presented as an epidural mass, causing spinal cord compression that produced constitutional symptoms such as fever, headache, and lab abnormalities. The result is sensory-motor dysfunction at the level of the lesion and sphincteric dysfunction. The laboratory tests in CD show an elevated erythrocyte sedimentation rate (ESR), anemia, hypergammaglobulinemia, luekocytosis, and thrombocytosis. A tissue biopsy will show one or more typical pictures of CD better than imaging. Plain radiography may be negative; magnetic resonance imaging (MRI) and computed tomography (CT) myelography will show an intraspinal space-occupying lesion, similar to intraspinal tumors.

54.6 Diagnosis

Diagnosis is based on:

The disease should be differentiated from rheumatoid arthritis, Rosai-Dorfman Disease (see sinus histiocytosis with massive lymphadenopathy entry), Sjogren syndrome, polyneuropathy, organomegaly, indocrinopathy, monoclonal gammopathy, skin changes syndrome, autoimmune disease, lymphoma, plasma cell granuloma, and Kaposi's sarcoma. For further details see Kachur, et al.

54.7 Management & Prognosis

Localized forms may be treated with local resection or radiation. Those that are multifocal are treated with radiation therapy as well as systemic chemotherapy and if possible surgery.

Localized forms are usually benign. Multicentric forms are usually aggressive and end fatally from infection. An increased risk of non-Hodgkin's lymphoma and Kaposi's sarcoma has been associated with the multicentric form of CD. The plasma cell type is associated in about 50 % of the patients with splenomegaly, lymphadenopathy, and chronic anemia. Patients with the localized form, presenting with a pseudotumor, may be cured with surgical resection.

References

Alper G, Crumrine PK, Hamilton RL, Albright AL, Wald ER. Unusual case of inflammatory spinal epidural mass (Castleman syndrome). Pediatr Neurol. 1996;15(l):60–2.

Eisenstat RS, Price DB, Rosenthal AD, Schuss AL, Katz DS. Thoracic epidural Castleman's disease. AJR Am J Roentgenol. 2002;178(1):208–10.

Kachur E, Ang LC, Megyesi JF. Castleman's disease and spinal cord compression: case report. Neurosurgery. 2002;50(2):399–402.

Lee HY, Lee SH, Kim SN. Castleman's disease: unusual case of inflammatory spinal dorsal epidural mass: case report. Neurosurgery. 2002;50(2):396–8.

Cruciate Paralysis 55

55.1 Definition

Cruciate paralysis (CP) is a condition characterized by bilateral upper extremity paralysis with minimal or no lower extremity involvement. Wallenberg, whose first detailed description, in (Wallenberg 1901), described the complex neuroanatomy of the corticospinal tracts at the cervico-medullary junction.

55.2 Synonyms

Wallenberg syndrome

55.3 Incidence

Hatzakis, et al. gathered 26 cases of CP and added one of their own, in (Hatzakis et al. 2000), for a total of 27 case reports.

55.4 Etiology

There may possibly be many causes of cruciate paralysis, namely:

- Odontoid fracture as mentioned by Bell; he attributed the paralysis to injury of the midline fibers of the upper portion of the pyramidal decussation.
- Atlantoaxial-subluxation (Dai et al.)
- Metastasis to the occipitocerivical junction (Faillace and Guthrie)
- Gunshot injuries to the anterior arch of the atlas (Marano et al.)

I.M. Eltorai, *Rare Diseases and Syndromes of the Spinal Cord*,
DOI 10.1007/978-3-319-45147-3_55

- Association to Arnold Chiari I malformation due to contusion of the cord and/or edema or an extending syringomyelia. (Erlich et al.)
- Hematomyelia extending proximalwards as a birth injury (Önal et al.) or antenatal injury (Berck et al.)
- Tuberculoma of the odontoid process (Nielsen)
- Infarction caused by systemic hypoperfusion or carotid obstruction or by embolism. According to Sage and van Uitert, systemic hypoperfusion (systolic blood pressure less than 50 mmHg for at least 5 min). The found brachial dipelgia in 11 out of 34 comatosed patients with hypoperfusion. They coined the term man-in-the-barrel syndrome (MIBS) for the condition described.

Other causes mentioned are vertebral artery dissection, polyneuropathy, motor neuron disease, central pontine myelinolysis, and ischemia of the anterior horns during septicemia.

55.5 Pathophysiology

According to Bell, he suggested midline injury of the ventral aspect of the junction of the medulla and the cervical spinal cord causing damage to the pyramidal tract where the corticospinal motor fibers subserving the upperlimb functions decussate. Most authors relate cruciate paralysis with selective damage to pyramidal decussation. The anatomy of the pyramidal tracts is important to mention. The fibers arise along with the Betz cells of the precentral gyrus of the cerebrum. The fibers descend to the spinal cord via the internal capsule, the crus cerebri, the pons, and the medulla oblongata. Finally, they form the corticospinal tracts, except for some fibers going to the brainstem forming the corticobullbar tract. The corticospinal tract subsequently divides into two parts: part one decussate at the junction of the medulla oblongata. The superior cervical spinal cord forms the lateral corticospinal tract. The undecussated make up the anterior corticospinal tract. The general concept is that the motor tract of the upper extremities crosses ventral to the medulla and that the lower extremities fibers cross lower down. When the fibers of the upper extremities at the pyramidal decussation are injured a specific clinical syndrome will be induced. This hypothesis has not been confirmed by neuroanatomist research.

Barnard and Woolsey, and Coxe and Landau traced the generating fibers from discrete lesions of the motor cortex of the cynomolegus monkey. As a result, they found no evidence for differential decussation of forelimb fibers in the monkey. Pappas et al. supported this; they concluded that the pyramidal tract in the monkey appeared to be uniformly distributed. They theorized that damage of the pyramidal tract decussation could not selectively influence the upper limb performance in humans unless human anatomy differs markedly from the primates. This latter statement the writer agrees, since primates use the four limbs for walking, which means the use of upper and lower extremities in the humans.

55.6 Clinical Picture

Cruciate paralysis is characterized by upper extremity deficits most commonly bilateral and symmetrical with minimal or absent lower extremity involvement. After spinal shock reflexes are hyperactive (upper motor neuron lesion) this kind of paralysis is named brachial diplegia. The man-in-barrel syndrome is used to describe paralysis of the upper extremity, due to supratentorial or medullary lesions. MIBS is now exclusively used to describe bilateral frontal lobe lesions, due to cerebral hypoperfusion resulting in ischemic lesions resulting in the appearance of the patient being confined in a barrel. The clinical pictures of MIBS and CP are similar. In the early phase of CP there may be some sensory change but they do not last. There may also be present transient respiratory insufficiency, urinary retention, and cranial nerve palsies.

55.7 Diagnosis

Brachial diplegia gives the picture of upper motor neuron paralysis of the upper extremities, with lack of disability in the lower extremity. The diagnosis can be confirmed by imaging and neurophysiological studies. It should be differentiated from central cord injury, which is characterized by more severe paralysis of the upper extremities than the lower extremities. Furthermore, due to the involvement of the gray matter the upper extremity paralysis can present a lower motor neuron dysfunction. There is no affection of the cranial nerves in central cord injury. Also, in central cord injury there is sensory deficit, bladder and bowel dysfunction.

55.8 Prognosis

Most of the reported cases have recovered partially or completely when treated early and the offending cause dealt with.

55.9 Management

Early management is important depending on the cause. The following are abstracted from the recorded cases:

- Atalanto-axial dislocation: open reduction and occipito-cervical fusion
- Odontoid fracture: occipital traction and plaster cast immobilization
- Atalanto-axial subluxation: occipital traction and plaster immobilization
- Fracture of C1 anterior ring and fracture of the odontoid: halo traction
- Hematomyelia: evacuated with good result in a birth injury child
- Metastatic cancer: halo traction applied, tumor debulking and long occipital spinal fusion to C7 using contoured Luque rods. Bone graft was performed and was

ended by stable spinal fusion. The tumor was a breast metastasis, which wa positive for estrogen receptors for which Tamoxifen was given in addition to radiotherapy. The primary source was dealt with a modified radical mastectomy. More details can be seen in Faillance and Guthrie's article

Variant

(abstracted from T. Yayama et al.)

A variant type of CP was described by Arseni and Maretsis, Dai et al. Nielsen, and most recently three cases by Yayama et al. Whereas characteristically patients with CP present with bilateral paraparesis or paralysis of the upper extremities without significant involvement of the lower extremities; the variant when the neural compression occurs predominantly on one side spastic palsy on the ipsalateral side of the upper extremity associated with spasticity on the contra-lateral side of the lower extremity. A condition described as hemiplegia cruciata. The paralysis is a result of a mechanical injury, metabolic disorder, or a complication with surgery at the cervicomedullary junction proximal to the pyramidal decussation. Various pathologies can result in neuroanotomical disorder of the corticospinal tracts at the cervicomedullary junction and the neurological presentations in this particular region may vary according to the location of the lesion involving the descending pyramidal tracts. The authors comment modern imaging techniques including 18 F-2-fluoro-deoxy-D-glucose-positron emission tomography to enhance detection of mechanically compressive lesion to the cord and the vertebral-cranial junction. Lesions affecting the proximal portion of the pyramidal decussation could affect cranial nerves IX, X, XI, XII and sometimes respiratory insufficiency. The presence of mechanical compressive lesion warrants surgical therapy, which needs a very careful consideration. Early diagnosis and appropriate surgery are very helpful; however, delayed surgery with prolonged palsy should have a negative affect on neurological outcome.

Reference

Yayama T, Uchida K, Kobayashi S, et al. Cruciate paralysis and hemiplegia cruciata: report of three cases. Spinal Cord. 2006;44(6):393–8.

References

Hatzakis Jr MJ, et al. Cruciate paralysis, hypothesis for injury and recovery. Spinal Cord. 2000;38(2):120–5.

Wallenberg A. Anatomischer Befund in einen als "acute bulbaraffection (embolie der Art. cerebellar. post. inf. sinister?)" beschrieben Falle. Arch Psychiatr. 1901;34:923–59. German.

56 Myelopathy Due To Gorham's Disease

56.1 Definition

Gorham's disease (GD) is extremely rare and a mysterious bone pathology with unknown etiology. Jackson first described it in 1838; in 1955 Gorham and Stout presented 24 cases with an overview and described it as progressive osteolysis associated with angiomatosis of the blood or lymphatic vessels. GD may originate in virtually any osseous structure. Other terms were introduced, such as: the disappearing bone, the phantom bone, primary lymphangioma, acute absorption of bone; Gorham and Stout called it massive osteolysis.

56.2 Incidence

Aizawa et al. reported in (Aizawa et al. 2005) that there were 28 cases with spinal involvement in the English literature; the authors added one case of their own. Nine of the cases (31.0 %) had myelopathy and two had neuropathy. The patients ranged in age from 5 to 72; the male to female ratio was 18:10. Girn et al. have reported case of GD of the skull base and cervical spine in a 2 year old. Though GD can arise at any level from the cervical spine to the sacrum, the thoracic and cervicothroacic was most frequently involved.

56.3 Etiology

The disease is of unknown etiology

Abstracted from Aizawa et al. (2005)

I.M. Eltorai, *Rare Diseases and Syndromes of the Spinal Cord*,
DOI 10.1007/978-3-319-45147-3_56

56.4 Pathology

Heffez et al. suggested the following criteria for pathological diagnosis:

- a positive biopsy for angiomatous tissue
- absence of cellular atypia
- minimal or no osteoblastic response and absence of dystrophic calcification
- evidence of local progressive osseous resorption
- non-expansible, non-ulcerative lesion
- absence of visceral involvement except the presence of chylothorax in thoracic spine involvement
- oseolytic radiographic pattern
- negative hereditary metabolic, neoplastic, immunologic, or infectious etiology

The first pathological stage consists of diffused intraosseous osteolysis, which may be accompanied by pathological fracture. This is followed by increasing deformity with loss of bone mass. In the third stage the cortex is disrupted with invasion of the surrounding soft tissue. The last stage consists of complete resorption of the bone. The appearance can be consistent with hemangiomatosis or lymphangiomatosis. The disease is polyostotic, so one or several vertebrae, up to ten as in Aizawa et al. can be involved. Cases have been studied showing destruction of the ribs and long bones; sometimes GD involves the skin. Microscopically there is regional to massive osteolysis to complete absorption of the bone. There is increased intraosseous capillary formation, which are ectatic, giving the appearance of hemangioma. Occasionally lymphangiectasis occurs causing chylothorax, which develops as a complication in 17 % of the cases. There is a large number of osteoclasts; it was suggested that perivascular cells are preosteoclasts. According to Gorham and Stout, there is a presence of fibrosis and osteoclasts may be absent in the area of bone resorption. There is absence of osteoblasts, as well as bone deposits. It does not metastasize nor is there neoplasia. Mechanical pressure caused by increased vascular tissue might act on bone absorption process. As GD progresses to the spine it causes a pathological fracture, deformity, kyphosis up to 100°, kyphoscoliosis and subluxation. Involvement of the spinal cord is mostly by pressure.

56.5 Clinical Picture

The picture varies with the level of involvement. The onset is insidious with dull pain in the affected area; however, a pathological fracture or even deformity of the involved area with neurological deficit may be found in the initial presentation.

56.6 Diagnosis

There is much difficulty in diagnosing the pathology of GD. Plain x-ray, computed tomography (CT) scan, and magnetic resonance imagining (MRI) confirm the diagnosis. To make a confident diagnosis of GD, one must conduct a bone biopsy. GD needs to be differentiated from other angiomatosis. Both entities are composed of hemangiomatosis or lymphangiomatosis or a combination of both. GD, unlike other angiomatosis, tends to result in complete resorption of bone and periostial cells with replacement of fibrous tissue. There is often a delayed diagnosis due to the fact that the lesion is not distinguishable from localized, nonsclerosing osteolysis.

56.7 Management

It is often difficult choosing a treatment for GD, with the possibility of spontaneous arrest, which has been reported in some cases. Hence it is recommended to follow a conservative treatment and surgical treatment should be performed as late as possible. Radiotherapy, medication, and surgical treatment were used alone or in combination for the management of GD of the spine, however most of them led to unsatisfactory results. Many authors stated that radiotherapy did not stop the progression of osteolysis; whereas, others reported favorable outcomes when used in conjunction with a brace or halo traction. Hagberg et al. prescribed clodronate and α-2b interferon after operation with radiotherapy, which ceased a progressive spinal deformity and decreased a pleural chylous effusion. Aggressive medical approaches have been tried, including: vitamin D, parathyroid hormone, androgen, calcium, calcitonin, adrenal extracts, vitamin B12, and biphosphonates. The surgical treatment of 8 cases 5 cases (62.5 %) could obtain stable spine. It was concluded that a total spondylectomy should be performed, if the number of involved vertebrae is small. With the case of Aizawa et al. since there were ten vertebrae affected, situ posterior fusion with hook and rod system and iliac bone grafts were performed, but after surgery, the patient had complete paraplegia. fSome cases may be stationary, but most advance to pathologic fracture and complete myelopathy. The data collected by Aizawa et al. there were nine deaths [32.1 %] ranging from 2 weeks to 11 years after treatment. According to Chong et al. of the eight cases, which involve the cervical spine, five [62.5 %] were reported to have been fatal.

Reference

Aizawa T, Sato T, Kokubun S. Gorham disease of the spine: a case report and treatment strategies for this enigmatic bone disease. Tohoku J Exp Med. 2005;205:187–96.

57 Hajdu Cheney Syndrome

57.1 Definition

Hajdu Cheney syndrome (HCS) is an idiopathic bone disease characterized by abnormal cranial shape, premature loss of teeth, acro-osteolysis and short stature. Its neurological manifestations are hydrocephalus, trigeminal neuralgia, basilar impression.

57.2 Incidence

The disease is rare about fifty cases are recorded (NORD statistics).

57.3 Etiology

There is the familial type due to autosomal dominant inheritance

Nonfamilial type is less common

57.4 Pathogenesis

This is unknown however theories include:

- Brown theory: abnormal osteoblasts leading to structural protein abnormality
- Nunzita et al.: concluded that the generalized osteoporosis was due to increased osteclastic activity leading to increased bone resorption. This activity is increased by osteoclast activating factors such as interleukins.

Abstracted from Tanimoto et al. (1996)

I.M. Eltorai, *Rare Diseases and Syndromes of the Spinal Cord*,
DOI 10.1007/978-3-319-45147-3_57

- Elias et al. theory: the bone marrow was replaced by vascularized intersepted fibrous nerve fibers that were

57.5 Clinical Picture

Only one case of jumbo-bursa developed and penetrated in ligmentum flavum epidurally and caused cauda equina symptoms as reported by Rajasekaran et al. and is the main source for this subject and from which the clinical picture is summarized:

A 50-year-old female presenting with chronic lower back pain increasing with activity and becoming progressive to neurologic claudication pain. Physical exam showed palpable steps at L3–L4 and L4–L5, which were tender. Paraspinal muscles were spastic on flexion.

Radiography showed Grade I anterolisthesis of L3 over L4 and Grade II L4 over L5.

MRI T2-weighted images: neoarthrosis between the spinous processes with interspinous bursitis, indicating Baastrup's disease. A cyst was seen in posterior epidural space at the same level with resultant spinal canal compromise mass. Minor disc degeneration was seen; no pressure was noted.

57.6 Management

Surgery was indicated to resolve the spinous process artherosis pain and to the intraspinal cyst. At surgery neoarthrosis was confirmed. The adjacent surfaces of the spinous processes were facetted with well-formed pseudoarthotic cavity, of which was formed by a thick fibrous wall and was found to have an hourglass communication intraspinally through midline cleft of the ligamentum flavum. The intraspinal cyst, thin walled, filled with fluid and tense was causing epidural compression. The spinous processes were removed, the cyst excised and vertebral stabilization done by posterior Moss-Miami fixation along with intertransverse fusion.

The result was relief of spinal pain and neurocladication. In other cases there may be a failure due to associated degenerative diseases, such as disc prolapse, osteoarthritis, spina bifida occulta, spinal stenosis, etc.

Gato et al. reported a case of cervical myelopathy caused by osteophytic lipping and pseudoarthosis between the posterior tubercle of C1 and the spinous process of C2

Reference

Tanimoto A, Tamaki N, Nagashima T, Nakamura M. Syringomyelia associated with Hajdu-Cheney syndrome: case report. Neurosurgery. 1996;39(2):400–3.

58 Holocord Myelopathy with Thoracic Stenosis

58.1 Definition

Holocord myelopathy is myelopathy of the entire spinal cord from the cervical-medullary junction to the conus medullaris.

58.2 Incidence

One case reported by CH Kim et al.

58.3 Etiology

The authors hypothesize that in spinal stenosis in general myelopathy is due to ischemia caused by mechanical pressure on the cord vasculature and it is localized to the site of stenosis and mostly irreversible. In their case the whole cord is involved. They found the disturbance of cerebral spinal fluid (CSF) flow dynamics as shown by MRI and Ciné MRI and that recovery was achieved after decompression.

58.4 Pathology

It was found by Klekemp et al. that altered dynamics of CSF leads to interstitial edema below the stenotic lesion due to the pressure gradient between the subarachnoid space (SAS) and the spinal cord. The same authors suggested that interstitial edema is a presyrinx state and that it may alter the extramedullary fluid dynamics.

Abstracted from Kim et al. (2003)

I.M. Eltorai, *Rare Diseases and Syndromes of the Spinal Cord*,
DOI 10.1007/978-3-319-45147-3_58

58.5 Clinical Picture

The patient was a 64 year old male presenting with paraparesis with sensory level at T10.

58.6 Diagnosis

Diagnosis is based on the following criteria:

- MRI: Intramedullary high signal intensity involving the whole spinal cord on a T2 weighted image and suspicious stenosis at T11 level. Ciné MRI showed obstruction of the CSF circulation at T11 level.

58.7 Management

Patient had posterior decompression procedure, which lead to improvement of neurological deficit, resolution of myelopathy and resumption of CSF circulation.

Reference

Kim CH, Chung CK, Kwon BJ, Kim HJ. Holocord myelopathy with thoracic stenosis: case report and hypothesis. Spinal Cord. 2003;41(12):696–9.

Myelitis due to Hypertrophic Dens

59

59.1 Definition

This is a condition of upper cervical cord compression due to hypertrophied dens, i.e. increased diameter (15 mm or larger). It is usually associated with atlantodental osteoartheritis and may have developmental narrowing of the atlas ring.

59.2 Incidence

This is a very rare entity. One case was recorded by Moskovich and Crockard and another by Okada et al.

59.3 Etiology

Etiological factors are abstracted from Okada et al.:

- Osteoarthritis of the antlantodental joint causes hypertrophy of the dens, similar to osteoarthritis of the extremities. At the same time, this will reduce the internal diameter of the atlas ring, predisposing the cord to compression. There is also slight increase in the thickness of the anterior arch of the atlas.
- Atlantoaxial subluxation in developmentally small atlas ring complicated by hypertrophic dens. Atlantoaxial instability may in time cause atlantodental osteoarthritis with subsequent dental hypertrophy.

  Both conditions are post-traumatic.

Abstracted and reported by Okada et al. (2000)

I.M. Eltorai, *Rare Diseases and Syndromes of the Spinal Cord*,
DOI 10.1007/978-3-319-45147-3_59

59.4 Pathology

This unique case reported by Okada et al. is the only source and one has to quote the pathology they reported:

"The sagittally cut section of the cranium 2/3 of the hypertrophic dens showed thickening of the cortical bone of the anterior and cranial parts of the dens. Distribution of the cancellous bony trabeculae was also dense in the anterior and cranial parts. The apical portion of the dens, where the ala ligaments was attached, showed marked degeneration of the enthesis, including irregularity or disruption of the tide marks and obscure Sharpey's fibers. Partially overlapped tide marks were observed. The ALA ligament showed diffused myxoid degeneration and many fissure formations. Fibroblastic cells or tenocytes in the ligament had severely ballooned. In the anterior part, the cartilage showed severe fibrillation with myxoid degeneration of the matrix. Multiple fissure, which extend into the basal layer of the cartilage, were also observed. Chondrocystes were arranged in a columnar fashion, although their nuclei and lacunar structures were frequently obscure. In the posterior part, where the cruciate ligament had supported the dens, the cortex was covered by fibrous tissue. The continuity of the cortex was partially disrupted, and dense fibrous tissue had proliferated with immature bone formation. There was no apparent calcification.

59.5 Case Report

The picture of upper cervical myelopathy is present with pain and limitation of neck movement, weakness of the upper and lower extremities, sensory loss, and hyperreflexia.

59.6 Diagnosis

Diagnosis is based on the following criteria:

- Clincal picture, history of trauma
- neurological exam
- radiographic series and frontal tomograms:
  - cobra-head-like hypertrophic dens
  - osteoarthritisof the atlantoaxial joints
  - the AP diameter of the dens is increase in the sagittal plane
  - the anterior arch of the atlas is thickened and sclerotic
  - the atlantodental space is increased
- MRI of the spinal cord shows upper cervical cord compression between the hypertrophied dens and the neural arch of the atlas.

59.7 Management

To relieve the myelopathy, the authors recommended decompression procedures, with or without occipitocervical fusion. Details can be seen in the article.

Reference

Okada K, Sato K, Abe E. Hypertrophic dens resulting in cervical myelopathy: histological features of the hypertrophic dens. Spine. 2000;25(10):1303–7.

Myelopathy due to Léri's Disease

60

60.1 Definition

It is considered relatively benign disease affecting the skeleton and adjacent soft tissue, but it causes much pain, deformity and considerable functional morbidity. Synonyms include melorheostosis, flowing hyperostiosis, osteopathia hyperostotica, or sclerosing bone dysplasia.

60.2 Incidence

Only a few cases have been reported affecting the vertebrae; according to Reznik and Fried, since the disease was described in 1922, about 400 cases have been reported.

60.3 Etiology

The cause of the disease is unknown. It is not hereditary and it affects genders equally. It is thought to occur as an embryonal metameric disturbance which causes a failure in intramembranes and to a lesser extent, endochondral ossification. Another hypothesis is that it is of neural origin (sometimes herpes zoster) associated with the sensory nerve roots with resultant scarring and hyperostiosis. It may occur with other types of bone sclerosis such as osteopoikilosis and osteopathia striata. According to Zeiller et al. (2005), abnormality of sensory spinal nerves enables the disease to affect its sclerotome, which is why the disease is almost always unilateral and affects single sclerotome more frequently than multiple ones.

Abstracted from Reznik and Fried (2005)

I.M. Eltorai, *Rare Diseases and Syndromes of the Spinal Cord*,
DOI 10.1007/978-3-319-45147-3_60

60.4 Pathology

According to Reznik and Fried: As a mesodermal disease Léri's disease tends to be segmental involving one or more sclerotomes, one bone (monostatic) or multiple bones (polyostatic). Skeletal abnormalities may be restricted to one side of the body (hemimelic) or to a single limb (monomelic), most predominately lower limb. The bones involved are the diaphysis of the long bones, pelvis, small bones of the hands and feet, rarely the ribs, vertebrae, skull, or facial bones. In the vertebrae the bone is markedly sclerotic, causing compromise of the spinal canal and compression myelopathy, and also foraminal stenosis leading to root compression. Extradural fibrolipomatous tissues were described by Graver and Raby also Vivian. Schellhammer et al. (2006), report a case of intraspinal lipoma associated with the disease (German). The disease is seen in early childhood and 40–50 % of cases are seen by 20 years.

60.5 Clinical Picture

Vertebral involvement leads to spinal stenosis and compression myelopathy manifested by: back pain (in mild cases may be the only symptom). With cord compression there will be sensory changes and motor weakness and eventually paresis. Hyperosteosis of the extremities may be detected, by swelling, hyperpigmentation, scleroderma, tissue calcification, muscle atrophy, and myosclerosis. Skin lesions, vascular anomalies and joint contractions may be associated with melorheostosis.

60.6 Diagnosis

Diagnosis is based on the following criteria:

1. Clinical picture, the age varies wildly from birth to 64 years.
2. Radiography shows hyperosteotic bone disease. The radiological appearance of wax flowing down a candle in longitudinal bones. For more details see Motimaya and Meyers (2006).
3. CT scan showed: block level
4. MRI of the spine: melorheostosis and reduced spinal canal with cord compression.
5. Bone biopsy: sclerosed bone matrix with narrow Haversian canals

60.7 Management

Surgery consists of:

1. Decompression laminectomy and root decompression.

2. Fusion may be needed in lumbar cases. See lumbosacral fusion by Robertson et al. (2003).

Rehabilitation consists of:

1. In absence of neurological manifestation–the uses of diphosphonates, non-steroidal anti-inflammatory drugs, local steroid injections, analgesics, bracing, and physical therapy.
2. For deformity of limbs— fasciotomy, tendon lengthening, capsulotomy, osteotomy may be needed and in uncorrectable deformities amputation may be considered as a last resort.

References

Motimaya AM, Meyers SP. Melorheostosis involving the cervical and upper thoracic spine: radiographic, CT, and MR imaging findings. AJNR Am J Neuroradiol. 2006;27(6):1198–200.

Reznik M, Fried GW. Myelopathy associated with melorheostosis: a case report. Arch Phys Med Rehabil. 2005;86(7):1495–7.

Robertson PA, Don AS, Miller MV. Painful lumbosacral melorheostosis treated by fusion. Spine. 2003;28(12):E234–8.

Schellhammer F, Rapp M, Saleh A. Melorheostosis of the HWS in an intraspinal lipoma. Rofo. 2006;178(8):822–3.

Zeiller SC, Vaccaro AR, Wimberley DW, Albert TJ, Harrop JS, Hilibrand AS. Severe myelopathy resulting from melorheostosis of the cervicothoracic spine. A case report. J Bone Joint Surg Am. 2005;87(12):2759–62.

Idiopathic Primary Spinal Myoclonus

61

61.1 Definition

Spinal myoclonus is a rare movement disorder, characterized by myoclonic involvement of a group of muscles supplied by a few contiguous segments of the spinal cord.

61.2 Incidence

Primary spinal myoclonus is extremely rare.

61.3 Etiology

The etiology is unknown and is coined as idiopathic. There are theories to its cause:

- Loss of inhibitory function of local dorsal horn interneurons.
- Abnormal hyperactivity of local anterior horn neurons.
- Aberrant local axon re-excitations
- Loss of inhibition from supra-segmental descending pathways.

61.4 Pathology

The condition has no detectable pathology. Pathophysiology is discovered by electrophysiological changes. In secondary category one or more of the following may be found:

- Spinal infection
- Spinal tumors

Abstracted from Campos et al. (2003)

I.M. Eltorai, *Rare Diseases and Syndromes of the Spinal Cord*,
DOI 10.1007/978-3-319-45147-3_61

- Vascular disease
- Demyelinating diseases
- AIDS
- Spinal anesthesia

61.5 Clinical Picture

From the case described by Campos et al. a female, 26 years old with negative history of neurological disease, drugs, trauma, etc. She developed involuntary, spontaneous synchronous myoclonic jerks of the anterior wall of the neck, submadible region, and the nape muscles resulting in neck extension. The contractions were bilateral and rhythmic at of 1 Hz. The contractions were not controlled by will and did not cease during sleep. They increased by emotion and neck extension. Tests that included MRI, neurological, immunodeficiency, metabolic, and endodermal tests were all negative. However, electrophysiologic studies showed needle elctromyelography (EMG) irregular bursts, discharges of the motor units with a rate of 1–3 Hz in the anterior cervical muscles and posterior paraspinal muscles excluding trapezius and sternomastoid. The affected muscles are the infrahyoid (geniohyoid, thyrohyoid, sternothyroid, sternohyoid, and omohyoid). Supplied by C1 and junction of C2-3, the paraspinal muscles involved are: semispinalis capitis, rectus capitis posterioris, obliquus capitis superioris, and splenius capitis, which all depend on the C2 segment. All the muscles tested by EMG showed burst charges.

61.6 Diagnosis

Diagnosis is based on:

1. Clinical picture
2. EMG
3. Negative MRI and all other tests (see Clinical Picture above)

61.7 Management

Since the condition has no detectable cause, Botox® block of the affected muscles resulted in relief, which stayed in their report for 5 months.

Reference

Campos CR, Limongi JC, Machado FC, Brotto MW. A case of primary spinal myoclonus: clinical presentation and possible mechanisms involved. Arq Neuropsiquiatr. 2003;61(1):112–4.

Idiopathic Retroperitoneal Fibrosis

62

62.1 Definition

Retroperitoneal fibrosis is a pathological condition, in which fibrotic tissue is formed in the retroperitoneal space leading to compression of various organs in that space. In most cases there is no detectable cause and is therefore termed idiopathic retroperitoneal fibrosis (IRPF).

62.2 Incidence

IRPF is a rare clinical entity. Spinal cord compression due to IRPF is still rarer, very few cases have been reported (Schoen E et al. 1975; De Sá et al. 1990); and Dorado-bouix et al. 2004., which is abstracted here.)

62.3 Etiology

In most cases the etiology is unknown; however, some causative factors are proposed especially when the disease is multifocal and is called multifocal fibrosclerosis:

- Ingestion of certain drugs e.g. methysegride, hydralazine
  - Vaso-active drugs: which act on the wall of the aorta and other arteries
- Collagen disease
- Chronic inflammatory disease: tuberculosis, histoplasmosis
- Neoplastic: reticulum cell sarcoma, Hodgkin's disease
- Lupus erythematosus, periarteritis nodosa, scleroderma, autoimmune disease amongst the multiple theories of the disease.

Abstracted from Dorado-Bouix et al. (2004)

I.M. Eltorai, *Rare Diseases and Syndromes of the Spinal Cord*,
DOI 10.1007/978-3-319-45147-3_62

62.4 Pathogy

The disease involves the retroperitoneal space, but it may be multifocal, involving the pelvis, the mediastinum, and separate organs including the gall bladder, bile ducts, liver, thyroid, testis, cranial artery, orbit etc. Pathologically, there are mutli-foci of fibrosis without anatomical continuity. Sometimes it forms masses of fibrosis. Histiologically, it consists of fibrous tissue, adipose tissue with lymphocytes and plasma cell infiltration. The retroperitoneal mass may spread to the spinal canal through the intervertebral foramena or intervertebral space to the epidural area and cause cord compression aggravated by increased vascular retention and venous congestion. The authors also call it mediastinitus fibromatosa and periaortitis cronica.

62.5 Clinical Picture

IRPF may be symptomless, symptoms of retroperitoneal organ compression e.g. the ureters, the aorta or its branches, the venous system may be manifested clinically. Compression myelopathy may be manifested by pain in the back or in the lower extremities, low grade fever, weakness of the limbs, urinary dysfunction, inability to walk, paraparesis, sensory changes. There may be associated signs of hydronephrosis and vascular compromise.

62.6 Diagnosis

Diagnosis based on:

1. Clinical picture
2. CT Scan and myelography show epidural mass with extension into the intervertebral foramena.
3. MRI shows deformity or displacement of the spinal cord or even partial atrophy. The mass is enhanced by gadolinium infusion.
4. Erythrocyte sedimentation rate (ESR) somewhat elevated
5. CSF increased protein level

62.7 Management

Surgical treatment according to De Sá et al. a laminectomy and removal of the mass compressing the cord extramedullary.

Conservative treatment according to Dorado-Bouix et al:

- Use of corticosteroids
- Chemotherapy cyclophosphamide, azathioprine etc. in cases resistant to steroids.
- Hormonal therapy by tamoxifen

They claim good response to medical therapy.

Updates

Abstracted by from Bell and Thomson (2012)

The authors report a case of retroperitoneal fibrosis causing spinal claudication. The case is a 47-year-old man complaining of claudication pains in both lower limbs after walking about 200 yards. The pain was aching in nature and more present in his left leg. The pain was worse when walking up an incline and was continued when walking was recommenced. The claudication distance was 50 yards.

The patient's pain ceased when walking was stopped and when he bends forward for a couple of minutes. The pain starts in the thighs, radiates down to the ankles and up to the buttocks and to the groins. There was no rest pain, no sphincter trouble and no sensory disturbance.

Medicine routinely taken were:

Ramipril 10 mg P.O. qd (for hypertension)
Sodium Valporoate: 800 mg bid (for epilepsy)
Co-Codamol: 30/500 mg up to eight times a day (analgesic). He also had a probable history of Perthe's disease in the left hip.

Physical exam showed marked varicose veins of both legs extending to the anterior abdominal wall. A left sided varicocele was found. The peripheral arterial systems were normal. There were no neurological deficits.

Ultrasonic exam showed marked refluxes in the peripheral veins bilaterally. The arterial tree was not sclerotic. A left varicocele was detected.

MRI of the lumbar spine showed minimal disc bulges at L3-L4 and L4-L5 without nerve compression. There was epidural spinal varicosity, and dilatation of subcutaneous veins in the lumbar area, mild hydronephrosis, and possible retroperitoneal mass.

CT scan of the abdomen showed retroperitoneal fibrosis involving both ureters causing right hydronephrosis. The left kidney was atrophic. The inferior vena cava (IVC) was involved in the fibrosis. The patient was referred to vascular surgery for decompression of the IVC and to urology for ureteric stent for hydronephrosis.

Reference

Bell S, Thomson S. Retroperitoneal fibrosis causing spinal claudication. Br J Neurosurg. 2012;26(4):564–5.

References

De sá J, Pimentel J, Carvalho M, Evangelista P, Martins P. Spinal cord compression secondary to idiopathic retroperitoneal fibrosis. Neurosurgery. 1990;26(4):678–81.

Dorado-bouix L, Millán-torné M, Capellades-font J, Gomà-gállego M, Olivé A. Spinal cord compression: an unusual clinical manifestation of retroperitoneal fibrosis. Rev Neurol. 2004; 39(12):1143–5.

Schoen E, Creissard P, Auquier L. [Cauda equina syndrome during retroperitoneal fibrosis: discovery of another coincidental etiology]. Ann Med Interne (Paris). 1975;126(4):297–302.

Isolated Spinal Neuro-Behçet Disease

63

63.1 Definition

Behçet disease (BD) was first described by a Turkish dermatologist Hulnsi Behçet in 1937. BD is a chronic relapsing multisystem disease. It commonly affects young adults an can invade the skin, mucous membranes, eyes, joints, vascular system, lungs, gastrointestinal tract, and the central nervous system (CNS). The focus of this paper will be on neuro-Behçet disease (NBD) with special description on involvement of the spinal cord.

63.2 Incidence

Prevalence, the disease is most common in the countries around the Mediterranean Sea, the Middle East, and the Middle Easter Asia, particularly in Japan. In Turkey the prevalence is higher in rural areas 37/1,000,000 in the United Kingdom 4/100,000. In hospital population, in Istanbul the prevalence is 5.3 %, in Casa Blanca it is 16 %, Alexandria 25 %, Iraq 3.3 %; in the United States according to Calamia there is a prevalence rate of 6.6 per 100,000. According to Abda BD affects the CNS in about 23 % of the United States patients. The age range is 16–61 (Al-Araji et al.); males are three times more like to get BD than females. NBD has a very variable prevalence in different countries from 2.2–50 % depending on the interest in the disease, the study group, the region, and the good of research. In Iraq's study, it was 14.3 %. The duration of the disease varies from 0.4 to 26 years. Family history was positive in 10 % of Iraq study.

Abstracted from S Cakirer (2003), Green and Mitchell (2000)

I.M. Eltorai, *Rare Diseases and Syndromes of the Spinal Cord*,
DOI 10.1007/978-3-319-45147-3_63

63.3 Etiology

The etiopathogenesis of the disease is still unknown however there are some theories:

- Viral: suggested when the disease was discovered in 1937, by Behçet. The viruses suggested were and reviewed with great interest
- Bacterial: streptococci were suggested, the inflammatory viral and bacterial theories waned
- Antigenic cross-reactivity and auto-immunity: Kurhan-Yauwz et al. looked at T-cell responses to synthetic peptide B27PD and the retinal S antigen patients with and without eye disease. The synthetic peptide shares common antigenic sequence with HLA-B molecules of the retinal S antigen. Patients with BD and retinitis had significant proliferative and cytokine response, suggesting that the immune response self antigen may be pathogenic in BD.
- T-cells: T-cells were found in peripheral blood of patients with BD increased in number and producing interferon-Y and tumor necrotizing factor alpha (TNF-α), suggesting that TNF-α, interferon-Y, and Th1 cytokines are important in the pathogenesis of BD.
- Cytokine Th 1: peripheral blood lymphocytes are considerably higher in peripheral blood of patients with BD. Conjoined with higher blood interleukin 12, which is a positive correlation with the progress of BD.
- Vasculitis: especially phlebitis, not excluding larger vessels, cerebral venous thrombosis is evidence.
- Cytokine activation: IL-1, IL-6, IL-12, SIL-2R, TNF, INF are all higher in BD and are involved in immune system activation.
- Genetic: In the Mediterranean HLAB51 is significantly higher in patients with BD, in Turkey it was found in 84 % of patients.

63.4 Pathology

BD is a multisystem disease with will be briefly presented, focusing more on the spinal cord.

System review

General Description

The disease is episodic, characterized by recurrent oral and genital ulcerations, with constitutional symptoms of malaise, fatigue, and loss of weight. The onset may be acute, subacute, or chronic with relapses. It may be missed.

- Cutaneous lesions: erythema no dosum, pustular eruptions, pseudofolliculitis, skin ulcer which resemble pus filled bumps, erythema no desum seen on the legs, ankles or toes. Skin involvement from Turkey study occurs in 84 % (following are from the same study).
- Arthritis or arthalgia: 56 %

- Thromophlebitis: 33 %
- Arterial lesions: 3.5 %
- Pulmonary involvement: 7 %
- Gastrointestinal involvement: 3 %
- CNS involvement:
  - Parachymal lesions at the mesencephalic function with the brain stem and diencphelon: 46 %
  - Pontobulbar lesions: 46 %
  - Hypothalamis thalamic lesions: 23 %
  - Basal ganglia: 12.8 %
  - Telencphelon: 5 %
  - Cerebellum: 3 %
  - Cervical spinal cord: 3 %
  - Non-parenchymal: increased intercranial tension due to venous thrombosis (aseptic meningitis is another manifestation)
  - Peripheral nerve involvement: optic nerve, 8th nerve
- Spinal cord BD: 5 cervical cases have been reported (Green et al.), a sixth case added by Kakirer. In autopsies up to 28 %. The thoracic cord is the most involved. Microscopically ther are multifocal necrotizing areas marked inflammatory cell reaction. Necrosis may affect both gray and white matter probably due to vasculitis.

63.5 Clinical Picture

- The association of cutaneous, oral, genital, and ocular manifestations of BD is characteristic
- Other system involvement
- Spinal cord pathology manifested by neurological deficits, both motor and sensory. This may be masked by brain stem involvement. There may be bladder dysfunction due to direct involvement and other CNS involvement, either cerebellar and/or cerebral.

63.6 Diagnosis

Diagnosis is based on:

1. History: suspicion in endemic areas
2. Physical exam: associated lesions in different systems, including EENT exam, genitalia, etc.
3. Laboratory tests: cerebral spinal fluid (CSF) will show elevated proteins and pleocytosis, lymphocytes especially in the acute phase. Pressure may be increased. CBC increased lymphocytes, ESR elevated, evoked potential studies

4. Electro-diagnostic tests: there is no diffuse mater axonal loss (for more details see Marciniak and Rosenfeld)
5. MRI of spinal cord and CT scan: usually negative. MRI should include the brain stem, as it may show some bulbar signs
6. Criteria of the international study group 2 of the following
   - Recurrent oral ulcerations
   - Recurrent genital ulcerations
   - Eye lesions
   - Skin lesions
   - Positive pathergy test
7. GI endoscopy for colon ulcerations
8. Pathological test: skin needle punctures result in a bump in a couple of days, but not always.
9. Immunological studies: Leukocyte antigen B51
10. A number of cytokines and makers of vascular disease are under investigation.

Neuro-Behçet disease needs to be differentiated from Ruter's disease, Crohn's disease, vasculitis, multiple sclerosis (MS), systemic lupus erythematosus (SLE), human immunodeficiency virus (HIV), syphilis, and other neurological diseases, especially of the brain.

63.7 Management

- Ophthalmous lesions treated with topical or intralesional cortisone, dapsone is another choice
- Thalidomide in male patients suppresses mucocutanieous lesions
- Calcium in more serious cases
- Calcium plus penicillin of use in mucocutaneous lesions and arthritis
- Azothroppin for young male patients with eye disease
- Interferon is useful in eye lesions
- Corticosteroids for acute cases, but it does not suppress CNS lesions and does not prevent blindness from posterior ureitits or retinal disease.
- Immunosupression using cyclophosphomide or chlorambucil for uncontrolled eye disease, CNS disease, large vessel vasulitis, and recurrent deep vein thrombosis (DVT). Chlorambucil leads to male infertility and possibly malignancy, but more useful to CNS lesions
- Heparin and cortisone are used for cerebral venous thrombosis

Treatment of the spinal cord

Moskau S et al. (2003) treated their patient with IV methylprednisolone for 6 weeks followed by oral steroid, which gave improvement to SCI lesion. In the case of Cakirer, paque lesions on MRI disappeared within 8 weeks with IV steroids, exact dosage and treatment not detailed. Green et al. treated a similar case with IV methylpredinsolone 1 gm/day × 3 days followed by prednisolone p.o. in decreasing doses. Patient's clinical condition resolved and complete resolution was achieved.

References

Cakirer S. Isolated spinal neurobehçet disease. MR imaging findings. Acta Radiol. 2003;44(5):558–60.

Green AL, Mitchell PJ. Spinal cord Neurobehçet's disease detected on magnetic resonance imaging. Australas Radiol. 2000;44(2):201–3.

Moskau S, Urbach H, Hartmann A, Schmidt S. Multifocal myelitis in Behçet's disease. Neurology. 2003;60(3):517.

64 Subacute Progressive Ascending Myelopathy (SPAM)

64.1 Definition

This is a condition of degeneration of the neurological deficit after spinal cord injury due to extension of the cord damage cephalad through four or more segments developing within 4–86 days, with median of 13 days.

64.2 Incidence

According to Hans Frankel this occurs after SCI in 1.5% of all cases. Planner et al. reported 11 cases over 15 years from Stoke Mandeville Spinal Center in the UK, which admits 175 patients per year. 80% are traumatic cord injury; age 18–50 (mean 35); males 9:11; cervical injuries 9:11. The injuries mostly due to motor vehicle accidents.

64.3 Etiology

The exact cause is not clear. Frankel hypothesized that subacute progressive ascending myelopathy (SPAM) is due to thrombosis or inflammatory changes at the injury site. Planner also exposed the possible etiological factors:

- In the cases stabilized by surgery:
- Arterial occlusion including fibrocartilaginous embolism
- Prolonged hypotension
- Infection
- Altered apoptotic cascade

Abstracted from Planner et al. (2008)

I.M. Eltorai, *Rare Diseases and Syndromes of the Spinal Cord*,
DOI 10.1007/978-3-319-45147-3_64

- Unregulated immune response
- Venous thrombosis
- Disturbance of the CSF producing a mass effect
- Possible intraspinal hematoma
- Possibly viral infection since the picture is similar to myelopathy following herpes simplex, Epstein Barr, or Coxsackie's viral infections. In SPAM some patients had fever and some lymphocytic rise in the CSF

64.4 Pathology

There is myelopathy cephalad to the cord injury invading from 4 to 11 segments with a mean of 6.2. There is expansion of the cord and central cord involvement. Planner et al. stated that pathologically no vascular occlusion is detected since ischemia is irreversible, while these lesions mostly improve within months. There is some degree of myelomalacia and there is no evidence of syrinx. In cervical cases the ascent may involve the brain stem, leading to death.

64.5 Clinical Picture

Some cases are subclinical and are diagnosed only by MRI. However, clinical neurological degeneration is usually evident. A rise of neurological deficit at least two segments cephalad is detected. There may be a complaint of shoulder pains and sensory changes and the patient of the 11 cases recorded had dysphagia and another patient had respiratory difficulties due to brain stem involvement, which ended fatally (6 %). The symptoms may remain subclinical but with MRI evidence. In few cases a history of fever may be obtained.

64.6 Diagnosis

Diagnosis is based on MRI: Abnormal signals within the cord were demonstrated in at least five segmental levels cephalad to the original injury. The maximal ascension found was 11 segments. There are high signals on T2-weighted images and minimal changes on T1-weighted images. There is cord expansion with minimal changes in the cord rim. In one case there was an extension into the medulla oblongata. Recovery to the original status was incomplete. Recovery was limited to a level cephalad to but not to the original level. There was no evidence of etiological factors so far (see etiology).

64.7 Management

No specific therapy. In cervical regions watch for respiratory difficulty and possible ventilator need. According to Planner et al. all cases recovered except the one death due to respiratory failure.

64.8 Prognosis

Ascending cervical lesions may involve the medulla; otherwise, incomplete recovery occurs.

Reference

Planner AC, Pretorius PM, Graham A, Meagher TM. Subacute progressive ascending myelopathy following spinal cord injury: MRI appearances and clinical presentation. Spinal Cord. 2008;46(2):140–4.

Idiopathic Spinal Cord Herniation

65

65.1 Definition

Idiopathic anterior spinal cord herniation (SCH) is a very rare condition causing progressive thoracic myelopathy.

65.2 Incidence

Idiopathic anterior spinal cord herniation is an increasingly recognized syndrome, causing progressive thoracic myelopathy in the middle aged. According to White and Tsegaye, in (White and Tsegaye 2004), the world literature is comprised of 37 publications, recording 61 cases reports. The incidence of spinal cord herniation is higher in females, affecting only 19 males. In (Sasani et al. 2009), Sesani et al. reviewed the English literature and found 100 cases reported. This increase is due to the use of MRI as a diagnostic tool, especially in patients presenting with Brown-Séquard syndrome; 67 of which were females.

65.3 Etiology

The exact cause of anterior spinal cord herniation is not very clear. There are theories to its cause, namely:

- Congenital anterior dural defect; against the theory is the late onset of the symptoms and in few cases the absence of congenital spinal deformity and dural defect incidental magnetic resonance imaging (MRI) before the onset of symptoms.

Abstracted from Sesani et al. (2009)

I.M. Eltorai, *Rare Diseases and Syndromes of the Spinal Cord*,
DOI 10.1007/978-3-319-45147-3_65

- Congenital duplication of the dura mater causes cord herniation through a single layer of the dura that was adherent to the posterior vertebral surface.
- Previous trauma, which may affect the dentate ligaments, helped by the anatomical curvature of the thoracic spine leading to the ventrally lying cord with subsequent erosion and prolapse.
- Thoracic disc herniation; this may precede cord adherence to the dura with disc resorption and subsequent dural pocket formation and simultaneous cord herniation.
- Intradural arachnoid cyst may cause pressure and erosion; against this theory is the negative computed tomographic myelogram (CTM).
- Erosion of the dura by herniated and calcified disc.

65.4 Pathophysiology

The herniation occurs in the thoracic region from T2–T10, most commonly. The spinal cord is displaced ventrally or ventrolaterally or just laterally. It may be sharply angulated within a few segments. That means the cord is tethered by the herniation. The subarachnoid space ventral to the displaced cord is obliterated due to the herniation itself or due to scarring. Initially there is involvement of the spinalthalamic tract, being disturbed within the margins of the dural defect. As the disease progresses more of the lateral funiculus herniates into the defect involving the corticospinal tract. The posterior columns are usually spared, which gives a predominant picture of Brown-Séquard syndrome. The herniation will result in cord lesion, vascular compromise and cord infarction, with subsequent atrophy.

65.5 Clinical Picture

The onset is slow, the course of the disease and its progression are over several years, with a range of 1–12 years. The sensory modality (spinalthalamic tract) is usually affected before the motor (corticospinal tract). Sphincter dysfunction may also occur. The symptoms are those of Brown-Séquard syndrome. It starts by weakness or muscle atrophy or spasticity or all, on the ipsilateral side. On the contralateral side sensory deficit is manifested by loss of temperature and pinprick sensation. The propioreception is preserved. There may be intermittent pain in the thoracic region, chest wall, or the lower extremities. If the condition is not treated it may progress to paraplegia, especially due to cord infarction. The reflexes on the weak extremity may be exaggerated and Babinski's sign may be positive. The senses of position and vibration are preserved. The condition should be differentiated from spinal cord injury or spinal tumors, disc degeneration, multiple sclerosis, arachnoid cysts, vascular malformations, etc. Careful history and imagining can easily diagnose the condition.

65.6 Diagnosis

Plain x-rays may show disc herniation or bony defect within the vertebral body and endplate at the disc level opposite the cord herniation; calcification may be seen at that level. MRI is diagnostic and may sow the following signs:

1. Anterior displacement of spinal cord
2. Enlargement of dorsal subarachnoid space
3. Atrophy of the spinal cord with decrease in spinal cord size and signal changes
4. The ventral subarachnoid space in front of the displaced cord is obliterated.

CTM is rarely needed, as it is invasive but may be used to rule out masses dorsal to the displaced cord or other pathological lesions; it also confirms the absence of subarachnoid space anterior to the cord. Wada et al. (2000), illustrates this in their article.

65.7 Prognosis

The condition is progressive if untreated. Surgical correction has a good outcome. On neglected cases spinal cord herniation will lead to paraplegia. As recurrence is possible, so are negative results after surgery.

65.8 Management

To avoid increase of the neurological deficit the spinal cord hernia should be reduced and the defect in the dura repaired. The approach is usually through a 3-level laminectomy centered over the hernia. The dura is opened in the midline to provide sufficient visualization of the herniation. Microsurgery is performed to release the adhesions between the pia of the herniated spinal cord and the circumferential dural defect; thus, letting the cord fall back into its normal position inside the dural sleeve. The dural defect is closed by duroplasty, using DuraGen® (artificial dura), it is gently slipped between the dural defect and the spinal cord and fixed in place with a couple of stitches; as described by Massicotte, et al. Other techniques are used by neurosurgeons. The dentate ligament may have to be divided laterally to facilitate reduction of the spinal cord to its normal position. If there is a bony defect in the body of the vertebra it is packed with bone chips taken from the laminectomy and then covered by the Neuropatch® graft (artificial dura); as described by White and Tsegaye. Sasani et al. described the original technique used by Masazawe. To obliterate the defect by muscle fascial flap, fat, lympholized dura and Gortex membrane. But they followed the technique of Makazawa, widening the defect to prevent cord strangulation. It is most feasible technique since the space is too narrow to pass the needle and risk cord damage, especially the anterior spinal artery.

References

Sasani M, Ozer AF, Vural M, Sarioglu AC. Idiopathic spinal cord herniation: case report and review of the literature. JSCM. 2009;32(1):86–94.

Wada E, et al. Idiopathic spinal cord herniation: report of three cases and review of the literature. Spine. 2000;25(15):1984–8. Review.

White BD, Tsegaye M. Idiopathic anterior spinal cord hernia: under-recognized cause of thoracic myelopathy. Br J Neurosurg. 2004;18(3):246–9. Review.

Spontaneous Spinal Epidural Hematoma 66

66.1 Definition

Spontaneous spinal epidural hematoma (SSEH) is a rare condition in which compression myelopathy is due to an epidural hematoma, the cause of which is unidentified.

66.2 Incidence

According to Kong and Mak (2003), 300 cases were found in the English literature review. The condition may occur in children or adults and the aged. According to Rosenburg et al. (2003), 25 % of the cases occur in children and they discovered 23 cases in 1994 and increased to 27 in 1998. In children above 2 years it is more common and in males. Male to female ratio is 1.5:1 and the commonest age is 50–80, accounting for 50 % of the total cases.

66.3 Etiology

SSEH is considered primary and idiopathic. It is unlike the secondary type, which is due to trauma, even minor epidural puncture, blood dyscrasias, use of anticoagulants, arteriovenous malformation (AVM), hemangiomas, tumors, leukemias, and excessive garlic ingestion (Rose et al.). A theory is known amongst many authors:

The epidural plexus of veins is valveless and quite numerous. Any sudden increase of the intravenous pressure such as by valsava's maneuver as trumpet blowing, increased intrathoracic or intra-abdominal pressure with forceful coughing, straining for micturation or defication, sexual activity, lifting heavy objects, and

---

Abstracted and reported by Kong and Mak (2003)

I.M. Eltorai, *Rare Diseases and Syndromes of the Spinal Cord*,
DOI 10.1007/978-3-319-45147-3_66

similar stimulations, such as labor will increase the intraspinal venous pressure leading to rupture and forming a hematoma. It has happened during sleep which weakens the above theory. In pregnancy five cases have been reported, possibly due to increased hemodynamics and hormonal association (Jea et al. 2005).

66.4 Pathology

The hematoma occurs most commonly in the cervicothoracic region and generally involves few segments of the cord, most commonly posteriorly (99 %). In the thoracic region the myelopathy is usually complete due to narrow space and watershed area leading to ischemia, especially between T4–T8 segments. The bleeding is almost always venous. Arterial bleeding is very rare. The hematoma, if not evacuated soon, can cause cord compression leading to ischemia, which is not recoverable. After decompression the hematoma may recur but very rarely if hemostatsis is complete. Spontaneous resolution is rare and only for minor hematomas.

66.5 Clinical Picture

The onset is sudden characterized by back pain associated with paresthesia of the upper and/or lower extremities, resulting in paraparesis or tetraparesis with sphincter dysfunction. Patient's history should be negative for trauma, anticoagulants, blood dyscrasias, etc.

66.6 Diagnosis

Diagnosis is based on the following criteria:

- Clinical history and findings.
- MRI of the spinal cord is superior to CT scan. It shows dorsal biconvex mass compressing the spinal cord, its vertical extent, and edema of the cord, since it has multiplanar capability. Sagittal MRI shows the biconvex dorsal epidural hematoma with well-defined contours. In the axial images it appears as convex or concave mass. The spinal intensity of the hematoma changes over time and that is why the age of the hematoma may be clearly determined by the MRI, blood degradation products have magnetic properties. In the acute phase the hematoma appears isointense on T1-weighted images and hyperintense on T2-weighted images, for more details see Kirazli et al. (Kirazli et al. 2004).

66.7 Management

The greatest majority of cases require emergent spinal cord decompression in order to reverse the neurological deficits. This entails laminectomy and evacuation of the hematoma and control of the source of bleeding. Chances of recovery are best when decompression is accomplished within 24-h, especially when neurological deficit is incomplete. Conservative management is rarely indicated. It must be tried in incomplete cases, where regressing and the size of the hematoma is small (Wagner et al.1996). Surgery should be resorted to on time in absence of regression or in cases of progression supported by MRI series. In case of reduction f hematoma size by MRI conservative treatment may be adopted.

References

Jea A, Moza K, Levi AD, Vanni S. Spontaneous spinal epidural hematoma during pregnancy: case report and literature review. Neurosurgery. 2005;56(5), E1156.

Kirazli Y, Akkoc Y, Kanyilmaz S. Spinal epidural hematoma associated with oral anticoagulation therapy. Am J Phys Med Rehabil. 2004;83(3):220–3.

Kong JK, Mak KH. Spontaneous spinal epidural haematoma--an unusual cause of spinal cord compression. Hong Kong Med J. 2003;9(1):55–7.

Rosenberg O, Itshayek E, Israel Z. Spontaneous spinal epidural hematoma in a 14-year-old girl. Case report and review of the literature. Pediatr Neurosurg. 2003;38(4):216–8.

Wagner S, Forsting M, Hacke W. Spontaneous resolution of a large spinal epidural hematoma: case report. Neurosurgery. 1996;38(4):816–8.

Tumoral Calcinosis of the Spine

67

67.1 Definition

Tumoral calcinosis (TC) is an uncommon pathological entity of obscure etiology, characterized by dystrophic calcification in periarticular soft tissue. The calcification usually takes the form of calcium hydroxyapatitic crystals surrounded by a foreign body giant cell histiocytic reaction. TC shows the following characteristics without common pathogenesis:

- Large size
- Juxta-articular locations
- Progressive enlargement over time
- Tendency to recur after resection
- Tendency to encase neighboring structure

67.2 Incidence

Carlson et al. (2007), reported one case and reviewed 21 reported cases of tumoral calcium pyrophosphate dihydrate deposition disease and 39 cases of TC. Kokubun et al. (1996) reported a case in the cervical and mentioned one previously reported case. Durant et al. (2001) reviewed 21 pathological specimens of tumoral calcinosis of the spine and stated, "several had radiculopathy in the distribution of the nerve roots that were being compressed. A few pateints presented with severe cord compression manifested by paraparesis, or sensory deficits."

Abstracted from Carlson et al. (2007)

I.M. Eltorai, *Rare Diseases and Syndromes of the Spinal Cord*,
DOI 10.1007/978-3-319-45147-3_67

67.3 Pathogenesis

This is not known. There are three categories:

1. Familial, inheritable disease
2. Patients on chronic renal dialysis
3. Sporadic

According to Durant et al. (2007) the following medical conditions were described as possible, contributing to the pathogenesis:

- Hypertension
- Osteoarthritis
- Rheumatoid arthritis
- Diabetes mellitus
- Trauma to the involved area
- Previous surgery on the spine
- Severely osteoporotic spine
- Scleroderma

In the familial group inherited, there is a frequent association of hyperphosphatemia in siblings.

67.4 Pathology

Tumoral calcinosis is characterized by small descrete calcified nodules, which coalesce into lobulated tumor. The calcium crystals are identical to hydroxyapatite. Scanning electron microscopy shows calcium pyrophosphate dehydrogenase (CPPD). Amongst the crystals collagen fibers are identified as they form septa, which are allahed peripherally to fibrous capsule. Microanalysis shows Ca and P1, the atomic ratio of CalP from 0.91 to 1.08. Around the tumor there is hystiocytes and foreign body giant cells. In the tumor may be some inflammatory cells and capillary vascularity.

67.5 Clinical Picture

Demographically, CPPD is more common in Japan, possibly due to higher incidence of spinal canal stenosis and older women are more predisposed. However, TC cases with history of minor local trauma, genetic influence (sibling), and metabolic disturbances are common. In Kukabin et al. the mass can be felt in the occipital region. There was pain and restriction of neck movement.

67.6 Diagnosis

Diagnosis based on:

1. Clinical picture
2. Plain x-ray may be visible, however may be too small in CPPD
3. CT Scan: Nodular calcified mass impinging on the spinal cord. The mass is spherical or oval in CPPD but in TC are irregularly rounded. Large masses of TC may be honeycombed or chicken wire.
4. MRI: in both conditions there is intermediate to low signal intensity on T1 and T2 weighted images. Enhancement is usually minimal or absent, cord compression is evident on MRI.

   Ultrasound or angiography most likely will not distinguish either case

67.7 Management

Surgery consists of:

1. Parathyroidectomy if needed
2. Removal of the mass
   (a) Laminectomy if small
   (b) Anterior approach if large, corpectomy, fibrilar struct and plate fixation

   Medical consists of:

1. Non-steroidal anti-inflammatory drugs
2. Dialysis patients: correction of abnormalities, e.g. phosphorus deprivation or use of low calcium dialysate
3. Treatment of tCPPDcdd in Japan with ethane-1-hydroxy-1-diphosphate.

References

Carlson AP, Yonas HM, Turner PT. Disorders of tumoral calcification of the spine: illustrative case study and review of the literature. J Spinal Disord Tech. 2007;20(1):97–103.

Durant DM, Riley LH, Burger PC, Mccarthy EF. Tumoral calcinosis of the spine: a study of 21 cases. Spine. 2001;26(15):1673–9.

Kokubun S, Ozawa H, Sakurai M, Tanaka Y. Tumoral calcinosis in the upper cervical spine: a case report. Spine. 1996;21(2):249–52.

Transient Cervical Myeloneurapraxia 68

68.1 Definition

Neurapraxia is a condition of temporary paralysis as a result of some kind of injury, which ends by rapid and complete recovery without degenerative changes.

68.2 Incidence

According to Torg et al. a survey on 503 schools participating in National Collegiate Athletic Association (NCAA) football in 1984 season found that 1.3 per 10,000 athletes had a history suggestive of neurapraxia of the cervical cord with transient tetraplegia

68.3 Etiology

- Individual with congenital stenosis of the cervical canal
- Congenital vertebral fusion
- Cervical instability due to ligamentous laxity
- Disc protrusion in association with a decrease in the anteroposterior diameter of the spinal canal.
- Acquired cervical canal stenosis due to spondylosis

Torg et al. proposed that hyperreflexia, axial loading and hyperextension in these patients will cause compression of the cervical cord causing transient sensory and motor loss.

Abstracted from Torg et al. (1995)

I.M. Eltorai, *Rare Diseases and Syndromes of the Spinal Cord*,
DOI 10.1007/978-3-319-45147-3_68

68.4 Pathology

The mechanism of neurapraxia is spinal cord compression. It is due to sudden approximation of the posterior inferior aspect of a vertebral body with the superior aspect of the lamina of the next vertebral body below. Resulting in sudden decrease in the anteroposterior diameter of the spinal canal thus compressing the spinal cord. This causes transient disruption of cell axonal membrane permeability resulting in reversible depolarisation (Torg et al. 1995)

68.5 Clinical Picture

After neck trauma, hyperextension or hyperflexion in young athelets may predue sudden sensory and motor loss below the cervical region, which is recoverable within minutes, especially in young adults and pediatrics. In older patients with spondylosis, central cord syndrome may develop with persistent neurological deficit. It may last up to 12 h. Tingling in the four limbs may be present for 30 min to weeks. Paresthesia may persist for weeks.

68.6 Diagnosis

Diagnosis is based on the following criteria:

1. History of hyperextension, hyperfexion, or axial compression
2. If seen on the spot, motor and sensory loss are detectable and soon recover.
3. Radiological exam:
   (a) Evidence of spinal stenosis:
   (b) Reduction of the sagittal diameter of the spinal canal, which may be exaggerated by osteophytes or disc protrusion. This is especially important between C3-6. It is critical since the cord is more mobile and fills most of the available space.
   (c) Torg's Ratio
   (d) This is the sagittal diameter of the spinal canal divided by the diameter of the vertebral body at the affected level. A ratio below 0.8 defines a significant spinal stenosis. This calculation eliminates errors due to different tube—target distance while taking the radiographs.
   (e) MRI
   (f) Measurement of the cord diameter between a disc and the posterior boney elements. Since Torg's ratio is not quite predictive, functional MRI are useful to determine the size of the cord at the level C3-6 and the functional reserve of the spinal canal (see Andrews 2002).
4. Neurophysiological study for persistent neurological changes

68.7 Management

The treatment of such injuries is dilated in view of their transient nature (Andrews 2002). Studies have shown cervical disc protrusion in 36 %, half of them were treated conservatively and the other half surgically. Patients who developed progressive neurological damage should be scheduled as emergency surgery after a through workup. Patients with a Torg ratio less than 0.8 have a risk of spinal cord injury and should be evaluated by an expert for decision-making. Athletes having more than one attacks of cervical neurapraxia should not go back to their practice without proper expert assessment.

References

Andrews FJ. Transient cervical neurapraxia associated with cervical spine stenosis. Emerg Med J. 2002;19(2):172–3.

Torg JS, Thibault L, Sennett B, Pavlov H. The Nicolas Andry Award. The pathomechanics and pathophysiology of cervical spinal cord injury. Clin Orthop Relat Res. 1995;321:259–69.

Part V

Infectious Cause of Myelopathy

69 Bacterial Meningitis in Adults

69.1 Definition

This is a spinal cord dysfunction due to acute bacterial meningitis in adults.

69.2 Incidence

According to Kastenbauer et al. (2001) 29 cases have been recorded having acute spinal cord dysfunction secondary to acute bacterial meningitis. Twenty-five of those patients were children and four were adults; the authors added three adult cases.

69.3 Etiology

Meningitis is due to the following organisms, *Streptococcus pneumoniae*, *Neisseria meningitides*, *Escherichia coli*, *Haemophilus influenzae*, *Streptococcus agalactiae*, *Klebsiella pneumoniae*, and *Coryneobacterium jeikeium*.

The possible causes of myelitis are

- Ischemia due to vasculitis especially with shock hypotension
- Venous infarct due to septic phlebitis or due to venous congestion due to spinal epidural arteriovenous fistula engagement
- Adhesive arachnoiditis constricting the cord and its vessels
- Edema of the cord and perivascular inflammation
- Facial hemorrhages

Abstracted from Kastenbauer et al. (2001)

I.M. Eltorai, *Rare Diseases and Syndromes of the Spinal Cord*,
DOI 10.1007/978-3-319-45147-3_69

69.4 Pathology

There is vasculitis, perivasculitis, venous congestion, capillary and arteriolar thrombosis, which lead to myelitis, necrosis of the cord, parenchyma especially the gray matter (myelomalacia) following scarring. There is also neuroradiculitis. Rarely the cauda equine may be involved (Bal et al. 2004). Syrinx may develop later. Associated cerebral complications may be detected, e.g. vascular thrombosis, sinus thrombosis, deafness due to the 8th nerve compression, hydrocephalus.

69.5 Clinical Picture

Fever, headache, nausea, vomiting, visual disturbances, followed by paraparesis or tetraparesis and sphincter dysfunction, usually within 3–4 days. Stupor and shock or coma may occur in severe cases. Of the 26 cases reported six died and only three of the survivors had neurological recovery. Patients are left with chronic disability.

69.6 Diagnosis

Diagnosis is based on the following criteria:

1. Clinical findings include: acute onset, fever, meningism
2. Kong's sing
3. Leukocytosis
4. Neurological signs
5. CSF: Increased pressure high cell count, increased proteins, sugar decreased, gram stain and culture results in the particular bacteria but may be sterile.
6. MRI: The spinal cord is shown by distinct intramedullary gadolinium enhancements. It may show hypo-intensive areas on T1 weighted images.

69.7 Management

- IV antibiotic therapy
- When myelitis is suspected steroid therapy is given 150 mgm IV QDX 3 days, 75 mgm IV per day until improvement of myelitis.
- Follow-up with neurological exam and MRI
- Rehabilitation program for the chronic cases.
- In the cases of meningitis the anterior sacral meningocele leading to cauda equina syndrome surgical excision was necessary.

Reference

Kastenbauer S, Winkler F, Fesl G, et al. Acute severe spinal cord dysfunction in bacterial meningitis in adults: MRI findings suggest extensive myelitis. Arch Neurol. 2001;58(5):806–10.

Bal S, Kurtulmuş S, Koçyiğit H, Gürgan A. A case with cauda equina syndrome due to bacterial meningitis of anterior sacral meningocele. Spine. 2004;29(14):E298–9.

Guillain-Barré Syndrome Following Allogeneic Bone Marrow Transplantation

70

70.1 Definition

Guillain-Barré Syndrome (GBS) is a clinical condition resulting from acute inflammatory demyelinating polyneuropathy (radiculopathy). It most frequently occurs after infection and immunizations and after malignancy. Allogenic bone marrow transplantation (BMT) is an important source.

70.2 Incidence

According to Tam et al. 2003 "Following the successful central and elimination of poliomyelitis in many regions of the world, GBS has become the most common cause of acute neuromuscular paralysis with estimated annual incidence ranging from 0.4 to 4 per 100,000 individuals in different populations."

70.3 Etiology

The majority of cases appear to have an infection as a trigger. The most common of these triggers is *campylobacter jejuni* infection. Evidence has accumulated linking GBS to campylobacter injection and Miller-Fisher syndrome. Miller-Fisher syndrome is a variant of GBS and comprises a clinical triad of ataxia, areflexia, and ophthalmoplegia autoantibodies against GQ1b have been considered archetypal anti-ganglioside auto-antibody-mediated neuropathy because the anti-GQ1b ganglioside antibody is detected in most patients with Miller-Fisher syndrome and decays with recovery. A related illness (Speed and Kaldor 1985; Jacobs et al. 1996; Rees et al. 1995) illustrated a link between *campylobacter* and

Abstracted from Hagensee et al. (1994)

I.M. Eltorai, *Rare Diseases and Syndromes of the Spinal Cord*,
DOI 10.1007/978-3-319-45147-3_70

serotypes in GBS were confirmed in Japan and in South Africa (see Tam et al. 2003). The mechanism is thought to be an autoimmune reaction against *c. jejuni* surface molecular with a structural similarity to gangliosides antigen on nerve endings (Hadden et al. 2001). Following *c. jejuni* infection the antibody level in the blood IgG isotype for up to 12 months, this is one of diagnostic criteria. In a Swedish study 30.1 cases of GBS per 100,000 confirmed *c. jejuni* cases. The same was found in England. In the U.S. *campylobacter* is one of the most common causes of diarrhea. About 15 cases are diagnosed each year per 100,000 population individuals. It is estimated that 1 million are infected annually in the U.S.; furthermore cases are not diagnosed or reported may be in addition. The bacteria are more isolated from infants and the young and more are males. It is estimated that probably a 100 persons die every year by *c. jejuni*. However, It is not know whether GBS in BMT subjects is equal to the GBS in the general population not definitive statistics are yet available

Two-thirds of GBS follow bacterial or viral infections. Lin et al. reported GBS after facial injuries and mentioned head injury as a possible precursor to GBS. It may follow general surgical procedures (see Merritt's Textbook of Neurology) and after delivery. GBS may follow allogenic BMT. This group of patients according to Wen et al. (1997) may have a higher risk of GBS. Neurologic complications are liable to develop in 50–70 % of patients having allogeneic BMT and less extent those having autologous BMT. Most of the complications are of central nervous system (CNS). Most of the peripheral nervous system (PNS) complications develop in the setting of graft-versus-host disease (GVHD). This includes chronic inflammatory demyelinating polyneuropathy as well as myasthenia gravis and polymyositis. GBS is acute inflammatory demyelinating disease of the peripheral nerves (polyneuropathy).

70.4 Pathology and Pathogenesis

The pathogenesis of GBS in patients after allogeneic BMT is not clear. It is believed to be a result of cellular immune response directed against components of the peripheral nerves. (Wen et al. 1997) According to Solare et al. GVHD is a frequent complication of allogeneic BMT; there is a possible relationship between neurological and MRI findings with a chronic GVHD. Solare et al., reported a case of allogeneic BMT resulting in central and peripheral neurological signs which correlates with chronic GVHD. Although rarely has this been confirmed in autopsy studies (Marosi et al. 1990; Mohrmann et al. 1990).

Pathology is the picture of chronic inflammatory demyelinating disease of the PNS. Histologically there is focal segmental demyelination with perivascular and endoneural infiltrations with lymphocytes and monocytes or macrophages. These lesions are scattered throughout the peripheral nerves, the roots and cranial nerves. There is segmental demyelination and axonal degeneration. During recovery there is regulation but lymphocytes remain.

70.5 Clinical Picture

The onset of the syndrome may be 10 days to 12 months after BMT (mean 3.8 months). According to Wen et al. (1997) GBS developed earlier in patients with autologous BMT. The same authors noted precipitating factors such as c. jejuni and cytomegalovirus. Before the onset there may be fever and GVHD. The CNS may also be involved. Solare et al. reported a case of cerebellar, pyramidal, and peripheral nerve involvement. The GVHD is manifested by skin rash and modest elevation of the liver function tests. GBS is characterized by acute onset of peripheral and cranial nerve dysfunction, which includes rapidly progressive weakness, loss of tendon reflexes, facial diplegia, esophageal and respiratory paresis, and impaired sensation in the hands and feet. The condition worsens in several days up to 3 weeks. The picture becomes stable for sometime and then improves gradually to normal or near normal condition. Sensory changes vary from normal to marked diminution in joint perception and vibration. There may be glove and stocking loss of pain and temperature sensation. The reflexes may be absent and occasionally transient positive Babinski's sign. Autonomic dysfunctions include hypotension, labile blood pressure, tachyarrhythmia, bradyarrhythmia, or resting tachycardia as well as cardiomyopathy as reported by Finkelstein and Melek 2006. Variants of GBS can be seen in Merritt's Neurology.

70.6 Diagnosis

Diagnosis is based on the following criteria:

1. History of BMT
2. History of respiratory or gastrointestinal infection
3. Neurological examination
4. Cerebral spinal fluid: Increased protein level, but may be normal early in the disease. Cytology is usually normal but monocytes may be high
5. Serological studies: Increased titres of IgG or IgA. GQ1b is a ganglioside antibody that is found in 90 % of Miller-Fisher syndrome
6. Symptoms of GVHD which are:
   (a) Anorexia
   (b) Diarrhea
   (c) Loss of hair
   (d) Leukocytopenia
   (e) Thrombocytopenia
   (f) Growth retardation
   (g) Sometimes death
   (h) The cause may be acute or chronic. The symptoms may develop 5–40 days after BMT in the acute form and after months in the chronic type
7. Nerve studies

70.7 Management

Methods adopted are:

- Plasmapheresis is helpful
- IV human immunoglobulin therapy as an alternative
- Steroid therapy is not so helpful
- Prevention of all kinds of infection in patients with BMT
- In severe GVHD immunosuppression may be considered

References

Finkelstein JS, Melek BH. Guillain-Barré syndrome as a cause of reversible cardiomyopathy. Tex Heart Inst J. 2006;33(1):57–9.

Hadden RD, Karch H, Hartung HP, et al. Preceding infections, immune factors, and outcome in Guillain-Barré syndrome. Neurology. 2001;56(6):758–65.

Hagensee ME, Benyunes M, Miller JA, Spach DH. Campylobacter jejuni bacteremia and Guillain-Barré syndrome in a patient with GVHD after allogeneic BMT. Bone Marrow Transplant. 1994;13(3):349–51.

Jacobs BC, Van doorn PA, Schmitz PI, et al. Campylobacter jejuni infections and anti-GM1 antibodies in Guillain-Barré syndrome. Ann Neurol. 1996;40(2):181–7.

Marosi C, Budka H, Grimm G, et al. Fatal encephalitis in a patient with chronic graft-versus-host disease. Bone Marrow Transplant. 1990;6(1):53–7.

Mohrmann RL, Mah V, Vinters HV. Neuropathologic findings after bone marrow transplantation: an autopsy study. Hum Pathol. 1990;21(6):630–9.

Rees JH, Soudain SE, Gregson NA, Hughes RA. Campylobacter jejuni infection and Guillain-Barré syndrome. N Engl J Med. 1995;333(21):1374–9.

Rowland LP, Pedley TA. Merritt's Neurology. Philadelphia, PA: Lippincott Williams & Wilkins; 2010.

Speed BR, Kaldor J. Guillain-Barré syndrome associated with Campylobacter infection. Aust N Z J Med. 1985;15(2):269.

Tam CC, Rodrigues LC, O'brien SJ. Guillain-Barré syndrome associated with Campylobacter jejuni infection in England, 2000-2001. Clin Infect Dis. 2003;37(2):307–10.

Wen PY, Alyea EP, Simon D, Herbst RS, Soiffer RJ, Antin JH. Guillain-Barré syndrome following allogeneic bone marrow transplantation. Neurology. 1997;49(6):1711–4.

Myelopathy due to *Cladosporium trichoides* or *Cladophialophora bantiana* 71

71.1 Definition

Cladosporium trichoides is also known as *Cladophialophora bantiana. C. bantiana* is a rare dematiaceous fungus, which is distributed worldwide (see McGinnis et al. 1986, for further details about the fungus).

71.2 Incidence and Etiology

Only one case, reported by Lopes et al., is summarized here. In the brain this infection is more common. This usually results in fungal brain abscess (see Raut et al., 2003 and Levin et al. 2004). Intracranial fungal infections occur in patients on long antibiotic and steroid therapies, low immunity, and debility are predisposing factors. The fungus is present in decaying vegetation, soil, and wood. Occupational exposure by inhalation of soil is important. Trauma may precede the infection (Dixon et al. 1989).

71.3 Pathology

This fungus route of entry is unknown. The most accepted theory is that the route of entry is through inhalation of spores. The fungus is abundantly found in skin, lungs, gastrointestinal tract, infection of the paranasal sinuses, and the ears has been reported. Hematogenous spread to the route of the central nervous system (CNS) infection. This may be parenchymal or meningeal.

In the case report the pathological report was as follows:

Abstracted from Lopes et al. (1989)

I.M. Eltorai, *Rare Diseases and Syndromes of the Spinal Cord*,
DOI 10.1007/978-3-319-45147-3_71

Morphology: an intradural granulomatous mass extramedullary fibrous tissue with necrotic foci, adherent to the distal medulla and to the upper cervical cord.

Microscopically: chronic inflammation with giant cells containing fungal fragments. Hyphae and spherical bodies are seen. The hyphae are segmented and stain golden yellow.

The fungus had a positive picture by using Grocott-Fontana-Masson technique. Its morphological and histochemical characteristics suggest the diagnosis of *c. bantiana*. Gomori-methenamine silver stain confirms the presence of fungal hyphae; cultures show *c. bantiana*.

71.4 Clinical Picture

The authors discuss the epidemiology and reviewed the cerebral infection cases. Their 25-year-old patient presented with progressive weakness and paralysis of all his extremities with sphincteric disturbances. Clinically he was tetraplegic without sensory loss and his reflexes were exaggerated.

71.5 Diagnosis

Diagnosis is based on the following criteria:

1. Clinical exam: A 25-year-old male, tetraplegic, with marked loss of weight and atrophy of the extremities.
2. Myelogram showed complete occipito-cervical block.
3. MRI was not included
4. Hydrocephalus was detected and shunted.
5. Lumbar and suboccipital puncture showed signs of infiltration i.e. increased lymphocytes, granulocytes, monocytes, plasma cells, and high proteins.

71.6 Management

1. Hydrocephalus: ventriculo-peritoneal shunt
2. High cervical compression: suboccipital decompression and laminectomy C1-C2

In general CNS fungal infections are serious and morbidity is high. The patient reported expired a few days post-op. Anti-fungal chemotherapy is still ineffective. Amphotericin B IV: intrathecally have been used as well as Fluorocytosine in brain abscess.

71.6.1 Another Picture of Spinal Cord

Shields and Castillo (2002) report a case of spinal involvement by *C. bantiana* causing transverse myelitis. A 53-year-old woman who is on steroids for sarcoidosis developed paraparesis with sensory level about T12. The case was diagnosed by cord biopsy, which showed *C. bantiana*. The lesion being localized (not diffused), excision biopsy and anti-fungal therapy gave a favorable result.

References

Lopes MBS, Barbosa RF, Vellasco O, Rosemberg S. Cervical cord compression due to Cladosporium trichoides. Anatomo-clinic obersvation [in French]. Ann Pathol. 1989;9(4):275–8.

Dixon DM, Walsh TJ, Merz WG, McGinnis MR. Infections due to *Xylophypha bantiana (Cladosporium trichoides)*. Rev Infect Dis. 1989;2:515–23.

McGinnis MR, Borelli D, Padhye AA, Ajello L. Reclassification of *Cladosporium bantianum* in the genus *Xylohypha*. J Clin Microbiol. 1986;23(6):1148–51.

Raut A, Muzumdar D, Narlawar R, Nagar A, Ahmed N, Hira P. Cerebral abscess caused by Cladosporium bantianum infection. Neurol Med Chir (Tokyo). 2003;43:413–5.

Shields GS, Castillo M. Myelitis caused by *Cladophialophora bantiana*. AJR Am J Roentgenol. 2002;179(1):278–9.

Levin TP, Baty DE, Fekete T, Truant AL, Suh B. Cladophialophora bantiana brain abscess in a solid-organ transplant recipient: case report and review of the literature. J Clin Microbiol. 2004;42(9):4374–8.

72 Coxsackie Transverse Myelitis

72.1 Definition

There are two principal groups of Coxsackie virus:

- Group A: these are divided into 24 serotypes
- Group B: these are divided into 6 serotypes

Acute transverse myelitis (ATM) is a rare clinical manifestation of Coxsackie virus infection which causes an acute and progressive debilitating illness associated with loss of spinal cord functions both motor and sensory.

72.2 Incidence

Acute transverse myelitis has been rarely associated with Coxsackie virus. There have been a few cases reported due to Coxsackie viruses. Coxsackie virus is associated with other diseases of the CNS: aseptic meningitis, encephalitis, Guillian-Barré syndrome, and poliomyelitis. Coxsackie A7, A9, A23, and Coxsackie virus B strains frequently cause encephalomyelitis often associated with transient or permanent paralysis (Gear 1984; Lemer and Finland 1961). One case of transverse myelitis was reported by Dery et al., in 1974, caused by Coxsackie virus type B4; B3 strain by Mathews and Bailey, in 1977. Other cases of coxsackie's ATM include the A9 strain by Graber et al. in 1994; the B4 strain by Ku and Lee in 1998; and the case by Minami et al., 2004, with the B5 strain. In 2005, Strarakis et al., reported a brief case of B2 Coxsackie virus causing ATM.

Abstracted from Minami et al. (2004) and Starakis et al. (2005)

I.M. Eltorai, *Rare Diseases and Syndromes of the Spinal Cord*,
DOI 10.1007/978-3-319-45147-3_72

72.3 Etiology

Various infectious agents have been described as the cause of ATM, 20–40 % of these are attributed to viruses, although a specific virus has been rarely identified (Ku and Lee 1998).

72.4 Pathology

Pathogenesis of ATM: according to Minami et al., there are three hypotheses for the pathogenesis of ATM:

1. cell mediated post-infectious autoimmune response
2. direct viral invasion of the spinal cord
3. acute vascular occlusion

Sometimes a raised Coxsackie virus antibody is detected in the serum. Rarely this virus is found in the CSF, but it may be detected in the stools. Sometimes it is difficult to distinguish between autoimmune reaction and direct viral invasion. Pathologically several spinal cord segments are usually involved. In some cases the process is mainly a demyelination in others necrosis involves all cord elements. There are perivenous lymphocytes with areas of demyelination and microglial reaction. Superimposed ischemia and possibly vascular spasm may play a role, but one necroscopy shows necrotizing anterior spinal elements and cystic myelomalacia (Tyler et al. 1986).

72.5 Clinical Picture

There may be a history of respiratory infection or diarrhea or other manifestations of Coxsackie viral disease, but not necessarily so. It might be rather acute onset of paraplegia with or without sensory loss and with sphincter dysfunction. It is manifested usually within hours, days, up to a week. The previous history of viral disease (flu) suggests an immune-mediated pathogenesis. There is flaccid paralysis with loss of the reflexes including the rectal and bulbocavernous reflexes. Sensory loss may be associated with the motor loss. The picture is not specific for Coxsackie viruses, but occurs with other viral infections, and sometimes ATM is idiopathic. The course of the disease is variable depending on the time of the diagnosis and the efficiency of the management. Early management may lead to complete recovery motor and sensory-wise within months, and occurs in one-third of the cases; one-third gets partial recovery and one-third become chronically disabled and some of them die. Poor prognostic signs include extensive paralysis, widespread abnormal changes in the cord in the MRI and abnormal findings in somatosensory evoked potentials. Other CNS viral infections add to the risks.

72.6 Diagnosis

Diagnosis is base on:

1. Neurological exam
2. MRI of the spinal cord: (from Ku and Lee, for further details see their report) MRI is considered the best diagnostic modality in the intramedullary space. Common MRI findings of ATM are fusiform swelling of the cord having increased signal intensity with occasional gadolinium enhancement in T2 weighted sagittal scan and centrally located hyper-intensity of the cross-sectional area of the cord with variable enhancement in T2-weighted axial scan. Long-term follow-up may show atrophy with increased sagittal intensity on T2 weighted sequence consistent with myelomalacia and gliosis.
3. Serology: may show antibodies raised against Coxsackie virus and can be demonstrated in serum.
4. Cerebral spinal fluid (CSF): There is increasing of Coxsackie specific antibodies in the CSF due to two possibilities, either diffusion from the serum or local production from CNS. There is increased γ-globulin in the CSF and lymphocytes. Diagnosis of Coxsackie virus in the CSF is possible in half of the cases. Serum ratio of neutralizing antibody titres can be used as serological test for diagnosis and follow up during convalescence by comparison. Ku and Lee think that eight fold or greater neutralizing antibodies titres is diagnostic.
5. Tissue biopsy, if available, may grow the virus
6. Myelogram may be needed to rule out extramedullary lesions; however, MRI is the gold standard
7. Electrophysiological studies are useful diagnostic measures and if the changes persist during convalescence this indicates poor prognosis.
8. Stools for Coxsackie virus

72.7 Management

There is no consensus in the literature regarding the best treatment of ATM. Steroids in low doses or other specific treatment has no influence on the outcome of the disease (Ku and Lee et al. 1998). Intravenous methylpredinsolone has an anti-inflammatory effect in vivo and in vitro. Combined with cyclophosphamide in ATM due to SLE gave better results than prednisolone alone. Methylpredinsolone seems to be safe and effective in ATM in children. As an example Minami et al., treated a child 6 years old by IV methylpredinsolone 1000 mg IV daily for three consecutive days per week for 3 weeks followed by oral prednisolone (1 mg/kg/day) after which the patient's neurological condition had improved. The serum titre for neutralizing Coxsackie antibody against Coxsackie virus rose from ¼ to 1/256 1 month later.

References

Gear JH. Nonpolio causes of polio-like paralytic syndromes. Rev Infect Dis. 1984;6(2):S379–84.

Ku B, Lee K. Acute transverse myelitis caused by Coxsackie virus B4 infection: a case report. J Korean Med Sci. 1998;13(4):449–53.

Lerner AM, Finland M. Coxsackie viral infections. Arch Intern Med. 1961;108:329–34.

Minami K, Tsuda Y, Maeda H, Yanagawa T, Izumi G, Yoshikawa N. Acute transverse myelitis caused by Coxsackie virus B5 infection. J Paediatr Child Health. 2004;40(1–2):66–8.

Starakis I, Marangos M, Giali S, Bassaris H. Acute transverse myelitis due to Coxsackie virus. J Clin Neurosci. 2005;12(3):296–8.

Tyler KL, Gross RA, Cascino GD. Unusual viral causes of transverse myelitis: hepatitis A virus and cytomegalovirus. Neurology. 1986;36(6):855–8.

Cytomegalovirus Myelitis 73

73.1 Definition

This is a condition in which there is loss of motor and sensory functions and autonomic and sphincteric dysfunctions associated with cytomegaly virus (CMV) infection.

73.2 Incidence

According to Fux et al., there is an incidence of 1.3–4.6 cases per million per year. The disease viscerally develops in immunocompromised patients. Fux et al., reviewed the literature and found only eight cases in Immunocompetent patients and added one case of their own.

73.3 Etiology

Acute transverse myelitis (ATM) is caused by many viruses, including CMV. Approximately 40 % of ATM are preceded by infection herpes simplex virus (HSV), varicella-zoster virus (VZV), Epstein-Barr virus (EBV), enterovirus, hepatitis, measles, mumps, *mycoplasma pneumoniae*, or CMV. The pathological changes occur due to direct viral infection and autoimmune mechanisms.

73.4 Pathology

The changes in the nerve tissue are due to:

Fux et al. (2003)

I.M. Eltorai, *Rare Diseases and Syndromes of the Spinal Cord*,
DOI 10.1007/978-3-319-45147-3_73

- Direct infection by the virus
- Autoimmune reaction
- According to Kerr and Ayetey (2002): there is an element of vasculitis and granulomatous formation.

There is intraparenchymal and perivascular cellular infiltration in the spinal cord resulting in demyelination and neuronal injury. According to Fux et al. (2003), the pathophysiologic changes include molecular mimicry and the fulminant activation of lymphocytes by microbial super-antigens. In addition high levels of circulating antibodies may cause ATM by immune complex deposition.

73.5 Clinical Picture

The disease starts with back pain followed by neurologic manifestations acutely or subacutely. The manifestations of ATM following fever and chills and flu like cough for 1–2 weeks are:

- Paraparesis
- Ascending sensory loss
- Autonomic dysfunctions and spinal shock of variable degree
- Sphincteric dysfunction usually urinary retention and obstipation
- Occasionally cerebral manifestations

73.6 Diagnosis

1. Clinical history in an autoimmune competent patient
2. Blood picture is usually normal except in the presence of atypical lymphocytes (7.5 %)
3. CMV antigen may be detected
4. Active CMV IgM and IgG are positive and elevated in serum
5. Infections with other viruses need to be ruled out, e.g. HIV, VZV, tick-borne encephalitis, measles, mumps, *mycoplasma pneumoniae, Toxoplasma gondii, Borrelia, Rickettsia, Treponema pallidum* were all negative.
6. CSF: pleocytosis mononuclear 98 %, proteins elevated, CMV antibodies may be negative, CSF polymerase chain reaction (PCR) may be in 40–50 % negative for CMV DNA, but being positive confirms diagnosis.
7. MRI shows inflammatory regions but it may be within normal limits in 40–50 % of patients.

73.7 Management

- Ganciclovir (5 mg/kg BID ×14 days)
- Methylpredinsolone IV (500 mg/QD ×5 days)

In immunocompetent patients there is reversal of the neurological deficits totally or subtotally.

In immunocompromised patients, chances are small with these two measures added to them in a few cases was plasma exchange.

Updates

Abstracted from Karunarathne et al. (2012)

Case Report

The authors only found only ten published cases of CMV associated transverse myelitis have been reported. They report a patient with clinical myelitis followed by previously unreported finding of cytomegalovirus deoxyribonucleic acid in CSF. A 40-year-old immunocompetent male presented with acute onset progressive bilateral lower limb weakness. His spinal MRI, CSF analysis, and clinical picture were compatible with transverse myelitis. Polymerase chain reaction of the CSF for cytomegalovirus was positive. He was treated with IV ganciclovir with partial clinical response.

Reference

Karunarathne S, Govindapala D, Udayakumara Y, Fernando H. Cytomegalovirus associated transverse myelitis in an immunocompetent host with DNA detection in cerebrospinal fluid; case report. BMC Res Notes. 2012;5:364–8.

References

Fux CA, Pfister S, Nohl F, Zimmerli S. Cytomegalovirus-associated acute transverse myelitis in immunocompetent adults. Clin Microbiol Infect. 2003;9(12):1187–90.

Kerr DA, Ayetey H. Immunopathogenesis of acute transverse myelitis. Curr Opin Neurol. 2002;15(3):339–47.

Degos Disease (DD) 74

74.1 Definition

Degos disease (DD) is a condition of angiitis of the small vessels leading to occlusive vasculitis initially involving the skin. It may, in its simple form, be limited to the skin or may be a lethal multi-organ systemic variant. The disease has multiple nomenclatures of these a few are mentioned: Kiohliner-Degos disease, Degos-Delert-Tricot syndrome, malignant atrophic papulosis, arteriolar cutaneo-gastrointestinal thrombosis, etc. Systemic DD is usually fatal in 1–2 years (Scheinfeld ct al. 2005)

74.2 Incidence

In the United States DD is rare; about 150 cases have been reported worldwide (Scheinfeld et al. 2005). Matsura et al., have recently reported a case of spinal cord and optic nerve involvement by DD.

74.3 Etiology

According to Schienfield et al. (2005),

In 2003, Ball et al. 2003, thought that DD might be a variant of lupus erythematosus. In 2005, Scheinfeld et al. (2005), adduced strong evidence that DD is a distinct condition, since it starts with photosensitivity, does not respond to steroids, and its systemic form is fatal in 1–2 years. Some authors think that DD is due to a defect in the vascular endothelium, resulting in thrombosis, but it has not been

Abstracted from Matsuura et al. (2006).

I.M. Eltorai, *Rare Diseases and Syndromes of the Spinal Cord*,
DOI 10.1007/978-3-319-45147-3_74

proven yet. Vasculitis is also remote since there are no pathological inflammatory signs in the vessel wall. Recent suggested theories:

- immunity disturbance
- viral infection
- abnormality in blood clotting

Familial autosomal dominance has not been proven.

74.4 Pathology

- Cutaneous lesions: These are raised papules with umbilicated porcelain centers and a surrounding erythematous rim. Microscopically, there are degenerated wedge-shaped collagens. There is interface dermatitis and there is squamatization of the dermoepidermal, function, melanin incontinence and epidermal atrophy. There are areas of dermal papillary sclerosis. See more details in Scheinfeld et al. (2005).
- Mesenteric vessels: Thrombosis leads to infarction and perforation microaneurysm have been encountered, gastrointestinal ulcerations and infarcted areas have been detected.
- Kidney: There is thickening in the glomerular arterioles and capillary basement membrane. Other organs may be affected as well
- Spinal cord: The lesions are mostly in the lateral and posterior columns showing demyelination and axonal loss, the same in the nerve roots. Vascular thrombosis and endothelial proliferation are noted. Similar changes are noticed in the brain and the optic nerve was degenerated. Vascular thrombosis is a basic phenomenon. In the case described involvement of the optic nerve preceded the spinal cord changes. There was also central retinal artery thrombosis.

74.5 Clinical Picture

Initially, the disease starts by characteristic skin lesions: erythematous or red skin papules, which heal leaving scars which are pathognomic with porcelain white atrophic center. The papules have a peripheral telangiectatic rim.

In system DD, the gastrointestinal tract is affected in 50 % of the cases. Infarction of the bowel with intestinal perforation and peritonitis are most common and are fatal complication. Other systems especially the central nervous system may be involved with lesions in the brain and the spinal cord. Systemic DD appears weeks or months or years after the manifestation of the cutaneous disease. In rare cases it precedes the skin pathology.

74.6 Diagnosis

Diagnosis is based on:

1. Physical exam: cutaneous lesions, skin lesions, papules, erythremia around a porcelain like center
2. Neurological exam: the brain and spinal cord
3. Laboratory tests: Hemogram for anemia with intestinal bleeding, elevation of the thrombi-antithrombin III complex, plasmin-α2-plasmin inhibitor complex, cytotoxic T-cell subset (CD8, CD11) illustrating the coagulation, fibrinolytic and immunologic implications of DD include proteins, CSF.
4. MRI of spinal cord: Shows high intensity lesions with saw-teeth appearance. There is also a high intensity signal with a moth-eaten appearance in the periphery of the cord. Patchy lesions from the periphery to the center are characteristic of DD of the cord. The longitudinal nerve fibers appear severed by the lesions.
5. MRI of the brain: Shows multiple infarcts and areas of hemorrhage.
6. MR angiography: shows stenotic or occluded vessels
7. EGG and electrophysiological studies
8. Laboratory tests: Hemogram for anemia with intestinal bleeding, elevation of the thrombin-antithrombin III complex, plasmin-α2-plasmin inhibitor complex, cytotoxic T-cell subset (CD8, CD11) illustrating the coagulation, fibrinolytic and immunologic implications of DD include high proteins in the CSF.

74.7 Management

- Medical (medications non-surgical)
- Corticosteroids, heparin, warfarin, clopidogrel, aspirin, dipyradimale, pentaxophybline, IV immunoglobulin, dextran, ACTH, etc.
- Topical Applications
- Surgery as indicated for intestinal infarcts, perforation, or GI bleeding.

References

Ball E, Newburger A, Ackerman AB. Degos' disease: a distinctive pattern of disease, chiefly of lupus erythematosus, and not a specific disease per se. Am J Dermatopathol. 2003;25(4):308–20.

Matsuura F, et al. Optic nerve and spinal cord manifestations of malignant atrophic papulosis (Degos disease). J Neurol Neurosurg Psychiatry. 2006;77:260–2.

Scheinfeld N. Degos' disease is probably a distinct entity: a review of clinical and laboratory evidence. J Am Acad Dermatol. 2005;52(2):375–6.

Dengue Myelitis

75

75.1 Definition

Dengue fever (DF) and Dengue hemorrhagic fever (DHF) are caused by Dengue virus (DV) serotypes 1–4. It is transmitted by mosquito (Aedes Aegypti) bites.

75.2 Incidence

Dengue fever is an important virus infection in tropical and subtropical countries. In the United States, the disease is not endemic since the vector is not present. From 1977 to 2004, 3806 suspected cases were reported. Epidemic cases six times in the southern Texas, northern Mexico, and Hawaii were detected. There was no mention of myelitis. In South America especially in Brazil where the disease is endemic, the CNS complications are mostly encephalitis, myelitis is very rare. A case presented by Leão et al. is presented. Chanthamat and Sathirapanya reported a case of acute transverse myelitis associated with dengue fever. According to the authors there have only been four previously reported cases of transverse myelitis associated with dengue infection.

75.3 Etiology

The pathogenesis of the CNS disease is not clear and still little understood. Frequently, dengue infection has been associated with encephalopathy followed by shock and hypoxemia of the CNS (Leão et al.). Some authors including Chimelli et al., Cordeiro, Cunha et al., and Miagostovich et al., and Patey et al. have shown

Abstracted from Leão et al. (2002) and Chanthamat and Sathirapanya (2010).

I.M. Eltorai, *Rare Diseases and Syndromes of the Spinal Cord*,
DOI 10.1007/978-3-319-45147-3_75

the criteria for breakdown of blood–brain barrier of the CNS. Lum et al., have supported the encephalopathy to be due to the dengue viruses. Ramos et al., have detected the antigen by immunohistochemistry, and DEN-4 RNA in neurons, astrocytes, microglia, and endothelial cells. For more details see Seet et al.

75.4 Pathology

Myelitis is caused by dengue viruses 1–4. Severe gray matter myelitis may occur in DV type 1. The myelitis may be exclusive as to be detected by MRI from the cervical region to the cauda. Sometimes myelitis appears after the infection subsides. The picture is involvement of the gray matter like poliomyelitis, but there is sensory involvement as well. Partial resolution may occur in DV types 2 or 3.

75.5 Clinical Picture

The condition starts by fever, muscular rash, or capillary hemorrhages. There is flaccid paralysis, paraparesis, or tetraparesis, pin-prick sensations is decreased. Sphincter dysfunction usually retention of urine; in some cases there is encephalopathy as well. High spinal involvement results in respiratory distress requiring ventilator assistance.

75.6 Diagnosis

Diagnosis is based on the following criteria:

1. History of patient in endemic area
2. Physical exam shows rash, fever or dengue hemorrhagic fever
3. Neurological exam: sensory changes, onset of flaccid paralysis
4. Laboratory tests
   (a) blood count shows thrombocytopenia,
   (b) Anti-DV IgM to IgG in the serum and CSF
   (c) Plaque neutralization assays for antibodies for DV types
   (d) Laboratory tests for other viruses
   (e) Cultures for bacteria, mycobacteria, and fungi
5. MRI: high intensity signals limited to the gray matter region in any region from the cervical to the lumbar on T2 weighted images
6. Electrophysiology: peroneal compound muscle action potentials (CMAP) were absent in the case reported.

75.7 Management

Patient in Kunishige et al., case report was treated with:

- IV methylpredinsolone
- IV immunoglobulin
- Non-specific antibiotics
- Plasmapheresis

In the authors' case a tetraplegic, the upper limbs improved but remained paraplegic. After treatment the laboratory tests changed, the elevated DV antibody index came down IgM/IgG in both serum and the CSF.

References

Chanthamat N, Sathirapanya P. Acute transverse myelitis associated with dengue viral infection. J Spinal Cord Med. 2010;33(4):425–7.

Leão RN, Oikawa T, Rosa ES, et al. Isolation of dengue 2 virus from a patient with central nervous system involvement (transverse myelitis). Rev Soc Bras Med Trop. 2002;35(4):401–4.

Dental Extraction

76

76.1 Definition

This is a paraplegia developing as a result of metastatic epidural abscess after dental extraction and is due to oral bacteria from poorly hygienic teeth.

76.2 Incidence

One case reported by Larkin and Scott.

76.3 Etiology

The bacteria found in the epidural abscess are:

Streptococcus salivarius
Mutans
Mitis

No prophylactic or post extraction antibiotics were given.

76.4 Pathology

The most common source of pyogenic infection of the spine is metastatic bacteriemia source oropharyngeal infections are recognized as primary sources for metastatic infection. The infection settles in the vertebral cancellous bone and if

Abstracted from Larkin and Scott (1994)

I.M. Eltorai, *Rare Diseases and Syndromes of the Spinal Cord*,
DOI 10.1007/978-3-319-45147-3_76

uncontrolled it spreads outwards and destroys the intervertebral disc. Epidural abscess forms and may compress the spinal cord.

76.5 Clinical Picture

The recorded case was 65 year old male who had dental extraction, developed back pain, which was treated by analgesic and bed rest. Five weeks post-extraction he developed paraplegia, spastic type, and with sensory level at T8.

76.6 Diagnosis

Diagnosis is based on the following criteria:

1. Neurological exam
2. Radiography of the spine showing degenerative changes at T8-T9
3. Myelogram showed complete block at T8-T9

76.7 Management

- IV antibiotics
- Surgery I: exploratory through a left costo-transversectomy, degenerated disc material was evacuated as well as the questionable bone.
- Surgery II: 4 days later through a laminectomy decompression and removal of septic granuloma.

  There was no neurological improvement perhaps due to delay.

Reference

Larkin EB, Scott SD. Metastatic paraspinal abscess and paraplegia secondary to dental extraction. Br Dent J. 1994;177(9):340–2.

Holospinal Epidural Abscess

77

77.1 Definition

This is a relatively rare condition in which epidural abscess extend form the cervical to the lumbar region.

77.2 Incidence

The authors reviewed the literature and found only 13 cases reported and added two of their own.

77.3 Etiology

Predisposing factors:

- Diabetes mellitus
- Low immunity, e.g. receiving chemotherapy

  Predisposing causes:

- Psoas abscess
- Crohn's disease
- Congenital sacral teratoma
- Osteomyelitis of the spine
- Idiopathic

Abstracted and reported by Lau et al. (2014)

I.M. Eltorai, *Rare Diseases and Syndromes of the Spinal Cord*,
DOI 10.1007/978-3-319-45147-3_77

77.4 Pathology

There is an abscess extending throughout the whole spinal canal from the cervical to lumbar region. There is compression of the spinal cord. There are marked neurological deficits. There may be osteomyelitis of the spine.

77.5 Clinical Picture

Fever, pain in the back, neck or all spine. Neurological deficits from paraparesis to tetraparesis with sphincter dysfunction. Here the first case reported is abstracted:

A 50-year-old diabetic man presented with fever, leukocytosis, and upper extremity weakness.

77.6 Diagnosis

Physical exam showed weakness of both deltoid muscles 1 out of 5; biceps and triceps 2 out of 5 and weak handgrips bilaterally. MRI holospinal abscess from the base of the skull to T5 ventrally and dorsally from T1 to L5. Spinal cord severe compression at C2-C3 and L3-L4 discitis and osteomyelitis.

77.7 Management

- IV antibiotics
- Emergency surgical decompression performed through transoral odontoidecotomy, removal of anterior arch of the atlas and partial corpectomy of C2 due to C2-C3 osteomyelitis.
- Six days later the patient underwent C3-C6 laminectomy and C1-C2 posterior fusion.

Follow-up showed slow recovery of motion.

The second case was a 45-year-old man with a holocord spinal epidural abscess involving the whole spinal canal.

Drainage was performed through L2-L3 laminectomy

Two days later the patient developed upper limb deficits for which C3-C6 and T6-T9 laminectomies for decompression. A rubber catheter was introduced to irrigate the area between the surgical sites. Slow neurological recovery occurred; the patient could not be followed-up.

Reference

Lau D, Maa J, Mummaneni PV, Chou D. Holospinal epidural abscess. J Clin Neurosci. 2014;21(3):517–20.

Imported Vaccine-Associated Paralytic Poliomyelitis

78

78.1 Definition

This is a condition of paralytic poliomyelitis in an unvaccinated individual who traveled abroad and was in contact with an infant recently vaccinated with oral polio vaccine (OPV).

78.2 Incidence

This is the first case in the United States since 1999. According to Kelly form Australia OPV can cause vaccine-associated paralytic polio (VAPP) with a frequency of approximately on case per 2.5 million doses of OPV distributed. According to the CDC to the mid-1990s approximately 8–10 VAPP occurred annually (Alexander et al.).

78.3 Etiology

Most VAPP occurred in OPV recipients rather than amongst contacts. In the 1990s, cases of contact VAPP occurred in 1 case per 13 million doses of OPV distributed. Vaccination was changed to inactivated polio vaccine (IPV) in 2000; thus eliminated VAPP in the United States. From Australia a child received OPV at the age of 4 months and developed immunity to serotypes 1 and 2 but not type 3 and developed acute transverse myelitis. Poliovirus type 3 was isolated from the stool and the throat specimens after the onset of myelitis. This was confirmed by ELISA and nucleic acid probe hybridization. It is accepted that poliovirus can cause acute

---

Abstracted from CDC's publication MMWR (2006)

I.M. Eltorai, *Rare Diseases and Syndromes of the Spinal Cord*,
DOI 10.1007/978-3-319-45147-3_78

transverse myelitis in 1:125 to 1:800 polio case or 1:300,000,000 to 1:2,000,000,000 doses distributed. Laboratory studies provide plausible evidence of a link between OPV and VAPP or acute transverse myelitis.

78.4 Pathology

Poliovirus is an RNA virus that is transmitted through the oral-fecal route or by ingestion of contaminated water. The virus multiplies in the nasopharynx and gastrointestinal tract, from which it spreads to the lymphoid tissue and the blood (viremia). The virus is neurotrophic and settles in the anterior horns and bulbar cells, whose destruction leads to flaccid paralysis. The incubation period is 5–35 days.

78.5 Clinical Picture

The case reported in the United States:

A 22-year-old woman had not been vaccinated against polio for religious reasons. She went to a study trip to Central America and she was healthy. She was in contact with the grandchild of her hosts. He was an infant 2 months old; who received his first dose of OPV 4 days after the woman came to live with the grandparents. After about 40 days she developed fever and general malaise. After 24 h she got neck and back pains 4 days later she got acute leg weakness and was hospitalized locally and 3 days later was air lifted back to the United States where both legs were paralyzed and areflexic and had respiratory failure needing intubation. The CSF showed high lymphocytic count, high protein, and normal glucose. It was thought to be Guillian-Barré syndrome and received steroids and plasmapheresis. Electrophysiological studies showed anterior horn cells or motor axons damage. MRI showed anterior horn involvement in the cervical and thoracic cord. Serological studies were positive for Sabin poliovirus type 2 and 3, with no other viruses. She recovered her respiratory function, but had weakness of both legs.

In the Australian case:

A 6 month old boy developed acute transverse myelitis 7 days after the receipt of OPV. He was seen age 9 years and was found to have developed immunity to poliovirus type 1 and 2 but not to type 3, which was isolated from his stool and throat specimens. He later developed immunity to type 3 later.

78.6 Management

Essentially the treatment is supportive:

- care of respiration
- swallowing
- bowel and bladder

Bulbar paralysis need a mechanical management, and anxiety medication to calm patient may indicate cerebral anoxia, which may precede respiratory problems. Physiotherapy starts in the convalescent stage; orthotics and surgeries in the chronic stage.

78.7 Prophylaxis

For individuals traveling to an endemic country or where it epidemic they should be vaccinated. If they were not vaccinated or if it s unknown they should receive two doses of IPV with and interval of 4–8 weeks and a third dose after 6–12 months. Individuals who were vaccinated should take a dose of IPV before departure as a single dose for lifetime. For more details consult the CDC

Reference

CDC. Imported vaccine-associated paralytic poliomyelitis – United States, 2005. MMWR. 2006;55(04):97–9.

79 Lemierre's Syndrome

79.1 Definition

Lemierre's syndrome is caused by an acute oropharyngeal infection with secondary septic thrombophlebitis of the internal jugular vein and frequent metastatic infections.

79.2 Incidence

The infection subsided after its description in 1936 when the antibiotics came later; however, there seems to be recent resurgence. Metastatic infection causing epidural abscess and spinal cord compression was recently described by Park et al., a manifestation that has not previously been reported.

79.3 Etiology and Pathology

The infection starts in the oropharynx as an acute oropharyngitis caused by the anaerobic *Fusobacterium necrophorum*. It leads to postanginal septicemia and septic thrombophlebitis of the internal jugular vein, from which septic emboli immigrate into the body causing sepsis. The only case described by Park et al., was complicated by epidural abscess and cord compression.

Abstracted from Park et al. (2006)

I.M. Eltorai, *Rare Diseases and Syndromes of the Spinal Cord*,
DOI 10.1007/978-3-319-45147-3_79

79.4 Clinical Picture

The only case described by Park et al., was a female subject 43 years old, who had a sore throat with acute cervical lymphadenitis and fever, for which she received antibiotic therapy. She developed confusion and weakness of lower extremities 3 weeks later ending in paraparesis. The presentation was fever, tachycardia, agitation and confusion. She had flaccid paresis of the lower extremities.

79.5 Diagnosis

Diagnosis is based on

1. History oropharyngeal and cervical infections, although many clinicians remain unaware of this syndrome.
2. Neurological assessment: flaccid paraparesis
3. Lab tests: neutrophilia and raised C-reactive protein (CRP)
4. MRI of spinal cord: showed a collection anterior to the spinal cord from C1-T5 and post-epidural collection from T3-T5 and another collection form T11-L3.
5. CT scan: showed bilateral pulmonary basal consolidation and pleural effusion also bilateral psoas abscess (all are pyemic infections)

79.6 Management

Laminectomy and anterior C3 foraminotomy, drained the abscess, and antibiotic fluconazole, metronidazole, and meropenem therapy continued. Rehabilitation program helped the patient recover movement in 1 year with residual one foot drop.

Reference

Park D, Rezajooi K, Sabin I. Lemierre's syndrome: an unusual manifestation of spinal infection. J Bone Joint Surg Br. 2006;88(2):261–2.

Listeriosis

80

80.1 Definition

Listeriosis myelitis is a type of neurolisteriosis caused by listeria monocytogenes, which is a gram-positive rod bacterium that has a predilection to the central nervous system (CNS).

80.2 Incidence

Neurolisteriosis affects mostly the immunocompromised subjects. Listerial myelitis is very rare. A case by Nguyen-Huu et al., and by Josephson et al., were all that were found in an extensive search of the medical literature, in English and other languages.

80.3 Etiology

Neurolisteriosis affects mostly immunocompromised subjects, but it also involves the healthy persons. In the cases of listeriosis infection of the nervous system is involved. There are 13 serovars of Listeria monocytogenes, the most virulent of which are serovar 4b, 1/2b, and 1/2a, and cause human and animal disease. Transmission occurs through the following reservoirs of infection which are soil and intestinal tract of asymptomatic animals, wild or feral, mammals (cows or sheep), birds, fish, milk, crustacean, urine, and uterine discharge of infected animals. Transmission is through food that is contaminated, whether animal or plant, venereal transmission, inhalation, transplacental or through the genital tract in labor.

Abstracted from Josephson et al. (2006)

I.M. Eltorai, *Rare Diseases and Syndromes of the Spinal Cord*,
DOI 10.1007/978-3-319-45147-3_80

Food transmission can be as follows, uncooked vegetables, cheeses, cold cuts, or ice cream. Listeria is resistant to freezing, heating (1–45°C) and can multiply in refrigerators; spoiled silage favors the bacterial growth.

80.4 Pathology

Neurolisteriosis is more common in patients with compromised immune systems, but less commonly it affects immunocompetent individuals. The elderly and pregnant women are susceptible and may abort their fetuses. Involvement of the brain is usually meningitis, meningocephalitis, brain abscess, or hydrocephalus. Spinal cord involvement is by listerial myelitis, which is rare.

80.5 Clinical Picture

Listeriosis has two different pictures:

- In immunocompromised individuals in debilitated elderly patients and in pregnant women. It has a serious picture: fever, septicemia, meningocephalitis, which may end by brain abscess, or hydrocephalus.
- In healthy individuals, the symptoms are mild. It starts as a flu like with skin rash, symptoms of gastroenteritis and may be self-limited as seen in veterinaries. Myelitis may develop in immunocompetent individuals (Josephson et al., Nguyen-Huu et al.). According to the last authors in immunocompromised patients one in four develops CNS listeriosis. In the cases descried there is listeriosis myelitis in the cervical region. A case described by Dhiwakar et al., had meningocephalitis ending by hydrocephalus and syringomyelia. The clinical picture is that of pain in the neck and shoulder and upper arm, followed by paresis of the arm and lower extremities, sensory loss was minimal. In one case hydrocephalus developed due to inflammatory material in the third ventricle and was drained.

80.6 Diagnosis

Diagnosis is based on:

1. History: contact with animals or birds or taking contaminated food material
2. Neurological exam
3. Laboratory tests: cerebral spinal fluid (CSF) will show elevated proteins and pleocytosis, of the neutrophils, PCR, immunochromatography, immunofluorescence, ELISA, immunomagnetic separation. According to the CDC serology is unreliable
4. Culture: CSF, cord, or brain biopsies will show the bacteria

5. MRI of spinal cord: shows enhancing area in the cord with reenhancing after gadolinium.
6. rDNA: according to Nguyen-Huu et al., universal Polymerase change reaction from the biopsy, followed by sequencing of the amplified rDNA gene is the confirmed diagnosis

80.7 Management

- Steroid therapy for the tissue edema
- Antibiotic therapy:
- 4 weeks of IV ampicillin and IV trimethoprim/sulfamethoxazole (TMP-SMX)
- 8 days of concomitant intrathecal gentamycin
- Surgery:
- Laminectomy and durotomy for decompression and possibly cord biopsy
- Hydrocephalus or syrinx: shunting

References

Josephson SA, Pillai DR, Phillips JJ, Chou D. Neurolisteriosis presenting as cervical myelitis in an immunocompetent patient. Neurology. 2006;66(7):1122–3.

Nguyen-huu BK, Thümler A, Weisner B, et al. Neurolisteriosis with acute myelitis. Nervenarzt. 2005;76(10):1255–8.

81 Melioidosis

81.1 Definition

This is an endemic disease in Sri Lanka causing transverse myelitis due to *Burkholderia pseudomallei.*

81.2 Incidence

Although the infection is endemic in Sri Lanka, this is the first case of transverse myelitis causing paraplegia.

81.3 Etiology

Melioidosis is an infection caused by *Burkholderia pseudomallei*; a gram negative saprophyte in the soil and fish water. It is endemic in tropical and subtropical zone and southeast Asia and northeast Australia. It is underdiagnosed in Sri Lanka, due to lack of knowledge and awareness of the disease. Also there is lack of diagnostic tools to confirm the disease. It has low prevalence. The disease is more common in males aged 40–60, rare in children and is more common in rural areas (farmers). The infection is transmitted through the skin inhalation, and ingestion. Predisposing factors are alcoholism, diabetes, and chronic disease.

Abstracted from Nandasiri et al. (2012)

I.M. Eltorai, *Rare Diseases and Syndromes of the Spinal Cord*,
DOI 10.1007/978-3-319-45147-3_81

81.4 Pathology

From the case reported:

It can invade any organ in the body. The disease may be dormant, invading phagocytic and non-phagocytic cells. It spreads from cell-to-cell through actin based motility and when very active is associated with high instability. The infection spreads throughout the body. It involves the skin, the subcutaneous tissues, the musculoskeletal system, the urogenital system, the lung, the brain, and the spleen. Neurological involvement is rare; 3 % in an Australian series. When it occurs, it causes brain abscess, brain stem encephalitis, meningoencephalitis, and rarely transverse myelitis. A 20 year prospective study in northern Australia, where the disease is endemic, and only 14 cases presented with neurological complications, two of which were myelitis. The case reported by the authors is the first case of transverse myelitis in Sri Lanka.

81.5 Clinical Picture

The case presented by the authors:

A 21-year-old man, from northern Sri Lanka, who health and worked in the farm, where he was exposed to contaminated water and soil. The day before, he had low grade fever, which resolved spontaneously. The day of presentation he had pain and numbness in the lower limbs ending by flaccid paraplegia with urinary retention. Exam showed normal vital signs. Neurological exam showed flaccid paraplegia with sensory loss at T10 level. Elevated WBC, ESR, CRP. Radiography and CT of the spine was normal, except left psoas abscess. MRI showed a left psoas abscess which was multiloculated and measures 29.7×5.7 cm in size, with a finger-like extension towards the spine. There was transverse myelitis at T4 with foci at T2 at T2 weighted images. The central canal of the cord was dilated in all its length.

81.6 Diagonsis

Diagnosis is based on laboratory tests. The pus cultured on blood agar and Macconkey agar on which non-lactose fermenting colonies. Further studies showed identification of *Burkholderia pseudomallei*. Other lab tests were negative. CSF studies were not performed, due to the risk of introducing organisms into the CNS.

81.7 Management

Emergency ultrasound aspiration of the psoas abscess produced 350 ccs of purulent fluid. IV ceftazidime followed by cotrimoxazole and oral doxycycline for a year. Residual neurological deficits, including paraplegia, complete sensory loss, and sphincter disturbance persisted.

Reference

Nandasiri S, Wimalaratna H, Manjula M, Corea E. Transverse myelitis secondary to melioidosis: a case report. BMC Infect Dis. 2012;12:232.

Mumps Viraemia

82

82.1 Definition

This is a condition of acute transverse myelitis (ATM) and Guillain-Barré syndrome (GBS) occurring in association with mumps viremia.

82.2 Incidence

Myelitis due to mumps virus as the first manifestation is very rare (Bansal et al. 1998 and Okada et al. 2002); whereas, neurological complication of mumps are common especially in endemic areas. Meningitis is the commonest and encephalitis occurs in less than 1 % of the cases. Rare manifestations are neural deafness, optic neuritis, cortical blindness, neuropathy, facial palsy, Guillian-Barré syndrome, cerebellar ataxia, and hydrocephalus are the neurological manifestations of mumps. Bajaj et al., reported a case of Guillian-Barré concomitant with acute transverse myelitis due to mumps viremia and was the second cases in the literature.

82.3 Etiology

The virus causes ATM and at the same time leading to sensorimotor axonal polyradiculopathy (GBS). These changes may be direct effects of the virus or immune mediated reaction.

Bajaj et al. (2001)

I.M. Eltorai, *Rare Diseases and Syndromes of the Spinal Cord*,
DOI 10.1007/978-3-319-45147-3_82

82.4 Pathology

Neurological complications of mumps are: meningitis, encephalitis, myelitis, cranial nerve palsies, and rarely GBS. The area of myelitis shows increased vascularity, perivascular demyelination, proliferation of glial cells, degeneration of the anterior horn cells, and perineural edema. These changes are not different from other viral myelitis. Acute transverse myelitis may occur, especially in the thoracic and lumbar regions, higher lesions are more accompanied by edema of the cord and more demyelination. Associated viral pathology apart from neuropathy changes are: parotitis, submaxillary sebadenitis.

References

Bajaj NP, Rose P, Clifford-jones R, Hughes PJ. Acute transverse myelitis and Guillain-Barré overlap syndrome with serological evidence for mumps viraemia. Acta Neurol Scand. 2001;104(4):239–42.

Bansal R, Kalita J, Misra UK, Kishore J. Myelitis: a rare presentation of mumps. Pediatr Neurosurg. 1998;28(4):204–6.

Okada Y, Fukasawa N, Tomomasa T, Inoue Y, Morikawa A. Atlanto-axial subluxation (Grisel's syndrome) associated with mumps. Pediatr Int. 2002;44(2):192–4.

Myelitis due to Sparganosis

83

83.1 Definition

According to Stedman's Medical Dictionary Sparganosis is an infection with the plerocercoid or sparganum of a pseudophyllidean tapeworm, usually in a dermal sore resulting from application of infected flesh as a poultice; infection may also occur from ingestion of uncooked frog, snake, mammal, or bird intermediate or transport host bearing the spargana, but not from fish with Diphyllobothrium larvae, inasmuch as sparganosis is an infection with nonhuman pseudophyllidean tapeworms, usually species of Spirometra. Sparganosis may also develop from ingestion of water containing procercoid-infected Cyclops.

83.2 Incidence

According to Kwon and Kim (2004) who reviewed the literature they found seven cases involving the spinal cord and added one case of their own. Another case was added by Bao et al. Six were males and three were females and the ages ranged from 10 to 59.

83.3 Etiology

See definition above. Human infection occurs by:

- Drinking untreated water containing infected pepods (first intermediate host)
- ingesting raw or inadequately cooked flesh of frogs or snakes that are infected with sparganum (second intermediate host)
- Applying the flesh of an intermediate host as a poultice to a wound.

Abstracted from Kwon and Kim (2004)

I.M. Eltorai, *Rare Diseases and Syndromes of the Spinal Cord*,
DOI 10.1007/978-3-319-45147-3_83

83.4 Pathology

The spinal cord is most probably infected via blood stream. The parasite excites chronic inflammation and a sort of parasitic granuloma with adhesions around it. The parasite may be detected as in the case by Kwon and Kim. The lesions may be extradural, intradural, intramedullary, or cauda equine.

83.5 Clinical Picture

The disease is most common in East Asia. Exposure to contaminated water or eating undercooked frog or snake meat or using the raw meat as poultices. The common symptoms are: back pain, paresthesia, anesthesia, paresis or paralysis (paraplegia) and sphincter disturbances especially incontinence.

83.6 Diagnosis

Diagnosis is based on:

1. Patient exposure and from endemic areas
2. Neurological assessment
3. Pleocytes: Eosinophils, monocytes, lymphocytes, occasionally plasma cells
4. Evoked potentials
5. Cerebral spinal fluid (CSF): increased protein level
6. enzyme-linked immunoabsorbent assay (ELISA): test for *sparganosis* antibodies is positive indicating that intrathecal production; IgG oligoclonal bands show high sensitivity
7. MRI of spinal cord: mass in the spinal cord, nodular, and with mild enhancement. The brain should be included to rule out its involvement. Other organs may be involved as well.
8. Biopsy: will show chronic inflammation and scar tissue formation

83.7 Management

Debulking the mass through laminectomy and removal of the parasite. Specific therapy Praziquantel has been used to treat cerebral sparganosis but its efficacy has not been documented (Merk Manual).

Updates

Abstracted from Oh et al. (2011)

Sparganosis is a rare parasitic infection caused by the migrating plerocercoid larva of the tape worm, *Spirometra mansoni*, which commonly invades the subcutaneous tissue, skeletal muscle, and viscera. The CNS involvement is rare. Few cases have been reported involving the thoracic spinal cord including their case.

Case Report

A 51-year-old man complaining of progressive paresthesia of all the limbs and left motor weakness of 4 months prior to coming in, he had a history of ingesting inadequately cooked frogs and snakes several years earlier. He was treated with cervical laminectomy at C2-C3. The dura and the arachnoid were thickened yellow-white discoloration, with adhesions to the cord. Aspiration of the compression fluid was done. Pathology revealed granulomatous inflammation, tunnel-like cavities with necrotic larvae of sparganum and psammoma like bodies and calcifications. Post-op praziquantel; left sided paresis improved.

Reference

Oh SI, Koh SH, Pyo JY, Lee KY, Lee YJ. Sparganosis mimicking an intramedullary tumor of the cervical cord. J Clin Neurosci. 2011;18(8):1128–9.

Abstracted from Boonyasiri et al. (2013)

The authors present a case of sparganosis of the spine with subarachnoid serpiginous-mass from the preponitine levels to the oblongata, C7, T2 to T8 and T12 until the end of the thecal sac and filling in the right S1 neural foramen.

Incidence

The parasite can be found everywhere in the body, only three cases have been reported in the cauda equina. Boonyasiri et al., added a case of their own, first diagnosed by molecular identification.

Case Report

A 52-year-old woman living in rural Thailand, presented with lumbodorsal pain for 1 month. Paraparesis and radiculopathy for 2 weeks; bladder and bowel disfucntion for 3 days. No history of ingestion of inadequately cooked frogs, snakes, or birds. Molecular diagnosis was performed. DNA was extracted from μm unstained serial sections, cut from the formalin-fixed paraffin-embedded specimen, attached to glass slides using DEXPAT kit (TaKaRa Bio Inc., Tokyo, Japan). The test was positive for *S. erinaceieuropaei.* Laminectomy at L1 and L2; a scar with cystic formation was noted and biopsied. The section showed larvae of cestode with the folding segments and eosinophils. Calcareous corpuscles were evident, which is a sign of cestode. The patient received corticosteroid therapy and praziquantel; however, the symptoms persisted.

Reference
Boonyasiri A, Cheunsuchon P, Srirabheebhat P, Yamasaki H, Maleewong W, Intapan PM. Sparganosis presenting as cauda equina syndrome with molecular identification of the parasite in tissue sections. Korean J Parasitol. 2013;51(6):739–42.

Reference

Kwon JH, Kim JS. Sparganosis presenting as a conus medullaris lesion: case report and literature review of the spinal sparganosis. Arch Neurol. 2004;61(7):1126–8.

Toxocara canis

84

84.1 Definition

Toxocara canis is a round worm of dogs, which can cause visceral larva migration syndromes in humans by ingestion of contaminated soil. *Toxocara canis* causes the visceral larva to migrans in the central nervous system (CNS), brain and spinal cord.

84.2 Incidence

In the United State *toxocara canis* (TC) is a health problem. In different communities the prevalence is directly proportional to the infection rates depending on the free access to dogs to public places. The incidence is higher in the south, Puerto Rico, and minority areas as shown by enzyme-linked immunoabsorbent assay (ELISA) test from 16 to 30 %. Involvement of the spinal cord is very rare, no definitive incidence is available.

84.3 Etiology

TC larva migrans induce TC syndrome, which involves the liver, lungs, skin, eyes, and rarely the CNS. In the spinal cord the larva migrans cause transverse myelitis or eosinophilic memingo-myelitis, cervical arachoiditis, meningo-encephalitis, menigo-encephalo-myelitis, radiculitis, and sometimes spinal abscess. As a parasitic infection, it causes eosinophilic reaction. The migrant larvae reach the cord through focal blood-spinal barrier disruption due to reactive inflammatory process.

Abstracted from Goffette et al. (2000)

I.M. Eltorai, *Rare Diseases and Syndromes of the Spinal Cord*,
DOI 10.1007/978-3-319-45147-3_84

84.4 Clinical Picture

The syndrome starts by fever, eosinophilia, hepatomegaly, and pulmonary symptoms, which usually have a limited course. The patient usually was exposed to TC eggs and develops dysesthesia, paresthesia, weakness of lower limbs, and mild sphincter dysfunction. A sensory level may be noted, the tendon reflexes are exaggerated, and Babinski sign is usually positive.

84.5 Diagnosis

Diagnosis is based on:

1. History especially initial stages of fever, hepatomegaly and respiratory symptoms.
2. Patient from a community where there is free access of the dogs to public places.
3. Neurological assessment
4. Pleocytosis: Esinophils, monocytes, lymphocytes, occasionally plasma cells
5. Evoked potentials confirm myelopathy
6. Cerebral spinal fluid (CSF): increased protein level
7. enzyme-linked immunoabsorbent assay (ELISA): test for *t. canis* antibodies is positive indicating that intrathecal production; IgG oligoclenal bands may be negative.
8. MRI of spinal cord: slightly hyper-intense foci within the cord on T-1 weighted images with slight contrast enhancement on post contrast T-1 weighted images at the level of the lesion. Transverse T2 weighted images show hyper-intense foci. MRI of the lesion is added evidence. For more details on the cerebral *t. canis* see Moreira-Silva et al. (2004).

84.6 Management

Goffette et al., treated giving methylprednisolone 32 mg daily and tapered over 2 weeks. Mebendazole up to 3 g daily, both for 30 days. During the antihelminthic treatment Hexheimer's reaction may develop and for that reason it is better to combine the antihelminthic with steroids in addition to its anti-inflammatory action.

A follow-up with the therapy is useful:

- The CSF will normalize its cytosis and protein level, disappearance of the IgG oligoclonal bands, and drop of the antibody titre.
- ELISA titre to *t. canis* in the blood may remain positive for months or years after recovery.
- MRI: the pre-contrast T1-weighted scan no longer shows abnormality, but a residual hypersignal on T2-weighted images may persist for sometime.
- Esinophilia drops down to normal
- Neurological recovery continues

References

Goffette S, Jeanjean AP, Duprez TP, Bigaignon G, Sindic CJ. Eosinophilic pleocytosis and myelitis related to Toxocara canis infection. Eur J Neurol. 2000;7(6):703–6.

Moreira-Silva SF, Rodrigues MG, Pimenta JL, Gomes CP, Freire LH, Pereira FE. Toxocariasis of the central nervous system: with report of two cases. 1. Rev Soc Bras Med Trop. 2004;37(2):169–74. Epub 2004 Apr 13.

Toxoplasmosis of the Spinal Cord

85

85.1 Definition

Toxoplasmosis refers to both asymptomatic and symptomatic infection due to *toxoplasma gondii* parasite. Infection when symptomatic is usually short lived, rather acute and self-limited. In the chronic form the parasite causes persistent or recurrent clinical manifestations. The disease has many clinical manifestations, which are beyond this paper. A few examples are:

- The congenital form is usually complicated by damage in the brain and eye
- The acquired form involves viscera, e.g. the heart, lungs, liver, brain.

We will focus this paper on spinal cord involvement.

85.2 Incidence

Toxoplasm of the central nervous system (CNS) is not uncommon in patients with immunodeficiency due to immunosuppression or AIDS. According to the Centers for Disease Control (CDC) toxoplasma infection in the United States is approximately 60,000,000 may be infected with the parasite, mostly are asymptomatic. According to National Health and Nutrition Examination Survey (NHANES) there are about 4000 symptomatic cases and more common in females. Brain involvement in 50 % of patients with toxoplasma and autoimmune disease; whereas spinal cord involvement is rare only sporadic cases.

Abstracted from Cosan et al. (2001) and Campbell et al. (2001)

I.M. Eltorai, *Rare Diseases and Syndromes of the Spinal Cord*,
DOI 10.1007/978-3-319-45147-3_85

85.3 Etiology

Toxoplasmosis occurs by:

- accidentally swallowing cat or dog feces
- eating contaminated food (pork, lamb, venison)
- contaminated drinking water
- organ or blood transfusions

Toxoplasma tissue infection is caused by cysts in raw meat or by oocysts in cat feces.

85.4 Pathology

The disease comprises the following:

- toxoplasmic lymphadenitis: reactive follicular hyperplasia with irregular clusters of epitheliod histiocytes, monocytoid cells can also be seen.T. gondii can be demonstrated.
- CNS: there is meningoencephalitis with necorsis and microglial cells. There are similar changes in the heart, lung, liver, kidney, all of which are beyond this paper.

Spinal cord involvement is in two pictures:

- Toxoplasmic myelitis: pathologically is due to tissue reaction
- Toxoplasmic arachnoiditis
  - Granulomatous arachnoidits
  - Adhesive arachnoiditis
  - Arachnoiditis ossificans
  - Arachnoiditis calcificans

These constrict and compress the cord causing ischemia and sometimes atrophy of the spinal cord.

85.5 Clinical Picture

In immunocompetent individuals toxoplasmosis may produce acute symptoms with flu like and focal or diffuse meningoencephalitis, which may subside. In chronic cases adult and infants with congenital toxoplasmosis there may be no symptoms. When symptoms develop there may be flu-like illness. In patients with immunodeficiency the disease will persist with manifestations of meningoencephalitis. As regards to the spinal cord myelitis it may develop in congenital toxoplasomosis leading to ascending flaccid paralysis (see report by Campbell et al.). In adults toxoplasma arachnoiditis of the spinal cord presenting with spinal paralysis (see Erhan et al.) due to toxoplasma adhesive arachnoiditis.

85.6 Diagnosis

Diagnosis is base on:

1. Serological tests: IgG and IgM are positive in the acute infection and may not be highly positive in the chronic infection. Indirect Florescent Antibody (IFA) and Sabin-Feldman tests are rarely used clinically. IgM toxoplasma antibody may not be detected in acute cases of immunocompromised patients. Compliment fixation test may be tried.
2. Pathological test: The demonstration of *T. gondii* tachyzoites and bradyzoites in tissue specimens. In body fluids by periodic acid-Schiff (PAS), IFA, immunohistiochemical studies by staining (NeoMarkers)
3. Cerebral spinal fluid (CSF): xathochroma and mononuclear pleocytosis
4. Fundus exam: may show chorioretinal scar
5. MRI of spinal cord: shows hyperintensive subarachnoid space thickened adhesive arachnoiditis and spinal cord atrophy. Plaques of calcification even ossification may be detected.

The case described is isolated spinal cord toxoplasmosis with no visceral or cerebral changes.

85.7 Management

- Medical treatment of the organism using sulfadiazine and pyrimethamine.
- Surgical treatment: decompressive laminectomy and debridement of the arachnoid scars and plaques.

References

Campbell AL, Sullivan JE, Marshall GS. Myelitis and ascending flaccid paralysis due to congenital toxoplasmosis. Clin Infect Dis. 2001;15(10):1778–81.

Cosan TE, Kabukcuoglu S, Arslantas A, et al. Spinal toxoplasmosis Arachnoiditis associated with osteoid formation: a rare presentation of toxoplasmosis. Spine. 2001;26(15):1726–8.

86 Trypanosomiasis

86.1 Definition

This is an inflammatory condition of the spinal cord caused in Africa, by a trypanosome transmitted by a fly tsetse in Africa; in South America, where it is commonly called Chagas' disease, it is transmitted by reduviid bug (called the kissing bug or the assassin bug).

86.2 Incidence

There is no definite statistics about the trypanosomal myelopathy. In Africa the disease is caused by a flagellate protozoon, the trypanosome which has two species of *T. brucei*, which involves the human disease. The others are *T. brucei gambiense* (West Africa) *T. brucei rhodesiense* (East Africa). The trypanosome which causes Chagas' disease is *T. cruzi*. It is estimated that 16–18 million persons are infected with *T cruzi* and death toll of 50,000 every year.

86.3 Etiology and Pathology

(From Meritt's Neurology) In the African form of the disease, the organisms retain their trypanososme form and multiply by longitudinal fission. They are transmitted from person to person by tsetse fly, or occasionally by other fleas, insects and by mechanical contact. According to Kibiki and Murphy, *T. brucei* invades ova, has marked tropism for the CNS giving rise to perivascular inflammatory lesions, immune complex formation and a generalized vasculitis. Demyelinating encephalitis is the terminal stage of the disease. A well described diffused meningoencephalitis is the usual dominant picture. The parasite itself may rarely be demonstrated in

Abstracted from Lury and Castillo (2005) and Kibiki and Murphy (2006)

I.M. Eltorai, *Rare Diseases and Syndromes of the Spinal Cord*,
DOI 10.1007/978-3-319-45147-3_86

the nervous tissue as in the case reported by Lury and Castillo of Chagas' disease. Miliary granulomas may be detected consisting of microglia with lymphocytic-plasmacytic perivascular and meningial infiltrates. The organisms may be found in glial and neurons. These lesions are scattered in the nervous system accompanied by patch reactions in the meninges and parenchyma.

86.3.1 Stages of the Disease

The African type passes in two distinct stages:

- Fever (hemalymphatic)
- Lethargic (meningoencephalitis)

The incubation period varies, from 1 week from the infection or may not be detected for months or years. The Rhodesian type usually has acute to subacute course, the Gambian type is usually more chronic. The fever is accompanied by exanthemia, lymphademitis, splenomegaly, arthrodyia, myalgia, and asthesia. This may last for months or years and the organisms are found in the blood. The first stage may pass imperceptibly to the second stage, in which these symptoms are exaggerated with CNS involvement producing tremors, incoordination, convulsions, paralysis, confusion, headache, apathy, insomnia, or somnolence followed by coma. The symptoms may last for a year and death ensues after intermittent infection.

86.3.2 The South American Type (Chagas' Disease)

The acute stage starts by fever, conjunctivitis, palpebral swelling (where the bug sticks) for blood sucking and they sometimes deposit their feces, which is rubbed by the individual for itching. Swelling of the eye at the bit site is called Romaña sign. The acute phase is uncommon and may last for a month. Fatigue, anorexia, nausea, vomiting, enlarged lymph nodes, liver and spleen enlargements. In infants and patients with AIDS, the phase may be fatal. This phase may subside without treatment. The second stage is the indeterminate stage, there may be no symptoms at all and this stage may last for years. The chronic stage starts 10–40 years after the acute stage; 20–30 % of the patients develop serious symptoms, for example: cardiac arrhythmias, cardiac failure, cardiomegaly, even cardiac arrest; Esophagostasis and colostasis leading to dysphasia and obstinate constipation. Acute exacerbations may develop and occasionally with meningoencephalitis. The parasites are found in the blood in the acute phase and may be transmitted to other people or to animals by the reduviid bug or other insects, also through the placenta, through blood transfusion, and organ transplants, or through breast fed infants and through eating uncooked food contaminated with the feces of the vector bug.

86.3.3 Neurological Manifestations

According to Lury and Castillo from MRI studies the brain shows lesions in the corpus callosum, periventricular white matter, deep white matter, and subcortical regions and the cerebellum. In the spinal cord, there are multiple intramedullary lesions. In the African trypanosomiasis there is demyelinating encephalitis in the terminal stage. In the spinal cord there is demyelinating myelopathy due to *T. brucei* which may be reversible with specific therapy.

86.4 Clinical Picture

The different stages of the African and the American trypanosomiasis have been referred to above. Specific picture for trypanososmal myelopathy:

- African trypanosomiasis: living under non-ideal conditions exposed to the tsetse fly, usually malnourished, and in poor hygienic conditions.
- American trypanosomiasis (Chagas' disease): Living in Southern America or the southern most part of the United States, living in non-hygienic homes, thatch style homes, which harbor the vector bugs. Many patients are poorly nourished and some have a lowered immune system, such as AIDS, etc. The skin signs may be present (Romaña sign) or skin nodules ("chagoma"). Splenomegaly, cardiomegaly, etc., maybe detected as well.

Neurological symptoms of the myelopathy include motor and sensory loss, sphincteric dysfunction, cerebral or cerebellar manifestations may be detected in both diseases.

86.5 Diagnosis

Diagnosis is based on:

1. Environmental conditions
2. Cutaneous manifestations: insect bites Romaña's sign, chagoma, etc.
3. Serum fluorescent antibody for trypanosome in a tissue biopsy
4. Blood test for the parasite
5. Parasite antibody in blood
6. CSF: positive for trypanosome antibody and trypanosomes may be found
7. MRI (abstracted from Lury and Castillo): multiple areas of enhancement in the spinal cord and contrast enhancement in T1-weighted images. Brain images show infra and supra tentorial lesions and tumor like masses.

86.6 Management

In the African case of trypanosomiasis, Kibiki and Murphy treated the patient with metronidazole, ciprofloxacin, ceftriaxone for infections. Supportive treatments include nutritional multivitamins. In the case of Lury and Castillo the patient with American trypanosomiasis was started on a treatment of nifurtimox however he continued to decline and subsequently died. Antiprotozoal agents, nifurtimox or benznidazole (not available in the United States) are used to treat infections caused by the protozoan *T cruzi*. According to the CDC the goals of pharmacotherapy are to eradicate the infection, to reduce morbidity, and to prevent complications. Medication administered in the acute phase of American trypanosomiasis is usually effective; however in the later, chronic stages it becomes less effective. There is no preventative therapy or vaccine for the disease.

References

Kibiki GS, Murphy DK. Transverse myelitis due to trypanosomiasis in a middle aged Tanzanian man. J Neurol Neurosurg Psychiatry. 2006;77(5):684–5.
Lury KM, Castillo M. Chagas' disease involving the brain and spinal cord: MRI findings. AJR Am J Roentgenol. 2005;185(2):550–2.

Compression Myelopathy due to Typhoid Spondylodiscitis

87

87.1 Definition

This is a condition of spinal infection by Salmonella typhi, resulting in spondylodiscitis and epidural abscess resulting in compression myelopathy.

87.2 Incidence

The authors reviewed the literature and found only nine reported cases and added one case of their own, which was the first in southeast Asia.

87.3 Etiology

Salmonella typhi is from an infected source (food) it passes the blood stream through the GI tract causing typhoid fever. Extraintenstinal infection is rare 5–10 %. Involvement in the spine is very rare and usually occurs in patients with poor sanitary hygiene and living in endemic areas. Debilitating causes were diabetes and sickle cell anemia.

87.4 Pathology

The organisms will cause spondylitis, discitis with or without epidural abscess. The level most commonly involved is the lumbar and lower dorsal region. One case was in the upper dorsal. One case had psoas abscess. In the presence of an abscess, the cord is compressed.

Abstracted from Suwanpimolkul et al. (2010)

I.M. Eltorai, *Rare Diseases and Syndromes of the Spinal Cord*,
DOI 10.1007/978-3-319-45147-3_87

87.5 Clinical Picture

A 57-year-old male diabetic not well controlled, ingested raw vegetables, which was contaminated. His symptoms included low back pain, paraparesis, bladder and bowel dysfunction. Physical exam showed tenderness at T12, tight paraspinal muscles, paraparesis, and sensory level at T12. Blood cultures were negative. Radiography showed mild thoracolumbar kyphosis, narrowing T11-T12 disc. MRI showed spondylitis of T11 and T12 and discitis, erosion of the adjacent vertebral endplates, extension of the infection to the epidural space causing cord compression.

87.6 Management

Surgery consists of:

1. Laminectomy T11-T12, discotomy and debridement of epidural abscess, culture showed S. typhi

   Medical consists of:

1. IV Ciprofloxacin and thimethoprim-sulfamethoxazole, followed by oral treatment for 5 months.

   Patient was doing well 2 months post-antimicrobial treatment.

Reference

Suwanpimolkul G, Nilgate S, Suankratay C. Typhoid spondylodiscitis: the first reported case in Southeast Asia and review of the literature. J Med Assoc Thai. 2010;93(1):137–41.

West Nile Virus Infection

88

88.1 Introduction

From Marciniak and Rosenfeld:

West Nile Virus (WNV) is RNA flavivirus of the Japanese encephalitis group that is widely present throughout Africa, the Middle East, parts of Europe, South Asia, Australia, and former Soviet Union. Epidemics were unknown in the United States until 1999. During that summer, New York had experienced 62 cases and seven related deaths, with migration of the virus throughout the U.S. in subsequent years. By 2003 reported cases increased to 9820 with 264 related deaths.

Although most of WNV infection are asymptomatic a total of 888 neuroinvasive diseases were reported in the US in 2004. Neuroencephalitis is the most common manifestation followed by 10% of hospitalized patients in New York had flaccid paralysis.

88.2 Definition

Acute flaccid paraplegia due to WNV is a condition in which anterior horns of the spinal cord are invaded by WNV. It has short or long-term illness and in some cases death, mostly due to respiratory failure.

Marciniak and Rosenfeld (2005)

I.M. Eltorai, *Rare Diseases and Syndromes of the Spinal Cord*,
DOI 10.1007/978-3-319-45147-3_88

88.3 Incidence

In New York epidemic, 10 % of hospitalized patients developed polio-like flaccid paralysis. In 2002 several cases have been reported by electro-diagnostic tests. Saad et al. (2005) described three patients with Acute flaccid paralysis due to WNV infection and review the clinical presentations of 56 patients with this complication derived from published studies.

88.4 Etiology

The most common mechanism is involvement of the spinal anterior horn cells producing poliomyelitis-like picture and rarely Guillain-Barré like syndrome and very rarely brachial plexus involvement. The exact pathological cause is not yet well known (myelitis only or myeloradiculitis)

88.5 Pathology

There is no damage to the anterior horn cells, which has different degrees and extent. It may involve the brain stem and may be complicated by encephalitis. There may be myelo-radiculitis or simple radiculitis. The pathological findings are sometimes contradictory to the clinical picture. In the anterior horns there is neurophagia and lymphocytic infiltration. In addition to motor neuron damage, there is also motor nerve demylination. (For further details on pathology see Leis, Stokic, and Fratkin, 2003, NEJM)

88.6 Clinical Picture

In Colorado epidemic of 2003 JJ Sejvar et al., (Emerging Infectious Diseases, 2005) found amongst 2947 cases reported to the Centers for Disease Control (CDC):

- 32 patients with acute paralysis to due WNV infection, 18 of which were males.
  The age range: 15–84
  All but one were Caucasians and three Hispanics
  18 (50 %) had encephalitis
  10 (31 %) had meningitis
  6 (19 %) had paralysis alone
- Poliomyelitis-like syndrome: preferably called by Sejvar as WNV poliomyelitis. The incidence was 3.7/100,000. There were systemic signs of infection except in four patients. Four patients developed weakness during the systemic disease manifestations. The mean period between the infectious disease and onset of symptoms was 3 days (range: 0–18 days).

- Paralysis: take different forms and usually asymmetrical e.g. upper monoplegia, generalized asymmetric tetraplegia, diplegia, or tetraplegia. 70 % had cranial nerve involvement; 84 % (27) patients had asymmetric weakness; 13 % had symmetric ascending weakness with sensory abnormalities, consistent with acute inflammatory demyelinating polyradiculopathy form of Guillain-Barré syndrome and one had scapular winging and shoulder abduction weakness, consistent with long thoracic nerve paralysis. Bowel and bladder dysfunction are sometimes present.

88.7 Diagnosis

Diagnosis is base on:

1. History: fever, chills, vomiting, confusion, and acute painless weakness of the arms and legs
2. Physical exam: asymmetric weakness, areflexic paralysis, usually no sensory changes, possible signs of encephalitis or meningitis
3. Laboratory tests: cerebral spinal fluid (CSF) will show elevated proteins and pleocytosis, lyphocytes or polymorphs. IgM titres are positive for WNV
4. Electro-diagnostic tests: there is no diffuse mater axonal loss (for more details see Marciniak and Rosenfeld)
5. MRI of spinal cord and CT scan: usually negative. MRI should include the brain stem, as it may show some bulbar signs.

88.8 Management

There is no specific treatment

- Plasmapharesis is useless
- Immunoglobulin does not help
- Steroids may be detrimental
- Medical supportive therapy, with close watch for respiratory deterioration, which may need intubation, and ventilator assistance. Rehabilitation program with followup with electro-diagnostic studies for recovery.

88.9 Update

Abstracted from Maramattom et al. (2014)

One patient had acute flaccid quadriparesis and florid meningoencephalitis; another two had acute asymmetric flaccid paralysis with fasciculations at the onset. MRI in the two cases showed prominent hyperintensities in the spinal cord and brain stem with prominent involvement of the gray horn (poliomyelitis). The CSF, polymerase chain reaction was positive for WNV in the index patient. All three cases had a positive WNV immunoglobulin M antibody in serum, CSF, and significantly higher titer of WNV neutralizing antibody serum, distinguishing it from Japanese encephalitis. The disease has been long in India and and is transmitted by Culex mosquitoes. The authors reported three patients age 53, 45, and 42 all men, all with positive lab tests. The treatment of WNV is supportive. There are some reports showing improvements with interferon alfa-2b at a dose of three million U S/C daily for up to 2 weeks. Four ribavirin has also been used. The patients presented one died, one had residual paralysis of the right leg, and the third made a near complete recover.

Reference

Maramattom BV, Philips G, Sudheesh N, Arunkumar G. Acute flaccid paralysis due to West Nile virus infection in adults: a paradigm shift entity. Ann Indian Acad Neurol. 2014;17(1):85–8.

References

Marciniak C, Rosenfeld EL. Serial electrodiagnostic studies in West Nile virus – associated acute flaccid paralysis. Am J Phys Med Rehabil. 2005;84(11):904–10.

Saad M, et al. Acute flaccid paralysis: the spectrum of a newly recognized complication of the West Nile virus infection. J Infect. 2005;51:120–7.

Zoster Myelitis

89

89.1 Definition

This is a condition of recurrent myelitis occurring shortly after the appearance of typical herpes zoster rash and the lesion in the spinal cord at the same segments as the skin lesions.

89.2 Incidence

The incidence of recurrent zoster infection in immunocompitent patients is less than 5 %; according to Gilden et al., myelitis occurs in less than 1:1,000. Recurrent zoster myelitis is very rare. According to Baik et al., one case of pure myelitis previously recorded by Nakano et al., and they added one case of their own. Recurrent myelitis associated with encephalitis is less rare (O'Donnell et al.).

89.3 Etiology

The cause of herpes zoster is the varicella zoster virus (VZV), which is an exclusively human herpes virus that causes chickenpox (varicella), becomes latent in cranial nerves and dorsal root ganglia and frequently reactivates decades later to produce shingles (zoster) and post-herpetic neuralgia.

Immunocompromised people and in immunocompotent elderly persons, VZV leads to CNS complications. Cranial involvement of the trigeminal nerve: ophthalmic, maxillary, and mandibular, the seventh nerve, the third nerve. Vasculopathy is an important complication; in the spinal cord, cervical zoster causes may lead to arm paresis, diaphragmatic paralysis, lumbosacral zoster leads to paraparesis, thoracic zoster may occur after spinal anesthesia.

Baik et al. (1997) and Gilden et al. (2000)

I.M. Eltorai, *Rare Diseases and Syndromes of the Spinal Cord*,
DOI 10.1007/978-3-319-45147-3_89

89.4 Pathology

The exact mechanism of zoster myelopathy recurrence is uncertain, theories include:

- Direct viral infection
- Immune mediated demylination
- Vasculitis resulting in cord ischemia
- Delayed hypersensitivity in case that did not respond to cyclovirus.

The histological picture is that of inflammation and neuronal loss in the ganglia that correspond to the dermatomal rash level. Normal inflammation may spread to the adjacent spinal cord with localized leptomeningitis and gray matter necrosis and demyelination.

89.5 Clinical Picture

The condition starts with pain parathesia of dermatomal distribution, a typical vesicular herpetic rash followed in 4–14 days by manifestations of myelitis, with sensory and motor losses depending on the level of the lesion; thoracic and lumbar will involve the lower limbs, whereas cervical involves the upper and lower limbs. There will be anesthesia, analgesia, allodynia pallesthesia, and sometimes paresis. There is close temporal and spatial relationship between the rash and the myelitis.

89.6 Diagnosis

Diagnosis based on:

1. Clinical history with a zoster rash
2. MRI: the cord lesion covers parts to the dermatomal rash area. A sagittal image shows a high signal intensity lesion with diffused swelling due to the edema. An axial image shows the lesion at the affected segment
3. CSF for VZV antibodies; for VZV DNA polymerase chain reaction (PCR); serum VZV antibody is of no value. See review by Gilden (2004).

89.7 Management

- Acyclovir IV (10 mg/kg Q80 ×7 days)
- Longer period of treatment is need for the immunocompromised patient. If the PCR is negative discontinue the therapy. Sam if VZV antibodies are negative.
- Predinsone (60–80 mg/PO ×3–5 days)

The cause of the disease is usually self-limited, but it may progress as to be fatal in the immunocompromised patient and may pass to chronicity. The key to recovery is early diagnosis and prompt treatment.

Updates

Abstracted from Anderson and Tummala (2013)

The authors present a case of herpes myelitis after thoracic spinal surgery. Herpes simplex or herpes zoster reactivation after spinal surgery is rarely reported. Patient was a 57-year-old man with a history of hypertension and tobacco use. He had progressive symptoms consistent with spinal cord tumor. MRI revealed an intradural intramedullary contrast-enhancing T2 hyperintense lesion from T8-T10. A laminectomy was performed and was medically treated with dexamethasone 10 mg/6 h and tapered 4 mg/8 h over the next 10 days; he was ambulatory and had full strength in his lower extremities. Pathological examination revealed an ependymoma. Eleven days post-op patient had a mild fever. Repeat MRI showed fluid collection. The steroid dosage was decreased to 6 mg/6 h. By day 22 the patient gradually became nonamublatory, developing a severe progressive paralysis of both lower extremities, dense numbness, and incontinence. Additionally, vesicular rash in an L1-2 dermatome. MRI showed T2 hypertensity at T8-11 and re-accumulation of the fluid collection. Another surgery for aspiration of fluid collection, which was evacuated. Lumbar puncture showed WBC 313/μL, RBC 4/μL, and protein 369/μL. Herpes simplex virus type I was detected in the CSF by PCR. IV acyclovir and increased doses of corticosteroids where his rash resolved; however at 6 month follow-up his lower extremity paralysis persisted and neurological deterioration did not reverse. The authors review the literature from 1980 to 2012, which showed 15 cases. VZV or HSV following surgery 9 of the 16 patients were women. The median age was 57 years. Sites of surgery were cervical = 3, thoracic = 6, and lumbar = 7. The median time to symptom onset was 6 days and diagnosis after surgery was 7 days.

Reference

Anderson MD, Tummala S. Herpes myelitis after thoracic spine surgery. J Neurosurg Spine. 2013;18(5):519–23.

References

Baik JS, Kim WC, Heo JH, Zheng HY. Recurrent herpes zoster myelitis. J Korean Med Sci. 1997;12(4):360–3.

Gilden D. Varicella zoster virus and central nervous system syndromes. Herpes. 2004;11 Suppl 2:89A–94.

Gilden DH, Kleinschmidt-demasters BK, Laguardia JJ, Mahalingam R, Cohrs RJ. Neurologic complications of the reactivation of varicella-zoster virus. N Engl J Med. 2000;342(9):635–45.

Part VI

Neoplastic Causes of Myelopathy

Adamantinoma of the Spine

90

90.1 Definition

This is a rare malignant neoplasm locally aggressive slowly growing and the has potential to metastasize.

90.2 Incidence

In the spine it is extremely rare. According to Dini et al., only five cases have been reported and they added the sixth. The first case is that of Nerubay et al. (1988), in 1988. In 1986, Moon and Mori collected 200 cases from world literature without any spinal cord incidence.

90.3 Etiology

The disease is of unknown etiology.

90.4 Pathology

The tumor is considered to be epithelial in origin. To the naked eye the tumor is rarely seen as a single cystic mass. It may be seen as a multi-cystic mass. According to Theros and Ishak, the more malignant the tumor the less distinctive the honeycomb appearance. The tumor was considered low malignancy and that was negated by the study of Theros and Ishak. Macroscopically the tumor is pale gray or white, cystic with watery yellow or hemorrhagic fluid. Microscopically, there are squamous

Dini et al. (2006)

I.M. Eltorai, *Rare Diseases and Syndromes of the Spinal Cord*,
DOI 10.1007/978-3-319-45147-3_90

and tubular patterns, epithelial cells joined cystic area growing in a reticulated appearance. They reported a mortality of 18 % due to metastasis. From Dini et al., there are two types of adamantinoma:

- Classic occurs in patients older than 20 years.
- Differentiated type in patients younger than 20 years.

In the classic type the cells form a tubular basaloid, squamous, or spindled pattern. The stroma consists of fibroblasts arranged in cartwheel appearance. Occasionally, the tumor contains tissue like Ewing's sarcoma like cells and in others like fibrous dysplasia.

90.5 Clinical Picture

The case presented showed a 55 year old man presenting with pain in neck and C8-T1 radiculopathy. He had swelling of the neck and mandible.

90.6 Diagnosis

Radiography films showed osteolytic tumor involving C6, C7, and T1 vertebrae extending into the lateral masses and the transverse processes. MRI and CT scan confirmed the osteolytic lesions in three vertebrae and the left mandible. Epidural compression was evident in explaining the radiculopathy. Immunohistochemical stain for CD99 was negative in the case presented. Adamantinoma should be differentiated from aneurysmal bone cyst, chondromyxoid fibroma, chondrosarcoma, fibrous dysplasia, hemangioendothelioma, osteofibrous dysplasia, eosinophilic granuloma, or simple bone cyst.

90.7 Management

In the case presented by Dini et al., a corpectomy of C6, C7, and T1 was performed through thoracic anterior approach. Spinal stabilization was accomplished by anterior approach, using an autologous iliac crest graft and osteosynthesis by an anterior plate. Chemotherapy was not used (see case report for more details).

References

Dini LI, Mendonça R, Adamy CA, Saraiva GA. Adamantinoma of the spine: case report. Neurosurgery. 2006;59(2):E426.

Nerubay J, Chechnick A, Horoszowski H, Engelberg S. Adamantinoma of the spine: case report. J Bone Joint Surg Am. 1988;70:467.

91 Amyloidosis

91.1 Definition

This a nodular mass of amyloid, without generalize amyloidosis.

91.2 Incidence

Solitary primary amyloidoma of the spine is very rare, 18 cases in the literature.

91.3 Etiology

The causative factors are unknown. There is a thought that the amyloidosis is a result of proliferating plasma cells, and macrophages.

91.4 Pathology

The amyloidoma is a focal mass of amyloid tissue within the spinal canal, epidurally leading to compression of the cord or cauda equina. It arises from the bone marrow of the ventral body without involving disc. It is extruded into the epidural space. It is more commonly found in the thoracic spine, followed by the cervical and lumbar. The amyloidoma may cause bone destruction and may lead to fracture. The mass is gray, nodular, firm, but may develop cyst formation. Interstitial hemorrhage may occur. The amyloidoma is a benign lesion and does not change to malignancy.

Haridas et al. (2005)

I.M. Eltorai, *Rare Diseases and Syndromes of the Spinal Cord*,
DOI 10.1007/978-3-319-45147-3_91

91.5 Microscopically

After Haridas et al., collection of eosinophilic material within fibrous and elastic tissue AL protein is the type found in primary amyloidoma. The material shows apple-green birefringence and congo-red staining and examination under polarized light. There are occasional areas of hemosiderin and mononuclear cells. Under light microscopy, amyloid appears as eosinophilic amorphous hyaline extracellular substance. Another picture from Aydin et al., fragmented cartilaginous tissue with lymphocytic and plasma cell infiltrate. Deposition of eosinophilic acellular mass around which foreign body giant cell response. In some foci blood vessel walls are thickened with deposition of eosinophilic material. Congo-red stain gave congophilic response in the acellular material and the vessel walls. There is no mark of future development of plasmacytoma. Under electron microscopy, according to Iplicoeioglin et al., amyloidoma deposits appear as composed of rigid 7.5–10 nm fibrils arranged in B-pleated sheets.

91.6 Clinical Picture

Primary amyloidoma is not accompanied by symptoms and causes systemic amyloidosis. The symptoms depend on the spinal segments involved. There is pain in the back, may radiate to the neck and arms in cervical lesions, to the chest in thoracic amyloidoma and sciatic distribution in lumbar lesions. It is accompanied by sensory changes, hypoesthesia, paraethesia, or sensory loss. There is weakness of the extremities, which may end in para- or tetra- plegia. There may be sphincter disturbances such as incontinence.

91.7 Diagnosis

Diagnosis based on:

1. Patient history
2. Physical exam, absence of systemic amyloidosis and its etiologies. There may be tenderness over the affected vertebra, soft tissue swelling or a deformity.
3. Neurological exam sensory and motor deficits, depending on the level of the lesion. There is hypoesthesia, anaestheisa, increased muscle tone, hyperreflexia, weakness, paresis, or paralysis.
4. Plain radiography shows no abnormality. Or it may show a lytic areas in a vertebral body or bone distraction or fracture.
5. CT scan shows osteolytic areas in the vertebra and paraspinal soft tissue calcification. Pathological fractures and bone destruction can be seen.
6. MRI usually shows low to intermediate signal intensity on both T1 and T2-weighted images. There is variable degrees of epidural mass enhancement due to contract

administration on T1-weighted images. It should be differentiated from metastasis, multiple myeloma, lymphoma, and chondrosarcoma.
7. Biopsy. Ultrasound or CT-guided biopsy or fine needle aspiration cytology with special staining techniques, Congo-red under polarized light microscope or electron-microscopy. Immunohistochemical studies may help diagnose amyloidoma.

91.8 Management

Primary solitary amyloidoma producing neurogenic symptoms and signs should be removed, since there will be neurological recovery and if totally removed there will be no recurrence. The surgical techniques vary according to the site of the amyloidoma. In general decompression, complete resection and stabilization are needed. In their case, Haridas et al., L3-L4 laminectomies were donc with complete resection of the amyloidoma. Abbas et al., had T9 vertebreotomy, which was collapsed and insertion of mass cage. In the case laminectomy was done as a second procedure with removal of the mass. The first procedure was just decompressive laminectomy. According to Haridas et al., if the mass is accidentally discovered and there are no neurological symptoms or signs the patient can be treated conservatively, with regular followup clinically and by imaging. As soon as neurological picture is seen, surgery should be performed.

Reference

Haridas A, Basu S, King A, Pollock J. Primary isolated amyloidoma of the lumbar spine causing neurological compromise: case report and literature review. Neurosurgery. 2005;57(1):E196; discussion E196.

Acute Paraplegia Secondary to Brown Tumor

92

92.1 Definition

Brown tumor is a lytic bone tumor caused by hyperparathyroidism, either primary or secondary. Synonyms: osteoclastoma, osteitis fibrocystica, Engel-vonRecklinghausen.

92.2 Incidence

Brown tumors are more common in primary hyperparathyroidism than in secondary. There is an increased risk in patients with end-stage renal failure, 1.5–13 % patients had brown tumors. In 2004, Vandenbussche, et al, in a review of the English literature reported eight cases with spinal involvement. All of the patients were women, and 6 out of 8 (75 %) were younger than 40 years old. Two (25 %) of the cases involved the cervical, the other six (75 %) involved the thoracic. Four (50 %) of the cases developed acute paraplegia.

92.3 Etiology

Primary hyperparathyroidism

- parathyroid adenocarcinoma in 85 % of the cases
- glandular hyperplasia associated with multiple endocrine neoplasia (Type I and Type II)
  - less than 0.5 % of cases are caused by parathyroid malignancies
  - 10–20 % of the cases are caused by inherited hyperfunction of multiple parathyroid glands

Abstracted from multiple sources

I.M. Eltorai, *Rare Diseases and Syndromes of the Spinal Cord*,
DOI 10.1007/978-3-319-45147-3_92

- Secondary hyperparathyroidism
- chronic renal failure (CRF) in long term dialysis

92.4 Pathology

CRF leads to osteodystrophy, which entails osteomalacia, osteitis, or osteosclerosis either alone or in combination with brown tumors. Brown tumors occur mostly in the maxilla, mandible, clavicle, ribs, sternum, pelvis, long bones- especially the femur and the vertebral column. there may be extra sklatal deposition of calcium and phosphate. The brown tumor is a non-neoplastic, which is not malignant. It appears as a reddish brown friable mass that replaces normal bone. Histiologically, there is loss of bone trabeculae with accumulation of giant osteoclastic cells within fibrous tissue containing hemosiderin deposits. the tumor is vascular with microhemorrages, there are microfractures of the trabeculae and with its eventual loss. Progressive bone absorption leases to microscopic cysts, which eventually coalesce, forming osteitis fibrosa cystica. The brown tumor is almost indistinguishable from a giant cell tumor. The tumor may continue to worsen despite a renal transplant. In the vertebral column it involves cancellous bone marrow and may progress slowly casing compression of the spinal cord, producing a space occupying effect. The cortex may be spared unless a pathological fracture occurs; in which case, it leads to acute paraplegia if it is in the thoracic spine or tetraplegia if is located in the cervical spine. The pathophysiology according to Fineman, et al:

In osteitis fibrosa a brown tumor mass results from secondary hyperparathyroidism that is manifested by hyperplasia of the parathyroid chief cells in which elevated serum parathyroid hormone (PTH) levels and osteoclast activation are produced. The pathogensis of secondary hyperparathyroidism is linked to:

1. phosphate retention
2. altered metabolism of calcitrol (vitamin D)
3. skeletal resistance to PTH
4. impaired degradation of PTH
5. altered feedback regulation of PTH by calcium

Phosphate retention reduces the concentration of ionized calcium in extracellular fluid due to increased binding of ionized calcium phosphate. there is also decreased renal production of vitamin D in response to increased serum phosphate concentration and decreased calcium mobilization from bone because of the direct effects of phosphate on bone.

Serum PTH levels are further elevated by reduced production of vitamin D. Elevated levels of phosphate inhibit the activity of the hyroxylase that is required for conversion of 25(OH)D_3 to 1,25$(OH)_2D_3$ (that is, calitrol, the active form of vitamin D), which is necessary for intestinal absorption of calcium. this leads to further decreased serum levels of ionized calcium and subsequent hyperstimulation of the parathyroid glands.

Skeletal resistance to PTH in patients with CRF is responsible for the additional reduction in serum ionized calcium. This results in further upregulation of parathyroid PTH production as an attempt to maintain adequate serum levels of ionized calcium.

Additionally, because parathyroid hormone is metabolized in the liver and the kidney, decreased renal function of end-stage renal disease may be responsible for increased serum levels of PTH due to slowed catabolism.

Lastly, feedback regulation of PTH production in the parathyroid gland caused by serum calcium is altered in cases of advanced renal disease that result from decreased sensitivity to calcium; this in turn, leads to further increases in serum levels of PTH.

92.5 Clinical Picture

Hyperparathyroidism may be asymptomatic, non-specific symptoms are lethargy, confusion, nausea, fatigability, bone pain and weakness. When symptoms occur the may be due to hypercalcemia and/or hyperparathyroid osteodystrophy. This is focused on acute paraplegia to brown tumor of the vertebral column. the paralysis may be a slow onset, due to slow invasion of the brown tumor into the spinal canal. The pathological fracture will present acute onset paraplegia. There will be loss of sensory motor function, as well as sphincter dysfunction.

92.6 Diagnosis

In primary hyperparathyroidism the diagnosis is based on persistant hypercalcemia, which is confirmed by repeated measurements of serum calcium concentration, and an elevated PTH level. Parathyroid localization is done by technetium-99 m (^{99m}Tc); although, sestamibi scanning is the most accurate test for localization of the parathyroid. In secondary hyperparathyroidism there is commonly CRF. there will be an elevation of creatinine, calcium, phosphate, Westergren sedimentation rate, and PTH. Diagnosis of the bony lesion is confirmed by computed tomography (CT) guided biopsy; other imgaing tests especially magnetic resonance image (MRI) will show spinal cord compression, and myelography may be indicated. Plain radiography will show generalized osteopenia, loss of the trabeculae, cystic formation and may show a pathological fracture.

92.7 Management

For patients with symptomatic primary hyperparathyroidism, a total or subtotal parathyroidectomy should be performed by an expert surgeon and is more than 90 % successful. For patients with secondary hyperparathryoidism one look at the medical treatment, which is:

1. initial control of serum phosphate by restriction of dietary phosphorus intake and phosphate binding antiacids
2. adequate calcium intake
3. vitamin D therapy

If the medical therapy fails to halt the progression of the brown tumors, a subtotal or total parathyroidectomy is performed to reduce the PTH levels. The indication for a parathyroidectomy are:

- vertebral lesion with or without cord compression
- persistant hypercalcemia
- intractable pruritis
- extraskeletal clacifications

However, parathyroidectomy may only slow the progression of symptoms, then one must look to spinal decompressive surgery. When the invading tumor is removed spinal fusion by hardware and bone grafts are performed. The approach can be either anterior or posterior; although, the latter is more favorable. Surgery should be done as soon as possible to prevent permanent paralysis. Embolization of very vascular brown tumors may be indicated before surgery.

Bibliography

Fineman I, et al. Chronic renal failure causing brown tumors and myelopathy. Case report and review of pathophysiology and treatment. J Neurosurg Spine. 1999;90(2):242–6.

Griffiths HJ, Ennis JT, Bailey G. Skeletal changes following renal transplantation. Radiology. 1974;113(3):621–6.

Sargent MA, et al. Bone cysts and haemodialysis-related amyloidosis. Clin Radiol. 1989;40(3):277–81.

Taniegra ED. Hyperparathyroidism. Am Fam Physician. 2004;69(2):333–9.

Vandenbussche E, et al. Brown tumor of the spine and progressive paraplegia in a hemodialysis patient. Spine. 2004;29(12):E251–5.

Myelopathy due to Chondroblastoma of the Spine

93

93.1 Definition

Chondroblastoma is a rare benign tumor of the epiphyseal region of the long bones and is very rare in the vertebral column. It is characterized by a sclerotic margin, intralesional calcification, rounded or polygonal chondroblast-like cells, cartilaginous intercellular matrix, and multinucleated giant cells.

93.2 Incidence

The most current statistics tabulated by (Vialle et al. 2005), 26 cases of spinal chondroblastoma have been reported in the past 50 years, only six of which were located in the lumbar region, they added two cases of their own. The cervical is the most common location affected. According to Lee et al., the age of diagnosis ranges from 9 to 59 years, with the majority in the second decade of life. As to the sex ratio men are more commonly affected.

93.3 Etiology

No causative factor was detected.

93.4 Pathology

The tumor is benign mimicking malignancy, but tends to local recurrence and irradiation may precipitate malignancy. The tumor arises from the secondary ossification center of the vertebra. The tumor has a chondroid appearance with cystic and

Abstracted from Vialle et al. (2005)

I.M. Eltorai, *Rare Diseases and Syndromes of the Spinal Cord*,
DOI 10.1007/978-3-319-45147-3_93

hemorrhagic areas. Its consistency varies from soft to gritty depending on the amount of calcification or ossification. Microscopically it consists of closely packed polyhedral cells separated by a scanty interstitial matrix, giving the chondroid appearance. Another classic feature is the presence of a lattice-like intercellular cellular calcification resembling chicken-wire or the picket fence and the multinucleated giant cells. There is no mitosis or atypia. Hemorrhages may be seen as well as sometimes aneurysmal blood cysts. When too big the tumor may extend to the soft tissues around (muscles) and may ulcerate. However, the tumor does not metastasize. When invading the spinal cord it causes compression myelo-radiculopathy without invading the dura.

93.5 Clinical Picture

The first symptom is pain usually in the neck and dorsal region, rarely in the lumbar region. The pain radiates depending on the site: in the cervical case the pain radiates to the upper extremities; in the thoracic region it radiates to the chest; and in the lumbar region it radiates to the abdomen and lower extremities. Sometimes the chondroblastoma has a sciatica picture.

Swelling in early cases may be visible or palpable. With large tumors a swelling on the back may be felt and it shows vascularity and pseudo-inflammatory signs. The consistency is heterogeneous, hard, firm, fleshy, and cystic in parts. Extraspinal soft tissue extension is also detectable in progressive cases.

Neurological signs in chondroblastoma vary; it is usually tetraparesis, paraplegia, or cauda equina syndrome depending on the site. In cervical cases extension to the neck in the supraclavicular region and involvement of the brachial plexus is possible. In the dorsal region may extend in the mediastinum and the lumbar region may cause hydronephrosis

93.6 Diagnosis

Diagnosis based on:

1. Clinical assessment
2. Plain radiography: bone destruction (osteolytic lesion) usually in the vertebral body and may be in the posterior elements, bone formation and calcification are usually detected
3. MRI: shows a bone tumor involving the vertebral body with soft tissue extension to the muscles nearby. Extension into the spinal canal causes compression myelopathy but the dura is not involved.
4. Gallium isotope scan: shows cystic fluid and also by ultrasounography.
5. Needle aspiration biopsy: confirms the nature of the tumor.
6. Neurophysiological studies: confirms neurological deficit.

93.7 Management

Because the tumor has a high tendency to recur wide excision and curettage are required. After thorough curettage, flush irrigation and hemostasis packing with polymethyl-methacrylate, may reduce recurrence rate. (Ramappa et al.) For extensive tumors combined anterior and posterior approach for corpectomy and removal of extracorporeal tissue, bone graft and hardware fixation. In recurrent cases another attempt may be taken or possibly followed by irradiation, the latter may precipitate malignant change. Early surgery is the key to avoid recurrence and may reverse neurological deficit.

Reference

Vialle R, Feydy A, Rillardon L, et al. Chondroblastoma of the lumbar spine. Report of two cases and review of the literature. J Neurosurg Spine. 2005;2(5):596–600.

Costal Osteochondroma Causing Compression Myelopathy

94

94.1 Definition

Osteochondroma may be a part of hereditary multiple exostosis (HME). It is rare for it to invade the spinal canal to cause compression myelopathy.

94.2 Incidence

Tang et al reported a case and review the cases from the literature; they found a total five cases, the male to female ratio being 2:3, and ranging in age 13–21.

94.3 Etiology

HME is a hereditary disease, which is transmitted as autosomal dominant trait.

94.4 Pathology

The tumor is benign and it consists of a bony part and a cartilaginous cap. Osteochondromas constitute almost half of all benign tumors; the incidence of costal osteochondroma had been estimated at 3 %; however, this figure may be underestimated, as costal osteochondromas are usually asymptomatic.

Abstracted from Tang et al. (1998)

I.M. Eltorai, *Rare Diseases and Syndromes of the Spinal Cord*,
DOI 10.1007/978-3-319-45147-3_94

94.5 Clinical Picture

Small tumors are usually asymptomatic, bigger tumors can cause pain and swelling. Extension into the spinal canal causes compression myelopathy, manifested by motor and sensory compromise and sphincter disturbances.

94.6 Diagnosis

Costal osteochondromas are confirmed by local exam of the osseous mass and the neurological signs. Plain radiography does not show the cartilage cap to the tumor. The intraspinous component of the tumor, the corticomedullary continuity between the rib and the tumor, and the continuity between the intraspinous and extraspinous components can only be detected on magnetic resonance imaging (MRI). Computed tomography (CT) scan can show the same, however cannot reliably detect the cartilage cap if it is less than 25 mm. CT myelography will demonstrate a block at the level of invasion, however the size of the intraspinal tumor may be underestimated.

94.7 Management

Surgery is done under general anesthesia and incision is done over the rib tumor and the adjoining spinal cord. The rib tumor is dissected towards the spine. A laminectomy is done and may require facetectomy to give better exposure. The dura is mobilized and the intraspinal component is traced to the intervertebral formina; the tumor is removed piecemeal to accomplish a complete decompression of the cord. There is no recurrence if it is completely removed.

Update

Abstract from Liu et al., 2013

We report the case of a 42-year-old man who presented with kyphosis resulting from a giant symptomatic costal osteochondromaaround the left fourth rib. The osteochondroma on the left side of the back was 56 cm × 47 cm × 33 cm and was painful. The size and growth of the tumor suggested a malignant transformation of a large costal osteochondroma. Multiple osteochondromas were also found on the legs. The patient's family history revealed hereditary characteristics. This patient was clinically diagnosed as a case of multiple familial osteochondromatosis. Complete removal of the tumor relieved the symptoms, and histopathologic examination confirmed malignant transformation of chondrosarcoma. There was no recurrence after 16 months of follow-up.

Reference
Liu W, Kong D, Tang J, Yu F. Giant costal osteochondroma in a man with multiple exostoses. Ann Thorac Surg. 2013;96(2):675–7.

Reference

Tang WM, Luk KD, Leong JC. Costal osteochondroma. A rare cause of spinal cord compression. Spine. 1998;23(17):1900–3.

Cutaneous Adenocystic Carcinoma 95

95.1 Definition

Adenocystic carcinoma is a malignant tumor, which arises from the major and accessory salivary glands. Cutaneous involvement may result from direct infiltration from salivary glands. Cutaneous adenocystic carcinoma (CACC) remote site of the salivary glands is very rare.

95.2 Incidence

The first and only case of CACC of the lumbar skin causing compression myelopathy by direct infiltration was reported by Gelber-González et al.

95.3 Etiology

Compression myelopathy is caused by direct spread of CACC. The tumor is locally invasive and may metastasize to the lungs, spine, and local lymph nodes.

95.4 Pathology

The tumor cells are arranged in tubular cribriform and adenoidal formation pattern, some have lumens and others are solid. The lumens are filled with mucinous secretions or filled with debris or they may be empty. The cells are monomorphic, with focal atypia and mitotic figures. The stroma is fibrous with mucinous changes.

Abstracted from Gelabert-González et al. (1999)

I.M. Eltorai, *Rare Diseases and Syndromes of the Spinal Cord*,
DOI 10.1007/978-3-319-45147-3_95

The other sites from which this type of tumor may arise e.g., lachrymal glands, the maxillary and sphenoid sinuses, the breast, the intestinal and genital tracts, and the bronchus.

95.5 Clinical Picture

The tumor usually arises in the elderly forming a cutaneous mass. In this reported case it was in the lumbar region invaded the spinal cord and caused lumbar and radicular pain for 5 year duration. Eventually the patient developed paraparesis with spasticity and sphincter dysfunction. The mass about two inches and was fixed in situ.

95.6 Diagnosis

Diagnosis is based on the following criteria:

- Clinical findings include: mass infiltration
- Neurological deficit
- Axial CT: L1 and L2 showed a voluminous isodense mass that extended subcutaneously to the spinal canal, occupying it and destroying the laminae and one pedicle. Severe ventral compression of the conus was noted.
- MRI: A subcutaneous isosignal intensive mass extending to the lumbar epidural space and compressing the conus.
- Tissue biopsy

95.7 Management

- Complete excision of the tumor down to the dura
- Post-operative radiation therapy: prevent recurrence
- Post-operative chemotherapy: not established however tumors consisting of tubular pattern of cells respond better than those made of sheets or solid pattern.

Reference

Gelabert-González M, Febles-Pérez C, Martínez-Rumbo R. Spinal cord compression caused by adjacent adenocystic carcinoma of the skin. Br J Neurosurg. 1999;13(6):601–3.

96 Myelopathy due to Intraspinal Desmoid Tumor

96.1 Definition

Desmoid tumor (sporadic aggressive fibromatosis) is a fibroproliferative tumor that has benign histologic features and does not metastasize. However, the tumor is locally invasive, has aggressive clinical behavior and often recurs after excision.

96.2 Incidence

The tumor is rare, estimated incidence is 2–4 per million population per year. Approximately 50 % occur in abdominal wall, mostly in women at third and forth decades of life, possibly related to hormone during child bearing years. Thirty-five percent occur in the limbs, head, and neck. At age less than 15 years, most of the tumors are extra-abdominal. There is only one case causing myelopathy recorded by Shindle et al.

96.3 Etiology

No know causative factors. Hormonal relationship is not definitive. Female to male ratio is 5:2; usually during or after pregnancy and normally in the third to fifth decade. The tumor arises from the connective tissues of the muscle and overlying fascia or aponeurosis.

Abstracted from Shindle et al. (2002)

I.M. Eltorai, *Rare Diseases and Syndromes of the Spinal Cord*,
DOI 10.1007/978-3-319-45147-3_96

96.4 Pathology

The tumor is locally aggressive and does not metastasize. It consists of spindle cells in loose collagenous matrix, having nuclei. Immunohistochemical stain for the S100 protein is negative and there is no mitosis. It tends to recur locally. In the case of myelopathy, the desmoid is paraspinal and causes scoliosis, and had intraspinous extension causing compression myelopathy resulting in paraplegia in 12-year-old girl

96.5 Clinical Picture

This is a unique case from which clinical data are abbreviated:

A 12-year-old girl premenarchal, who had back pain and spasms of the legs followed by numbness and weakness followed by paresis and sensory level at T1 and sacral sparing. The reflexes were exaggerated and Babinski's sign was positive. Radiography of the spine showed scoliosis 70° thoracolumbar region. CT with IV contrast showed a mass 11 cm in diameter in the left hemothorax extending from the cranium to the left kidney and was invading the neighboring vertebra. MRI showed the mass invading the spinal canal and compressing the spinal cord. MRI is very important to define tumor border. Surgery was done post-decompression intralesional anterior excision and anterior fusion. In a second stage T9-T10 laminectomy was done and intraspinal part of the tumor was debulked down to the dura. The wound was closed. The patient was put in right lateral decubitus and through a T7 thoracotomy a tumor 5 × 10 cm, was found subpleurally and wrapping around the ventral body. The tumor was completely removed and anterior fusion conducted. The pathology showed typical desmoids. Two weeks later, a spinal fusion was done for the scoliosis, using rods and bone graph. Neurologic recovery progressed; she had radiotherapy 50.4 Gy. Nine years later she was free from recurrence.

96.6 Management

- Surgery: wide resection
- Wide resection followed by radiation when the margin is not secure
- In the pediatric population, radiation is a hazard to growth centers are followed by contractures and potentially causative of malignancy
- Chemotherapy may be useful adjuvant and is indicated in children with inoperable tumor and in progressive tumors is slow its growth until the child reaches bone maturity and the risk of irradiation is decreased
- Surgery and close observation at 2–3 months

The procedure followed by Shindle et al:

- Posterior decompression
- Anterior resection
- Anterior spinal function to correct deformity
- Post-op radiation for 5 weeks

The tumor is slow growing and extensive in growth, usually painless, giving it a chance to invade the spinal canal and causing myelopathy.

Reference

Shindle MK, Khanna AJ, Mccarthy EF, O'neill PJ, Sponseller PD. Desmoid tumor of the spinal canal causing scoliosis and paralysis. Spine. 2002;27(12):E304–7.

97 Intramedullary Ectopic Adrenal Cortical Adenoma

97.1 Definition

Myelopathy secondary to ectopic adrenal cortical neoplasm.

97.2 Incidence

Cassarino et al. (2004), report the first male case of intramedullary adenoma with oncocytic features. Two cases of extramedullary oncocytic spinal tumors occurring in females has been previously been reported.

97.3 Etiology

Ectopic adrenal cortical neoplasms are extremely rare and only a few cases have involved the central nervous system (CNS). Etiology is unknown. According to Cassarino et al., The term *Oncocytoma* was first coined by Hamperl in 1931; oncocytomas have been described in the kidney, adrenals, thyroid, and salivary glands, among other locations. Adrenal cortical oncocytomas have rarely been demonstrated outside of the adrenals, including examples in the retroperitoneum, spinal nerve roots, and subdural space. Oncocytic tumors involving the CNS are highly unusual, although oncocytic meningiomas and oncocytic paragangliomas of the spinal cord and cauda equina have been described.

Abstracted from Cassarino et al. (2004)

I.M. Eltorai, *Rare Diseases and Syndromes of the Spinal Cord*,
DOI 10.1007/978-3-319-45147-3_97

97.4 Pathology

To the naked eye the tumor has a tan to brown color; microscopically the tumor is composed of sheets and large nests of bland polygonal cells with abundant granular eosinophilic to clear cytoplasm. Non-atypical cells were found, but no necrosis identified. Cassarino et al., performed electron microscopy (EM) on material collected from paraffin-embedded tissue showed numerous mitochondria with tubular and lamelliform cristae, stacks of endoplasmic reticulum (ER), lipid vacuoles, and lipofuscin—all consistent with adrenocortical cell origin. In the immunohistochemical (IMHC) confirmation, the cells were positive for inhibin, melan-A, and synaptophysin, and negative for GFAP, EMA, cytokeratins, S-100, HMB-45, and chromogranin.

97.5 Clinical Picture

Intramedullary neoplasm manifested by pain followed by hormonal changes. The patient presented with weakness of the lower limbs, ambulatory loss, paresthesias of the feet, and sphincter dysfunction. There was analgesia, anesthesia, increased reflexes and spasticity on the neurological exam.

97.6 Diagnosis

Diagnosis is based on:

- Patient history
- Clinical exam, hormonal changes.
- Immunohistochemical testing: see Pathology
- Laboratory abnormalities: CSF high cellularity, low glucose, high protien

  CT was inconclusive.

97.7 Management

In the case presented blockade of the dye column at the conus medullaris level with obliteration of sacral nerve roots on lumbosacral myelogram. Surgery was performed and an intramedullary tumor was identified and removed in pieces. The patient is currently doing well with no evidence of recurrent disease approximately 1 year later.

Reference

Cassarino DS, Santi M, Arruda A, Patrocinio R, Tsokos M, Ghatak N, Quezado M. Spinal adrenal cortical adenoma with oncocytic features: report of the first intramedullary case and review of the literature. Int J Surg Pathol. 2004;12(3):259–64.

Spinal Tanycytic Ependymoma 98

98.1 Definition

Tanycytes are the peculiar ependymal cells that are lining the ventral part of the third ventricle in the mature selachian brain. Normal tanycytes are long non-branching unipolar or bipolar cells that extend between the ventricular surface and the cortex. These cells in the spinal cord surround the central canal. The cells radiate from the ependyma of the central canal into the gray matter. Although the origin of the tanycytes is unknown, electronmicroscopy has identified features suggestive of secretion and/or chemical transportation. Tanycytic ependymoma is subtype of ependymoma, which is recognized formally as a pathological entity in the latest WHO classification of CNS tumors. The term "tanycytic"[1] was used because the morphology mimics a distinct type of embryologic ependymal cells that develops in parallel with epithelial ependymocytes. Because of this morphology this type of tumor may be misinterpreted for astrocytoma or other tumors with elongated cells, such as schwanoma or fibroblastic menigioma.

98.2 Incidence

This tumor is very rare, a very small number has been reported (13 cases) of which six cases were pure tanycytic.

[1] The name tanycyte comes from the Greek word "tanus" meaning elongated to stress the shape of these bipolar cells. Their functions are still in debate.

Abstracted and reported by Sato et al. (2005).

I.M. Eltorai, *Rare Diseases and Syndromes of the Spinal Cord*,
DOI 10.1007/978-3-319-45147-3_98

98.3 Etiology

Etiology is not clear. The association with neurofibromatosis type 2 (NFT2) makes one think that the gene of NFT2 may be involved in the genesis of the tanycytic ependymoma but not proven. Extensive investigation showed that inactivation of NFT2 is involved in tumor genesis of other tumors, viz: schwannomas, meningiomas, mesotheliomas, and ependymomas. Mutation of NFT2 was detected in only 10–35 % of ependymomas whereas in schwannoma was 50–70 %. This relationship is higher in spinal lesions suggesting a significant link between spinal ependymoma and NFT2. The explanation needs more molecular genetic data.

98.4 Pathology

These are elongated cells with highly fibrillary processes forming a fascicular architecture and perivascular areas with inconspicuous pseudorosettes. The tumor cells show immunopositivity to S-100 protein and occasionally to glial fibrillary acidic protein. Electron micrograph shows characteristic ependymal features, e.g. intracytoplasmic intermediate filaments, prominent intercellular junctions and microvilli lined lumina, all compatible with tanycytic ependymoma. A case of tanycytic ependymoma associated with hematomyelia was described by Sato et al.

98.5 Clinical Picture

The condition is usually associated with NFT2. The symptoms are sensory and motor changes depending on the site of the tumor. MRI shows hypointense mass on T1 and T2 weighted images in the center of the spinal cord as an intramedullary tumor.

98.6 Diagnosis

The prediction of the nature of the tumor preoperatively is hard. The MRI of tanycytic ependymoma is not frequently reported. The solid part of the tumor is usually enhanced after gadolinium injection and it is frequently associated with syrinx. The final diagnosis is based on immunohistochemical and ultrastructural studies (see Sato et al.)

98.7 Management

The tumor is removed through laminectomy and median myelotomy. Removal is usually subtotal to prevent neurological damage. Postoperatively sensory worsening may develop, but this is usually resolved in a few months and there is no recurrence.

For tanycytic ependymoma radiotherapy is another option if the diagnosis is certain, which is hard to confirm without surgical biopsy; whereas, other intramedullary tumors such as schwannomas or astrocytomas are not radiologically treated.

Updating

Article by Karabagli et al. (2010).

Incidence

Twenty-five cases of tanycytic ependymoma have been described in the literature of which fourteen cases were in the spinal cord and seven of them were pure in nature. The authors tabulated the spinal cord cases, most of them were in the cervical cord. Associated syrinx occurs in 45 % of the cases and in 40 % of them the syrinx cephalad and caudal to the tumor.

Pathology

From the authors' case:

The tumor has poor cellularity; the cells are markedly elongated spindle cells with round to oval nuclei, showing the salt and pepper speckling, arranged in dense fascicles, no rosettes were seen, nor Rosenthal fibers. Immunohistochemical studies showed the tumor cells were immunopositive for S-100 protein and glial fibrillary acidic protein. The Ki-67 (MIB-1) labeling index was 3 %.

Case Presentation

A 51-year-old female for 10 months had progressive sensory disturbance and weakness of both hands. Neurological exam showed positive bilateral Hoffman sign, exaggerated tendon reflexes in all the limbs. MRI showed an enhancing tumor at C2 and C4 and syringomyelia from C1 to C2 and from C4 to C5. Surgical exposure through C2 to C4 laminectomy and the tumor was totally resected. Follow-up showed the hand weakness recovered gradually. MRI 2 years later showed no recurrence or syringomyelia.

Reference

Karabagli H, Karabagli P, Hakan T. Rarely encountered spinal tanycytic ependymoma and concominant syringomyelia. J Neurol Sci [Turkish]. 2010:27(2):244–9

Article by Ishihama et al. (2011).

Abstract

Tanycytic ependymoma has been recently classified as a variant of ependymoma by the WHO. Twenty-five cases have been reported including the authors' case. Seventeen of them in the spinal cord almost always intramedullary, only three cases were extramedullary. The intramedullary tumors are mostly cervicothoracic. The extramedullary were thoracolumbar. The tumors are low grade in character, so near total resection is not followed by recurrence. They are frequently associated with a syrinx and sometimes with a hematoma (hematomyelia) sharing these with schwannoma. Histologically it is similar to pilocytic astrocytoma, making the differential diagnosis a challenge; both give positive reaction to GFAP. (See the histochemistry differential diagnosis in the article.)

Case Presentation

A 40-year-old female had low back pain and numbness in the legs. Neurologically she showed slight weakness of the leg muscles, sensory deficit at T10 on the left and hyperexcitability of the tendon reflexes on the right. Autonomic functions were normal. MRI showed a dumbbell tumor at T10-T11. MRI also showed low intensity on T1-weighted-images and hyperintensity on T2-weighted-images and heterogeneity after gadolinium. A small cyst was seen in the tumor. The cord at T10-11 was compressed and displaced. The tumor was decompressed by Cavitron ultrasonic surgical aspiration (CUSA) and then was carefully dissected from the dura and it originated from T10 root, which was sacrificed to remove the entire tumor. Pathology confirmed tanycytic ependymoma. The patient's symptoms resolved and MRI up to 16 months was negative for recurrence.

Ishihama H, Nakamura M, Funao H, et al. A rare case of spinal dumbbell tanycytic ependymoma. Spine. 2011;36(9):E612–4.

Article by Funayama et al. (2012)

Abstract

The authors present a case of tanycytic ependymoma of the cauda equina associated with multiple endocrine neoplasia type I (MEN-1). Statistically there are only five cases of ependymoma associated with MEN-1. The authors present the first cases of tanycytic ependymoma of the cauda equine associated with MEN-1.

Multiple endocrine neoplasia type I (MEN-1) is a rare autosomal syndrome with an estimated precedence of 1–17.5 per 100,000 inhabitants or 1 per 30,000 individuals.

MEN-1 is:

- Neoplasia of the parathyroids
- Neoplasia of the anterior pituitary
- Endocrine pancreas

It is correlated with mutations in the MEN-1 gene on chromosome 11q13. Other endocrine and non-endocrine tumors with lower frequency have been reported including adrenal cortical tumors; foregut and neuroendocrine tumors of the GI tract, the thymus, bronchi; facial angiofibromas; collagenomas; limpomas; and leiomyomas. Although many tumors are associated with MEN-1, CNS tumors are rare except intracranial meningiomas. Ependymomas associated with MEN-1 are very rare only few cases. Tanycytic ependymomas is a rare subtype of ependymoma. The authors presented a case of tanycytic ependymoma of the cauda equine associated with MEN-1.

Case Report
A 53-year-old man presented with nocturnal pain in the back, numbness in the perineum and intermittent claudication for 1 year. The years earlier he had weakness in both legs, which disappeared 1 year after the onset. MRI of the spine showed intradural large mass from T12 to L2 vertebral level.

Diagnosis was MEN-1 with pancreatic gastrinomas at the age of 51. At the age of 20 he had resection of pituitary adenocarcinoma; recurrent duodenal ulcer at the age of 25; he had total parathyroidectomy and immediate autotransplantation of the forearm at 43; and then the transplants were removed at the age of 51.

There was bowel and bladder dysfunction. Tendon reflexes and bulbocavernosus reflexes were reduced.

Management was open door laminoplasty T12 to L1 and L2. After opening the dura, the tumor was seen and dissected from the conus and cauda nerves and was removed *en bloc* with a portion of the filum terminale. Closure was done in standard technique.

Pathology: The tumor was tanycytic ependymoma class II of the WHO.

Post-op: symptoms except for bladder symptoms. Eight months follow-up showed no recurrence.

For histopathology details please see the original article and the histological challenge by Krisht and Schmidt. The authors stress the follow-up very carefully clinically and radiologically.

Reference
Funayama T, Sakane M, Yoshizawa T, Takeuchi Y, Ochiai N. Tanycytic ependymoma of the filum terminale associated with multiple endocrine neoplasia type 1: first reported case. Spine J. 2013;13(8):e49–54.

Krisht KM, Schmidt MH. Tanycytic ependymoma: a challenging histological diagnosis. Case Rep Neurol Med. 2013;2013:170791.

Reference

Sato K, Kuboto T, Ishida M, Handa Y. Spinal tanycytic ependymoma with hematomyelia. Neurol Med Chir (Tokyo). 2005;45:168–71.

99 Follicular Dendritic Cell Sarcoma (FDCS)

99.1 Definition

Follicular dendritic cell sarcoma (FDCS) of the spinal dura mater is an extranodal malignant tumor of the focal dendritic cells with a characteristic histological picture and immunohistochemically the cells are strongly positive for follicular dendritic cell markers CD21 and CD35. For more details see pathology.

99.2 Incidence

These tumors are rare. In the head and neck are uncommon. Nineteen cases have been reported recently, Biddle et al. In the spinal dura the first case is reported by Choi et al.

99.3 Etiology

The etiology of the disease is unknown. According to Choi et al.,

The cells giving rise to these tumors are currently divided into:

- Follicular dendritic cells (FDCS), interdigitating dendritic cells and indeterminate cells
- Langerhan's cells

Abstracted from Choi et al. (2006)

I.M. Eltorai, *Rare Diseases and Syndromes of the Spinal Cord*,
DOI 10.1007/978-3-319-45147-3_99

99.4 Pathology

There are two types of sarcoma arising from these systems

- Proliferation o spindle to oval cells showing the morphological and phenotypic features of FDCS, which involves ½ to 2/3 of all lymph nodes
- Extranodal involves the tonsils, oropharynx, mediastinum, and abdominal cavity. Amongst these the dura mater of the spinal and was involved in only one case.

  The pathological studies showed:

- Histology: diffused and dense infiltration of small lymphocytes and sheets of histocytes with formation of reactive germinal centers. The tumor cells are arranged in nodules, sheets, and interlacing fascicles with arborizing blood vessels.
- Histochemistry: the tumor cells were positive for CD21 and CD35. For more details and techniques please see Choi et al., and Biddle et al.

99.5 Case Report

A 68-year-old male with negative past history, complained of lower back pain radiating to the right lower extremity. Neurologically the motor power was intact, no sensory loss. MRI showed relatively well enhancing and diffusely infiltrating mass in the fourth and fifth lumbar vertebrae and extending into the right epidural space and completely encased L1 nerve root. Diagnostic and therapeutic curettage of the mass was performed which confirmed the diagnosis of FDCS. Radiotherapy was applied. Two months later patient came back with pain in the lower extremities. MRI showed a mass effect on the dural sac; ultrasound guided aspiration of the fluid, which was negative for neoplasia 7 months later. There was no lymphadenopathy.

99.6 Diagnosis

Diagnosis is based on

1. MRI findings
2. Pathology report and histiochemical studies

99.6.1 Differential Diagnosis

Other space occupying lesions in the spinal canal:

- Non-neoplastic lesions: tuberculosis
- Other inflammatory lesions
- Neoplastic lesions
  - Metastasis
  - Lymphoma
  - Lymphoplasmacyte-rich meningiomas
  - Langerhan's cell histiocytosis
  - Interdigitating dendritic cell sarcoma
- Hyaline-vascular Castleman disease

99.7 Management

1. Mass debridement
2. Local radiotherapy

Reference

Choi JW, Lee JH, Kim A, Kim CH, Chae YS, Kim I. Follicular dendritic cell sarcoma arising in the dura mater of the spine. Arch Pathol Lab Med. 2006;130(11):1718–21.

Left Atrial Papillary Fibroelastoma 100

100.1 Definition

Fibroelastomas are benign tumors which may arise in the cardiac chambers or on the valves. About 14 % develop on nonvalvular surfaces. They may arise on the cardiac valves, in the atria or in the ventricles, the atrial septum, the interventricular septum, and the ventricular outflow tract, or the chordae tendinae. They may be multiple and appear like bacterial vegetation. They may be shaggy and have irregular surface of projecting fimbriated elements, they may be too large to occupy the whole atrium. Emboli usually reach the brain but also the left anterior descending coronary artery causing sudden onsent. Pulmonary or central retinal embolisms can occur.

100.2 Incidence

According to Friedman et al. (2001), there was no report of cord embolism from fibroelastoma, although two cases from cardiac myxoma were reported.

100.3 Etiology

Tumor embolism may be difficult to differentiate from thromboembolism, or atheromatous emboli.

Abstracted from Friedman et al. (2001)

I.M. Eltorai, *Rare Diseases and Syndromes of the Spinal Cord*,
DOI 10.1007/978-3-319-45147-3_100

100.4 Pathology

The embolus causes ischemia and necrosis (an infarction). The embolus reaches the cord through the spinal arteries or the artery of Adamkiewicz.

100.5 Case Report

A 84-year-old woman developed band-like anterior chest pain followed by weakness of the leg passing to paraplegia of lower motor neuron type. EKG and cardiac enzymes were normal. MRI showed no gross abnormality. Transesophageal echocardiogram showed a sessile 1 cm mass attached to the left atrium on the ridge between the left upper pulmonary vein and the left atrial appendage. The rest of the heart and aorta were unremarkable.

100.6 Management

Cardiac surgery accomplished removal of the tumor whose pathology was papillary fibroelastoma (central myxoid stroma covered with endothelial cells). On discharge the patient had some weakness of the legs but could walk with a walker.

Updating

Abstracted from Pello & Ashkenazi (2011)

Abstract
The authors present a case of aortic valve fibroelastoma accompanied by spinal cord infiltration, only one case previously described.

Case Report
A 61-year-old woman presented with acute paraplegia and urinary incontinence. Neurologically paraplegia was areflexic and with T10 sensory level. MRI of the thoracic spine using echo planar imaging showed an intramedullary T2-hyperintense lesion that involved the part of the gray matter of the cord and part of the white matter extending from T8 level to the conus medullaris. Diffusion weighted-images (DWI) showed restricted diffusion in that area. There were also hyperintense areas at the posterior aspect of T11–T12 vertebrae likely to be due to ischemia. The CSF showed no abnormality. These findings suggest spinal cord infarction in the distribution of the artery of Adamkiewicz. Blood total cholesterol of 268 mg% and LDL 176 mg% (both high). Aortic aneurysm was ruled out by CT scan. Transesophageal echocardiogram showed a mobile oscillating mass of the left leaflet of the aortic valve consistent with fibroelastoma: Because of the hypercholesteremia and the

infarction the patient was put on Simvastatin® and aspirin. Patient refused surgical removal of the fibroelastoma. She was put on standard antiocoagulation medication. In 3 weeks the motor deficit was not corrected. There was no followup.

Reference

Pello SJ, Ashkenazi A. Spinal cord infarction in a woman with cardiac fibroelastoma. Neurologist. 2011;17(1):47–8.

Reference

Friedman GR, Pappas TW, Colangelo R, et al. Unusually located left atrial papillary fibroelastoma with probable embolization to the spinal cord. Echocardiography. 2001;18(6):523–6.

Gliofibroma 101

101.1 Definition

Gliofibroma is a neoplasm of mixed mesenchymal and glial components, which develops in the CNS.

101.2 Incidence

22 cases of gliofibroma have been reported in the CNS, 15 cases in the brain and seven in the spinal cord: three cervical, three thoracic, and one thoracic to conus. The male to female ratio is 3:4 and commonly occurs in the first two decades of life.

101.3 Etiology

The origin of the tumor is not clearly known there are theories about the origin:

- prenatal: as demonstrated by Iglagias 11 day old boy and by Windisch et al of an intramedullary tumor in a 5 month old boy.
- Transformation of preexisting hamartoma, suggested by Reinhardt and Nahser, however late onset tumors have the same biological features of neonatal tumors.
- Iglasia-Rozas proposed and aberrant metaplasia in glial cells resulting into mesenchymal cells.
- Cerda-Nicholas and Kepes postulate that the neoplastic astrocytes produce the connective tissue fibers similar to the prescence of glial and sarcomatous

Abstracted from Matsumura et al. (2002)

I.M. Eltorai, *Rare Diseases and Syndromes of the Spinal Cord*,
DOI 10.1007/978-3-319-45147-3_101

elements of gliosarcoma having the same genetic alteration of monosomy in chromosome 10 and 17.

More details of molecular genetic analysis can be seen in the work of Louis et al.

101.4 Pathology

In the spinal cord the tumor is intramedullary well demarcated, most soft yellowish, grayish causing syrinx rostral and caudal. The tumor usually has no extradural extension or new adhesion to the dura. Microscopically, the tumor consists of dense mixture of astrocytic and fibroblastic elements of the mature composition. The nuclei of the tumor cells are round or oval with particular chromatin network. In the care of the tumor there is deposition of retinbin-positive collagenous matrix. Between the gliomatous and fibrous elements the reticulin-positive fibromatous component is clearly separated from the gliomatous component. Histochemical studies can be seen in the reference paper by Matsumura et al. The tumor is usually a benign astroglial variant.

101.5 Clinical Picture

The tumor is usually encountered in the young. In the spinal cord it behaves like other intramedullary tumors. There is sensory loss of pain and temperature, motor weakness and paresis.

101.6 Diagnosis

Diagnosis is based on:

1. Clinical history
2. Neurological exam
3. MRI of spinal cord: The glial are fibrous elements can be seen as hypo- or iso-intense mass on T1 enhanced images. The center part of the tumor has hypointensity on plain images and markedly enhanced with gadolinium. The glial portion at the periphery shows hypointensity on plain images and slight enhancement with gadolinium. Other routine tests are done especially MRI of the brain.

101.7 Management

The tumor is removed through laminectomy, posterior myelotomy and microdissection. In cases of recurrence or malignant transformation, radiotherapy is to be done. If pathology shows malignant cells radiation is recommended.

Reference

Matsumura A, Takano S, Nagata M, Anno I, Nose T. Cervical intramedullary gliofibroma in a child: a case report and review of the literature. Pediatr Neurosurg. 2002;36(2):105–10.

Glioneuronal Tumor

102

102.1 Definition

This is a tumor composed of two distinct histologic components: one with uniform neurocytes forming rosettes and/or perivascular pseudorosettes, the other component is astrocytic and resembles pilocytic astrocytoma.

102.2 Incidence

There are 19 cases reported in the fourth ventricle, whereas Anan et al. (2009) reported the first case in the spinal cord.

102.3 Etiology

Unknown etiology: the tumor may be derived from the gray commissure or the middle motor nuclei in the middle or lower thoracic cord.

102.4 Pathology

The tumor has two components—neurocytic and astrocytic. The neurocytic component has moderate cellularity. The neurocytes formed neurocytic rosettes; the nuclei are round and small without atypica or mitosis. The cytoplasm has bipolar processes and sometimes joined neighboring rosettes together. At the center of the rosette there is an eosinophilic cell with absence of vessels. The astrocytic component

Abstracted from Anan et al. (2009)

I.M. Eltorai, *Rare Diseases and Syndromes of the Spinal Cord*,
DOI 10.1007/978-3-319-45147-3_102

shows low to moderate cellularity. The nuclei are round or oval, without atypia or mitosis. The tumor cells have bipolar and spindle processes. No foci or necrosis. For more details about histochemistry see Anan et al. (2009), where the authors discuss and analyze the fourth ventricle cases.

102.5 Clinical Picture

The cases described was a 44-year-old female presenting disassociate sensory changes of the lower limbs with gradually extending to the upper limbs with weakness in all the extremities over a 15 year period. She had two shunts for cervicothoracic syringomyelia. Neurological findings showed spastic tetraparesis below C7, dysthesia of all senses, and a neurogenic bladder.

102.6 Diagnosis

Diagnosis is based on the following criteria:

1. MRI of the spinal cord: syrinx between C2 and C4. A solid tumor showed low signal intensity on T1- weighted images and high signal in T2-weighted images between C2 and T4. A ring enhanced lesion with gadolinium at T4 intradural level. No calcification or lesion in the fourth ventricle.

102.7 Management

C4-T4 laminectomy was performed; the tumor was removed all intramedullary, except a small portion at T4 was extramedullary. Follow-up showed slight neurological deterioration, without recurrence at 14 months.

Reference

Anan M, Inoue R, Ishii K, et al. A rosette-forming glioneuronal tumor of the spinal cord: the first case of a rosette-forming glioneuronal tumor originating from the spinal cord. Hum Pathol. 2009;40(6):898–901.

103 Myelopathy in Primary Spinal Epidural Mantle Cell Lymphoma

103.1 Definition

Mantle cell lymphoma was regarded as a variant of intermediate lymphocytic lymphoma that proliferated as wide mantles around non-neoplastic appearing germinal centers. It is a non-Hodgkin's lymphoma can affect the central nervous system (CNS) either primarily or with late stage when the disease behavior is aggressive and widespread.

103.2 Incidence

Spinal cord compression occurs in 10.2 % of cases of non-Hodgkin's lymphomas, which are aggressive. Primary spinal epidural malignant lymphoma is rare and accounts for 3.3 % of all lymphomas and 9 % of all spinal epidural tumors. Primary mantle cell spinal lymphoma is extremely rare, three cases have been reported. Mantle cell tumors account for 2.5–4 % of all non-Hodgkin's lymphomas. Men are more affected than women 4:1. The median age is 60.

103.3 Etiology

The disease is of uncertain etiology.

103.4 Pathology

The tumor occupies the spinal epidural space with cord compression. Microscopically, it is made of malignant lymphoid tissue containing "naked" germinal centers surrounded by diffuse proliferation of neoplastic lymphocytes, small or medium with

Abstracted and reported by Barnard et al. (2000)

I.M. Eltorai, *Rare Diseases and Syndromes of the Spinal Cord*,
DOI 10.1007/978-3-319-45147-3_103

irregular indented nuclei containing dense chromatin and occasional nucleoli and frequent mitoses. Immunohistochemically expressed B-cell markers CD19 and CD20 and expression of T-cell marker CD5. More details can be found in the article by Barnard et al. In the mantle cell tumor, small lymphoid cells that are atypical grow in the mantle zone in a nodular or diffuse form. The lymphoma cells surround benign or germinal centers, with the normal lymphocyte cuffs. It is thought that the tumor arises in epidural lymphoid rests, but it is not proven.

103.5 Clinical Picture

In the secondary epidural lymphoma there is the full blown picture of lymphoma: lymphadenopathy, splenomegaly, and bone marrow infiltration, etc. In the primary lymphoma it is manifested by cord compression: sensory and motor loss, spasticity, hyporeflexia or areflexia, and sphincter dysfunction. However, after biopsy or excision of the tumor recurrence and full picture will be manifested. The prognosis is poor in either case.

103.6 Diagnosis

Diagnosis is based on the following criteria:

Confirmation is made with tissue biopsy and by other sites of lymphomatous deposits. If the lesion is primary as it is entitled it is a challenge for diagnosis until tissue examination. MRI shows epidural mass usually lumbosacral, the vertebra may be involved, so also paravertebral soft tissues. The mass described in this third reported case was of homogeneous signal intensity and exhibited mild diffused enhancement with gadolinium. After incomplete resection there was recurrence and open picture of mantle cell lymphoma.

Neuroradiologically the tumor may simulate metastasis, plasmacytoma, epidural schwannoma and other tumors; therefore, thorough differential diagnosis needs to be performed.

103.7 Management

- Surgery: Laminectomy and resection for histopathology
- Radiation therapy
- Chemotherapy using cyclophosphomide, vincristine, and prednisone.

This tumor has aggressive behavior and poor response to therapy and therefore poor outcome.

Reference

Barnard M, Perez-Ordoñez B, Rowed DW, Ang LC. Primary spinal epidural mantle cell lymphoma: case report. Neurosurgery. 2000;47(5):1239–41.

Malingnant Eccrine Poroma

104

104.1 Definition

Malignant sweat gland tumors are extremely rare, representing less than 0.01 % of all primary skin lesions. Malignant eccrine neoplasms can be divided into two main categories:

- Eccrine adenocarcinoma developing de novo in normal skin
- Eccrine adenocarcinoma arising in pre-existing sweat gland benign tumor (less common)

The first group is subdivided into five categories as follows:

1. malignant eccrine porocarcinoma
2. syringoid (tubular) eccrine carcinoma
3. mucinous eccrine carcinoma
4. clear cell carcinoma
5. microcytic eccrine carcinoma

Eccrine porocarcinoma is the most common constituting for approximately half of all eccrine adenocarcinoma.

104.2 Incidence

Magdum et al., reported the first case of myelopathy secondary to malignant eccrine poroma.

Abstracted from Magdum et al. (2001)

I.M. Eltorai, *Rare Diseases and Syndromes of the Spinal Cord*,
DOI 10.1007/978-3-319-45147-3_104

104.3 Etiology

The cause of carcinoma is not known, it is theorized that it may be develop after irradiation

104.4 Pathology

The tumor is usually ulcerated and nodular arising from the epidermis and growing into the dermis. It is usually composed of anastomosing trabeculae of epithelial cells embedded in glycosaminoglycan-rich matrix. In many areas the cells show ducts containing periodic acid-Schiff-positive material strongly suggestive of eccrine nature. This histiopathology is seen in both the skin tumor and its metastasis in the vertebral column, namely malignant eccrine poroma. The tumor shows up in patients around 60 years of age, only five cases below forty. Ten percent metastasized to the lymph nodes. It usually presents as localized nodule, a plaque, a verucous ulcer. The skin lesions frequently arise from the limbs, head, and neck, with itching, bleeding, and pain.

104.5 Clinical Picture

From Magdum et al., case Patient was a 57-year-old male, who had a history of chronic back pain and urinary hesitancy. Patient had an episode of psychosis and was subsequently diagnosed with hydrocephalus, which a ventriculoperitoneal shunt was made. The skin showed an ulcer over the left mandible, which bled on touch. Cerebral spinal fluid (CSF) showed malignant cells, he then developed weakness of the lower limbs. Magnetic resonance imaging (MRI) showed metastasis in T4 and L3 and compression. Decompression laminectomy was performed with a pedicular fixation. The bone biopsy and skin tumor which was of the same nature, i.e. that of malignant eccrine poroma. Patient developed pulmonary infection and died 2 months later. No autopsy was performed. The tumor was not radiosensitive. A new therapy is suggested isotretinoin and α-interferon for the treatment of the metastatic lesions.

Conclusions

Patient had malignant eccrine poroma in the neck that metastasized, leading to malignant meningitis, resulting in obstructive hydrocephalus and causing compression myelopathy. This suggests that malignant skin lesions should be dealt with as soon as possible, before metastasis to the central nervous system, which can produce a fatal outcome.

Reference

Magdum S, O'Brien D, O'Reilly G, Crooks D. Malignant eccrine poroma with spinal and cerebral-spinal fluid matastases: case report. Neurosurgery. 2001;49(4):1004–7.

Melanoma

105

105.1 Definition

Melanomas are tumors that arise in the organs or structures that have melanin producing cells.

105.2 Incidence

To date there is less than 60 cases of primary malignant melanoma of the spinal cord. Before 1968, 26 cases of primary malignant melanomas. An average of one case every 2 years. The mean age in the first twenty cases before 1960 was 50 years (range 15–80 years). Later, the mean age was 46 years (25–71 years. it involves more females than males, male to female ratio: 1:1.36. Thoracic is commonest, followed by cervical.

105.3 Etiology

Melanomas can arise in any organ which contains melanin-producing cells, e.g. skin, chromaffin tissue, leptomeninges, etc. Melanocytes are cells that arise from the neural crest during embryogenesis, and migrate to the skin, mucosa, and CNS. The exact etiology is not clear, theories include:

- Primary melanoma of the CNS arises from melanoblasts accompanying the pia sheets or vascular bundles

Abstracted from Yu et al. (2012)

I.M. Eltorai, *Rare Diseases and Syndromes of the Spinal Cord*,
DOI 10.1007/978-3-319-45147-3_105

- Melanoma may arise from the neuroectodermal cells during embryogenesis. More authors are in favor of this theory, since it suggests genetic origin and may suggest a genetic therapy, but this is only hypothetical.

105.4 Pathology

From the case reported:

The mass was subdural, measuring 5.3 × 1.8 × 1.1 cm with some adherence to the pia mater, the mass was black with intact capsule. Microscopically, fusiform and epithelial cells with deposition of melanin granules, growing around vessels. After depigmentation, vesicular nuclei and red staining nucleoli were seen. The cells stained with S100 protein and malignant melanoma monoclonal antibody HMB45.

105.5 Clinical Picture

The case presented by the authors:

A 48-year-old Chinese man presented with progressive numbness of the upper and lower extremities for 6 months. He had neck and shoulder pain for 1 month. Physical exam was normal except for hypothesia C3-T1 bilaterally. MRI of the cervical spine showed a space occupying lesion, C2-C6 with hyperintense lesion on T1 weighted image and hypointense signal on T2 weighted image. After gadolinium injection, hyperintense lesion T1 weighted images and showed cord compression. MRI of the brain lesion showed multiple lesions, especially on the surface and in the cisterna magna and the sula, hyperintensive on T1 weighted images. There was no mass effect and edema of the brain.

105.6 Management

Surgery consists of:

1. Laminectomy of C2–C6, duratomy, black mass was identified and was incompletely removed. Frozen and permanent sections sowed malignant melanoma.

   The case was considered terminal and the patient died 2 months later.

Updates

Hering et al. 2016

Only four cases of primary intradural extramedullary spinal cord melanoma (PIEM) have been reported. No previous reports have described a case of PIEM located in the lower thoracic spine with long-term follow-up. Demonstrating an unusual, extremely rare case of melanoma manifestation.

The authors report a case of a 57-year-old female suffering from increasing lower extremity pain, left-sided paresis, and paraesthesia due to spinal cord compression caused by PIEM in the lower thoracic spine. Extensive investigation excluded other possible primary melanoma sites and metastases. For spinal cord decompression, the tumor at level T12 was resected, yet incompletely. Adjuvant radiotherapy was administered 2 weeks after surgery. The patient was recurrence-free at 104 weeks after radiotherapy but presents with unchanged neurological symptoms. Primary intradural extramedullary melanoma (PIEM) is extremely rare and its clinical course is unpredictable.

Reference

Hering K, Bresch A, Lobsien D, Mueller W, Kortmann RD, Seidel C. Primary Intradural Extramedullary Spinal Melanoma in the Lower Thoracic Spine. Case Rep Oncol Med. 2016;2016:3815280.

Reference

Yu J, Zhao DD, Chen S, Zhang JM, Xu J. Primary melanoma of the cervical spine with cerebral metastases: case report and review of the literature. J Int Med Res. 2012;40(3):1207–15.

106 Intramedullary Meningioma of the Cervical Spinal Cord

106.1 Definition

This is a meningioma within the structure of the spinal cord.

106.2 Incidence

Five cases have been reported and the authors added the sixth. Of the six reported cases five were female. Salehpour stated, "Has a predilection to the female gender during the fifth to seventh decade of life."

106.3 Etiology

The causative factors are not clear; however, possible risk factors include:

- Genetic mutations
- Trauma
- Viral infection
- Irradiation

106.4 Pathology

The tumor arises mostly in the cervical cord, is well defined with edema around it. Histopathology shows syncytial tumor, WHO classification grade I meningioma. Histochemical studies show positive staining for epithelial membrane antigen and

Abstracted from Salehpour et al. (2008)

I.M. Eltorai, *Rare Diseases and Syndromes of the Spinal Cord*,
DOI 10.1007/978-3-319-45147-3_106

S100 protein. The reported tumor were cervical proximally, one invaded the medulla oblongata, and one started at the cervicomedullary junction. Their pathology was diverse: one agioblastic psammomatous, papillary fibroplastic, transitional, clear cell, and one meningiothelial (syncytial).

106.5 Clinical Picture

Symptoms varied from burning pain in the neck, in the upper limbs, dysthesia of the upper limbs, paresthesia in the four limbs, numbness in the limbs, spastic gait, and hemiparesis or spastic paraplegia. Sensory changes of spinothalamic or posterior column compression and sphincter dysfunction.

106.6 Diagnosis

Diagnosis based on:

1. Clinical picture and neurological exam
2. MRI (from Salehpour et al.): a sagittal T2 and T1 weighted-images of the cervical cord revealed isointense and isointense to hyperintensive intramedullary C1-C2 tumor related expansion of the cord and a developed syringomyelia. Edema of the cord at the distance between the tumor and the syrinx. Sagittal T2 weighted-images at the cervicomedullary junction showed extension of the tumor. The tumor is homogenous enhanced.
3. Electrophysiological studies

106.7 Management

Total resection of the tumor is ideal to prevent recurrence. However, its intramedullary position and extension into the medulla oblongata makes it not ideal outcome. The case recorded was approached through combined suboccipital craniotomy and C1–C2 laminectomy. Microsurgical techniques were utilized and the tumor was subtotally removed by applying Cavitron ultrasound surgical aspirator. Three years post-op there was no recurrence, the authors recommended close followup with MRI annually after a period of 2 years with closer observation every 3–6 months.

Update

Abstract from Perven et al. 2015

A 52-year-old man with a 7-year history of progressive weakness, gait problems, and pain in his extremities presented with subacute worsening of his symptoms. Examination revealed weakness in all four extremities, increased tone, hyperreflexia, and sensory deficits. MRI of the cervical spine showed an area of signal abnormality and abnormal enhancement within the cervical cord at the C5–C6 level. The patient initially underwent biopsy followed a few days later by a debulking surgery. Postoperatively, the patient showed improvement in strength as well as ambulation. Intraoperatively, the lesion was confirmed to be intramedullary without any dural attachments. Histopathological examination revealed an extensively hyalinized tumor with sparse collections of cells that were immunopositive for both cytokeratin and GFAP, and immunonegative for EMA and progesterone receptor. This is an unusual pattern of expression, with cytokeratin immunopositivity suggesting a meningioma and GFAP immunopositivity suggesting a glioma. Considering the combination of extensive hyalinization with cytokeratin positivity the tumor was thought to be most consistent with a hyalinized meningioma with GFAP positivity. GFAP-positive meningiomas are rare, and these include the recently described 'whorling-sclerosing' variant. Only three cases of this tumor have been previously reported, all of which were intracranial. This is the first reported case of an intramedullary whorling-sclerosing meningioma.

Abstract from Piazza et al. 2016

Reference

Perven G, Entezami P, Gaudin D. A rare case of intramedullary 'whorling-sclerosing' variant meningioma. Springerplus. 2015;4:318.

Spinal meningiomas are typically extra-axial, slow-growing, benign tumors that arise from the arachnoid cap cells. Intramedullary spinal meningiomas are exceedingly rare with few cases reported in the literature. A 64-year-old man with a history of grade I thoracic meningioma at the T4 level resected initially in 1989 and who required reoperation in 2013 for intradural, extramedullary recurrence of tumor presented again in 2015 with gait difficulty. Magnetic resonance imaging revealed a soft tissue mass at the T3 to T4 levels on the left side of the canal that was mildly enhancing on T1 contrasted sequences. The patient was taken to the operating room, where a purely intramedullary recurrence was discovered without extramedullary extension or a dural-based attachment. The intramedullary tumor was completely resected, and postoperatively the patient recovered well and was at his neurologic baseline. The patient ultimately underwent proton beam radiotherapy because this tumor, although benign, had recurred twice. Intramedullary spinal meningiomas, particularly intramedullary low-grade recurrence of a previously extramedullary tumor, are rare phenomena. Although the pathogenic mechanisms are not well understood, intramedullary recurrence as described in this patient may reflect extrinsic factors related to prior surgical resections in addition to histologic progression. When operating on recurrent extramedullary lesions, aggressive arachnoid dissection may predispose patients to unusual patterns of recurrence.

Reference

Piazza MA, Ramayya AG, Geiger GA, et al. Intramedullary Recurrence of a Thoracic Meningioma-Presentation of an Unusual Case and Review of the Literature. World Neurosurg. 2016; Feb 4. pii: S1878-8750(16)00161-3.

Reference

Salehpour F, Zeinali A, Vahedi P, Halimi M. A rare case of intramedullary cervical spinal cord meningioma and review of the literature. Spinal Cord. 2008;46(9):648–50.

Metastatic Retinoblastoma (Pediatric) 107

107.1 Definition

This is a condition of intraspinal metastatic retinoblastoma causing compression myelopathy.

107.2 Incidence

Extra ocular retinoblastoma metastasis to the central nervous system (CNS) is in general not rare. However, compression myelopathy caused by metastatic tumor is very rare. Tubran et al., reported 207 cases treated between 1991 and 1999 that had extra-ocular disease, but none of them involved the spinal cord. Kao et al., studied 96 retinoblastomas cases treated between 1978 and 2000 and found 27 had CNS metastasis, but again none involved the spinal cord. In another study spinal cord compression (SCC) from other malignancies is not rare. Chang et al., reviewed the literature from 1966 to 2004 and found only 5 cases of SCC and added two cases of their own, although one case was very limited.

107.3 Etiology

Retinoblastoma is a rare tumor caused by an autosomal dominant mutation (about 6 %). The gene product of the retinoblastoma gene is a tumor suppressor that interacts with transcription factors such as to block transcription of growth regulating genes. The Rb gene plays a role in normal development, not just that of the retina.

Abstracted from Chang et al. (2006)

I.M. Eltorai, *Rare Diseases and Syndromes of the Spinal Cord*,
DOI 10.1007/978-3-319-45147-3_107

107.4 Pathology

The tumor cells are poorly differentiated composed of dense and small oval cells bearing hyperchromatic nuclei and scanty cytoplasm. In the spinal canal the tumor forms a mass that causes compression myelopathy. The tumor may be epidural or intradural.

107.5 Clinical Picture

In the six reported cases Chang et al., found spinal cord compression (SCC) in 4 girls and 2 boys. None of which had a family history. The age ranged from 6 months to 4 years. SCC developed 4–12 months after enucleation. The thoracic spine is most commonly involved, followed by the lumbar and the sacral. Two of the six patients also had brain metastasis. The symptoms are usually weakness of the legs (paraplegia), sensory loss, and urinary or defecative disturbances. Survival in their two cases was 4 and 19.5 months.

107.6 Diagnosis

1. History of enucleation
2. Plain radiography for bone metastasis
3. Bone scan
4. MRI: diagnostic of the mass, brain inclusion in MRI is important

107.7 Prognosis

Survival in Chang et al., two cases was 4 and 19.5 months.

107.8 Management

- Surgical removal, laminectomy
- Dexamethasone
- Systemic and intrathecal chemotherapy: Methotrexate, cytarabine
- local irradiation over the spinal lesion

Reference

Chang CY, Hung GY, Hsu WM, Kao SC, Hwang B, Hsieh YL. Retinoblastoma with spinal recurrence presenting as spinal cord compression. J Formos Med Assoc. 2006;105(6):497–502.

Infantile Myofibromatosis

108

108.1 Definition

Infantile myofibromatosis (IMF) is a congenital disease characterized by formation of benign tumors either single or multiple, arising form cells supporting and binding the tissues of the body as well as smooth muscle tissues. The potentially massive tumors arise from the skin, subcutaneous tissues, muscles, bones, and viscera.

108.2 Incidence

According to Tamburrini et al. (2003), it is the commonest fibrous disorder of infancy and childhood. According to Wada et al. (1998), six cases of spinal canal involvement were reported and added a case of their own. Tamburrini et al., reported the first solitary case of spinal canal IMF.

108.3 Etiology

The condition is congenital. Extensive search did not show the genetics of this tumor.

108.4 Pathology

The tumor is benign, but it tends to be massive and has a tendency to regress with age. It is either solitary or multicenteric. It involves many tissues e.g. skin, subcutaneous tissues, muscles, bones, central nervous system (CNS) and viscera. It is

Tamburrini et al. (2003) and Wada et al. (1998)

I.M. Eltorai, *Rare Diseases and Syndromes of the Spinal Cord*,
DOI 10.1007/978-3-319-45147-3_108

encapsulated. Histologically it consists of spindle shaped cells without mitosis, lymphocytic infiltration, collagen bundles, and a prominent vascular pattern simulating hemangipericytoma in the central pattern. According to Wada et al., immunohistiochemistry shows immuo-reactivity for vimentin but desmin, neurofilament, neuron-specific enolase and leukocyte common antigen are negative. They report gross necrosis hemorrhage and dystrophic calcification. The paravertebral tumor, in the case by Wada et al., extended into the spinal canal and through the intervetebral foramen. The pelvic tumor compressed the ureter leading to hydronephrosis. There was bone involvement. They referred to nine intracranial involvement cases usually epidural calvarial masses causing compression. Adickes et al., 1985,reported a case of multicenteric tumors on the spinal epidural surface and within the parenchyma of the spinal cord.

108.5 Clinical Picture

IMF may be detected after birth (congenital) or within the first few weeks during which the tumor is becoming hypertrophic or it may initially appear within the first 2 years of life. Small non-visceral tumors may be asymptomatic. Generally there is a period of rapid growth, then stabilization and then regression. Small or residual tumors may eventually regress completely. Multicenteric progressive visceral tumors are life threatening due to complications. The spinal cord may be involved by compression in the presence of a paravertebral tumor or the tumor may intramedullary as in the case reported by Tamburrini et al. In either case there is paralysis of the lower extremities and bladder dysfunction. It may be associated with cerebral symptoms due to intracranial involvement. In some cases peripheral nerves or viscera maybe involved. Intrapelvic tumors give rise to pressure on ureter resulting in hyperureter and hydronephrosis. Osseous lesions give rise to pathological fractures. Dimmick and Woods reported a case with cervical myofibromatosis leading to tetraparesis, at the same patient had a parietal mass. Adickes et al, reported a case of spinal and cerebral involvement.

108.6 Diagnosis

Diagnosis is base on:

1. Clinical history from parents
2. Neurological assessment
3. The presence of mass especially paravertebral ones
4. X-ray: may show extremity fractures
5. CT scan: shows paravertebral tumor invading the spinal canal

6. MRI: shows involvement of the spinal canal and rarely intraperichymatous involvement of the spinal cord.
7. Brain studies: show epidural intracranial mass
8. Histopathology: CT guided needle biopsy will show the pathology as mentioned above.

It should be differentiated from disseminated neuroblastoma, soft tissue sarcoma, histiocytosis X, lymphangiomatosis and neurofibromatosis.

108.7 Management

- Small non-visceral asymptomatic masses may be left alone with frequent monitoring, since spontaneous regression is possible.
- Involvement of the spinal cord: in the presence of paralysis mass reduction is indicated, the residual mass will usually regress.
- Intrapelvic mass maybe resected if causing visceral pressure such as hydronephrosis.
- Chemotherapy and/or radiotherapy have been tried in children with unresectable or rapidly progressive disease. (Stewart et al. 1989; Davies et al. 1994; Coffin et al. 1995)

Update

Abstracted from Kim et al. 2013

Abstract

Infantile myofibromatosis (IMF) involving the spinal cord is rarely reported. Ten cases have been found in the literature. Three cases of the solitary form and one case involving the spinal cord. The congenital type is extremely rare, one case has been reported with involvement of the spinal cord. The second case is presented by the authors: a case of paraplegia detected at birth.

The case presented an 8 month old girl, presenting with weakness of both ankles and toes, progressing since birth with a decreased MRC Grade of 1/5. Nerve conduction studies showed no peripheral nerve involvement. MRI showed a cystic and solid mass from the mid-thoracic to sacral region and compression of the spinal cord. The main location of the mass was ventral to the cord and had strong wall enhancement. Abdominal ultrasonography was negative.

Management T12-L4 laminoplastic laminotomy; the dura mater could not be identified below L1, because of the purplish mass was intermingled with it. Median durotomy above L1 was done, a thickened pinkish membrane was found dorsal to the cord; intermingled ventrally and caudally with the dura. The mass was solid and hypervascular; it was partially removed because of its adhesion to the cord and nerve roots. Duroplasty and laminectomy ended the procedure.

Histopathology revealed the tumor sheets of monotonous primitive and abundant collagen in the background. Focally meningothelioma-like whirling of tumor cells were found. Melanin pigment-containing melanophages were positive for smooth muscle cells with actin and vementin. They were negative for epithelial membrane antigen, S100 protein, desmin, myoglobin, myogenin, CD34, CD31, and GFAP.

Followup

Paresis persisted 8 days post-op: MRI showed the residual tumor from lower thoracic to sacral level. The patient continued to be observed without adjuvant radiotherapy and chemotherapy; 19 months showed unchanged residual lesion with decreased enhancement. At 38 months patient showed improvement MRC Grade 3/5; however she could not walk and incontinence; without kyphosis

The authors state that correct diagnosis, decompression, observation may improve the neurological outcome.

Reference

Kim EJ, Wang KC, Lee JY et al., Congenital solitary infantile myofibromatosis involving the spinal cord. J Neursurg Pediatr 2013;11(1):82–6.

References

Coffin CM, Neilson KA, Ingels S, Frank-gerszberg R, Dehner LP. Congenital generalized myofibromatosis: a disseminated angiocentric myofibromatosis. Pediatr Pathol Lab Med. 1995;15(4):571–87.

Davies RS, Carty H, Pierro A. Infantile myofibromatosis--a review. Br J Radiol. 1994;67(799):619–23.

Stewart RE, Grossman DM, Shulkin BL, Shapiro B. Iodine-131 metaiodobenzylguanidine uptake in infantile myofibromatosis. Clin Nucl Med. 1989;14(5):344–6.

Tamburrini G, Gessi M, Colosimo Jr C, Lauriola L, Giangaspero F, Di Rocco C. Infantile myofibromatosis of the central nervous system. Childs Nerv Syst. 2003;19(9):650–4.

Wada H, Akiyama H, Seki H, Ichihara T, Ueno K, Miyawaki T, Koizumi S. Spinal canal involvement in infantile myofibromatosis: case report and review of the literature. J Pediatr Hematol Oncol. 1998;20(4):353–6.

Myopericytoma of the Thoracic Spine Causing Myelopathy

109

109.1 Definition

Myopericytoma (MPC) is a recently described tumor with perivascular myoid differentiation. It was described for the first time by Granter in 1994. In 2002 the WHO classified amongst the perivascular myoma (Fletcher). This neoplasm is ubiquitous in the skin and subcutaneous soft tissues, especially in the lower extremities.

109.2 Incidence

In 2003 Cox and Giltman reported the first case of MPC in the thoracic spine causing myelopathy in a 70 year old man. In 2009, Brunschweiler et al. reported a case of the thoracic spine causing osteomalacia, which removal cured the condition.

109.3 Etiology

There are no known causative factors.

109.4 Pathology

In the case reported by Cox and Giltman, the tumor was in the body of T3 with an extradural to the side and surrounding the cord on the right side. Microscopic exam of the specimen showed a concentric periluminal proliferation of bland round-to-ovoid cells, which lacked a clearly demarcated cell membrane. The cells showed a myoid differentiation as demonstrated by strong smooth muscle actin

Abstracted and reported by Cox and Giltman (2003)

I.M. Eltorai, *Rare Diseases and Syndromes of the Spinal Cord*,
DOI 10.1007/978-3-319-45147-3_109

immunoreactivity. Other immunostains including S-100 protein, epithelial membrane antigen, factor VIII,[1] and pancytokeratin tested negative in the lesional cells. The lesion was considered locally destructive but not metastasizing.

According to Hunald et al. 2008: The perivascular cells are contractible with oval eosinophilic cells, which are slow growing. Generally, the neoplasm is benign but there are reported malignant cases (McMeanann and Fletcher).

109.5 Clinical Picture

MPC may develop at any age, most commonly in the fifth and sixth decades. The case of spinal MPC was a man at 70. He complained of weakness of the right lower extremity, frequent falls, and weakness of both upper extremities, and was confirmed by clinical exam.

109.6 Diagnosis

CT myelography diagnosed a metatstatic lesion in T3 vertebra with extradural extension to the right and surrounding spinal cord. Myopericytoma should be differentiated from chondrosarcoma, lymphoma, chordoma, neurofibroma, and although it has some features suggestive of hemangiopericytoma MPC is a separate entity.

109.7 Management

Spinal cord decompression and curettage of the bone tumor. The frozen perspective sample diagnosed as large cell carcinoma. The total specimen confirmed the diagnosis of MPC. Recovery was attained and the patient received 45 gray radiotherapy and physical therapy. There was follow-up every 3 months and at the end of 32 months there was no recurrence and no muscle weakness.

Reference

Cox DP, Giltman L. Myopericytoma of the thoracic spine: a case report. Spine. 2003;28(2):E30–2.

[1] Factor VIII (FVIII) is an essential blood-clotting protein, also known as anti-hemophilic factor (AHF).

Natural Killer T-Cell Lymphoma of the Cauda Equina

110

110.1 Definition

This is a tumor of the cauda equina, consisting of nasal natural killer/T-cell lymphoma (NKTCL) of the cauda equina. According to Aozasa et al., nasal NKTCL is an uncommon disease, but usually shows in highly aggressive clinical course. The disease is much more common in Asian and Latin Amercan countries than in Western countries. It is usually associated with Epstein-Barr virus (EBV) infection. In the disease rapid destruction of the noes and midline of the face was first described by McBride in 1897.

110.2 Incidence

According to Morita et al. primary lymphoma of the cauda equina is extremely rare. Only eight cases have been reported. The authors report the first case of nasal type NKTCL of the cauda equina, although spinal involvement in advanced malignant lymphoma is not uncommon.

110.3 Etiology

According to Aozasa et al. epidemiological studies in Kore in the frequency of the disease. Case studies showed that the exposure to pesticides and chemical solvents could be causative of NKTCL. The etiological role of EBV studies showed consistent association of NKTCL with EBV. Almost all NKTCL in Korea and Japan had type A of EBV. Type B or EBV was found in NKTCL in immunocompromised patients. Molecular biological studies of NKTCL have been detail in this paper.

Abstracted from Morita et al. (2009)

I.M. Eltorai, *Rare Diseases and Syndromes of the Spinal Cord*,
DOI 10.1007/978-3-319-45147-3_110

Analysis of gene alteration in NKTCL showed P53, K-ra, C-kit, and B-catanin (see Aozasa). Epidemiological studies show the disease is common in Korea, Japan, China, Indonesia, and rare in Europe and United States. Lifestyle and environmental factors the disease is more frequent in Asian countries and closely associated with EBV. There are differences in frequencies of P53 and C-kit gene mutations in patients with NKTCL in Japan, China, and Korea. There is one familial case of a father and one of six children using large amount of pesticides. The use of pesticides and organphosphates in individuals who have titres of EBV antibodies are more susceptible. These findings suggest causative role for some genetic, environment, and lifestyle in the development of NKTCL

110.4 Pathology

The NKTCL of the cauda equina showed medium sized and large lymphoid cells with irregular nuclei, diffused proliferation among the necrotic nerve fibers, coagulative necrosis, angiocentric infiltration of lymphoma cells. There are inflammatory cells: neutrophils, macrophages, plasma cells, and eosinophils

110.5 Immunohistochemistry

Lymphoma cells were positive for CD3 and CD56. EBV early RNA-1 was detected in the nucleus of the lymphoma cell.

110.6 Clinical Picture

A 67-year-old man had 2 month history of severe leg pain, bowel, and bladder dysfunction, inability to walk. Neurological exam showed weakness of the distal muscles of the legs, sensory impairment of the perineal areas and loss of reflexes of both legs.

110.7 Diagnosis

Diagnosis based on:

1. Confirmation of clinical picture
2. MRI shows lumbar stenosis at L4 and L5, a mass occupying the entire thecal area at L3-L4 and L5 and normal demarcation of the cauda. The mass had marked homogenous enhancement after gadolinium injection. Myelography showed complete block at L3-L4. The brain and the rest of the spine were normal.

110.8 Management

Bilateral laminectomy L3-L5, duratomy and the tumor was reddish-gray infiltrating and adherent to the canal. The tumor was removed carefully. Post-op the pain disappeared, he could walk, but sphincter disturbances persisted.

Reference

Morita M, Osawa M, Naruse H, Nakamura H. Primary NK/T-cell lymphoma of the cauda equina: a case report and literature review. Spine. 2009;34(24):E882–5.

111 Myelopathy in Neurocutatneous Melanosis

111.1 Definition

The neural crest is the common embryonic origin of both the melanotic cells of the skin and the letomeninges. According to these authors neurocutaneous melanosis (NCM) is a congenital syndrome characterized by the development of congenital melanocytic naevi and benign or malignant melanotic tumors of the CNS. NCM is considered a rare complication of giant congenital meano-cytic-naevus (GCMN).

111.2 Incidence

The risk of developing begnin or malignant melanotic tumors in carries of GCMN is unknown; just over 100 cases were reported (2001). Involvement of the brain will not be discussed. Myelopathy is the subject of this presentation.

111.3 Etiology

NCM is thought to be due to an error in the embryogenesis of the embryological neuroectoderm.

111.4 Pathology

There is melanotic pigmentation of the spinal arachnoid and adjacent leptomeninges. Cord compression is usually due to development of melanotic arachnoid cyst or to direct infiltration or syringomyelia. The chance of malignant progression and

Abstracted from Holmes et al. (2001)

I.M. Eltorai, *Rare Diseases and Syndromes of the Spinal Cord*,
DOI 10.1007/978-3-319-45147-3_111

prognosis are unknown. Twenty percent of cases show or display widespread pigmentation and thickening of the full length of the spinal cord meninges. Malignant transformation in the CNS is estimated to be up to 50 %.

111.5 Clinical Picture

Patients with GCMN on the extremities never develop NCM. Posterior axial nevi are more subject to NCM. CNS involvement excluding intracranial lesions may be asymptomatic. Cord compression or infiltration will give the picture of myelopathy. Radicular syndrome is also common.

111.6 Diagnosis

Diagnosis is based on:

1. Congenital nevi
2. Neurological findings
3. MRI: for symptomatic patients and all asymptomatic patients with large multiple lesions of the head and neck or lesions of the posterior midline.

111.7 Management

Close observation of these lesions regularly by the dermatologist. There is no therapy for leptomeningial melanotic changes. Space occupying lesions may be approached neurosurgically.

Reference

Holmes G, Wines N, Ryman W. Giant congential melanocytic naevus and symptomatic thoracic arachnoid cyst. Australas J Dermatol. 2001;42(2):124–8.

112 Anaplastic Oligodendroglioma

112.1 Definition

This is an anaplastic dendro-glimoa of the spinal cord secondary to primary lesion of the brain.

112.2 Incidence

According to Mcbryde et al. less than ten cases have been reported in world literature. Oligodendroglimoa accout for 5 % of all primary brain tumors and 30 % for all intracranial glioma

112.3 Etiology

The causative factor(s) of this tumor are not known.

112.4 Pathology

The primary lesion brain lesion shows:

- Macroscopically, hemorrhages cystic formation and calcification
- Microscopically, tumor cells are homogeneous and have a characteristic "fried egg" appearance, showing a clear perinuclear halo surrounding a central nucleus as a result of fixation artifact.

Abstracted from Mcbryde et al. (2003)

I.M. Eltorai, *Rare Diseases and Syndromes of the Spinal Cord*,
DOI 10.1007/978-3-319-45147-3_112

This typical appearance is less common in anaplastic oligodendroglioma. The neoplastic cells may be in lobules, separated by branching vessels, forming a "chicken wire" pattern, with mucinous accumulation may be noted. The anaplastic form shows mitosis, endothelial proliferation, mitotic activity and necrosis. Metastases of oligodendrogliomas are rare due to:

- Blood brain barrier
- Absence of lymphatics in the brain
- Short survival of the patients

Immunohistochemistry is positive for glial fibrillary acidic protein and S100. Details of immunohistochemistry can be seen in Choon and Raepke. Only one case had intramedullary metastasis and the rest had meningeal involvement. It is believed that tumor cells reach the spinal cord via the CSF by the ependymal epithemlium or the pia mater.

112.5 Clinical Picture

A previous history of brain oligodendroglioma operated upon and metastasis to the spinal cord may be due to CSF leakage during surgery. Spinal metastasis in the cases recurrence occurred from 3 months to 6 years after initial brain surgery. Tumors were grade 2 or 3. The clinical picture is that of paraparesis.

112.6 Diagnosis

Diagnosis based on:

1. History of brain surgery and pathological report

   MRI, CT scan, CSF cytology are all performed

112.7 Management

Surgery consists of:

1. Debulking or excision

The patient received radiotherapy; the same treatment is applied to epidural anaplastic oligodendroglioma.

Updates

Yuh et al. (2015)

Primary spinal cord oligodendrogliomas are rare tumors comprising two percent of all spinal cord tumors. Although a treatment guideline has yet to be established, maximal surgical resection is primary in the treatment of spinal cord oligodendrogliomas. Adjuvant radiotherapy has remained controversial, and it is unclear whether chemotherapy adds any benefit. In this case report, the authors present a 24-year-old male who had a 7-year history of left leg weakness and a radiating pain in both legs. Magnetic resonance image (MRI) showed an intramedullary mass at the T4-T8 level. He underwent subtotal removal of the tumor and pathologic diagnosis revealed a WHO grade IIoligodendroglioma. The patient was treated with radiotherapy postoperatively and followed up with MRI annually. Clinical and radiological status of the patient had been stationary for 4 years after the surgery. The 5-year follow-up MRI showed an increase in the size and extent of the residual tumor. Despite radiological progression, considering that symptoms and the performance status of the patient had remained unchanged, further treatment has not been performed. Given the clinical outcome of this patient, close observation after subtotal removal with adjuvant radiotherapy is one of the acceptable treatment options for WHO grade II spinal cord oligodendrogliomas.

Reference

Yuh WT, Chung CK, Park SH. Primary spinal cord oligodendroglioma with postoperative adjuvant radiotherapy: a case report. Korean J Spine. 2015;12(3):160–4.

Reference

Mcbryde CW, Hamid NA, Mitchell RD. Anaplastic oligodendroglioma with metastasis to the spinal cord. Br J Neurosurg. 2003;17(4):364–6.

Oncocytoma in Melanocytoma

113

113.1 Definition

This is a benign neoplasm composed predominantly of monotonous sheets of plump oncocytes. By electron microscopy, the cytoplasm of the oncocyte is packed full with mitochondria. Focal areas of the tumor contain spindle cells with abundant intracytoplasmic granular deposits of brown melanin pigment that contains melanosomes.

113.2 Incidence

This is the first case described by Gelmen et al. Oncocytoma is extremely rare in the CNS. Oncocytic variant of meningioma has been described in six cases and one malignant spinal paraganglioma.

113.3 Etiology

The majority of oncocytomas probably have an epithelial origin. Because the prevalence of oncocytoma increases with age it is widely accepted that oncocytomas are the result of an aberrant metaplasia occurring during cell senescence.

Abstracted from Gelman et al. (2000)

I.M. Eltorai, *Rare Diseases and Syndromes of the Spinal Cord*,
DOI 10.1007/978-3-319-45147-3_113

113.4 Pathology

Oncocytomas are benign neoplasms. They occur most commonly in the kidney. They may appear in neoplasms as single cells or as a substantial portion of the tumor or ma constitute the whole tumor. Oncocytic transformation of a tumor of over 50 % then it is labeled as oncocytoma.

113.5 Histopathology

Sheets of plump polygonal cells containing abundant granular eosinophilic cytoplasm many areas around the blood vessels, spindle cells with intracytoplasmic granules, which by Fontana-Masson technique proved to be melanin; more detailed description of the histology and histochemistry can be seen in the original work of Gelman et al. 2000.

113.6 Clinical Picture

The patient described is a 71-year-old female who had episodes of lower back pain for 28 years. This extended to the legs and became worse, not responding to analgesics, urinary and fecal incontinence. The back pain then radiated to the buttocks and thighs, mild facial paresis. The reflexes were absent.

113.7 Diagnosis

Diagnosis is based on the following criteria:

1. Clinical history
2. MRI: intracanalicular (medullary) mass from L3 to S1.

113.8 Management

Laminectomy L3-L5 revealed the mass in the cord; removal by microsurgical technique *en bloc*. Recovery was uneventful and no recurrence 4 years later

Reference

Gelman BB, Trier TT, Chaljub G, Borokowski J, Nauta HJ. Oncocytoma in melanocytoma of the spinal cord: case report. Neurosurgery. 2000;47(3):756–9.

Osteosarcoma

114

114.1 Definition

Osteosarcoma is the most common nonhemtalogica primary malignancy of bone and is commonly reported in the appendicular skeleton.

114.2 Incidence

Primary osteosarcoma of the vertebral column is rare. Primary vertebral osteosarcoma (PVOS) accounts for 4 % of all osteosarcoma. Females outnumbered males. The age 8–80 years (mean 34.5 years); the cervical spine is the least affected; the site of origin arises most commonly from the posterior elements and involved the body of the vertebra. The spinal canal is involved in 84 % of reported cases.

114.3 Pathology

The tumor shows pleomorphic cells with abundant cytoplasm and atypical nuclei with mitosis. Osteoblastic giant cells are encountered with osteoid and fibrocollagenous tissue. The tumor may be osteoblastic or osteolytic.

114.4 Clinical Picture

The case reported was a 60-year-old female had 3 week history of the lower limbs and sphincteric disturbances. No history of fever nor trauma. Neurological exam showed upper limbs normal proximally but weak grip. Lower limbs were 2/5, deep

Abstracted from Makhdoomi et al. (2010)

I.M. Eltorai, *Rare Diseases and Syndromes of the Spinal Cord*,
DOI 10.1007/978-3-319-45147-3_114

tendon reflex of the lower limbs were brisk, Babinski's was positive. Sensory level was T2, hematology was normal.

114.5 Diagnosis

Diagnosis based on:

1. MRI shows destruction of vertebral bodies C7-T1 and cord compression with the tumor around. The paravertebral muscles were infiltration. The posterior elements were destroyed by the tumor. The tumor was firm and somewhat vascular.

114.6 Management

Laminectomy at C7 and T1 by removing the tumor with the posterior elements and near total decompression was achieved. Anterior extension was noticed and but nothing was done on the vertebral bodies. There was no subdural involvement. Post-op radio-chemotherapy was given. Confirmed primary osteosarcoma, metastatic tumor were ruled out by immunohistochemical studies. Five months post-op she gained motor power 4/5 and was ambulatory with one cane.

Update

Abstract from Dekutoski et al. (2016)

Primary spinal osteosarcomas are rare and aggressive neoplasms. Poor outcomes can occur, as obtaining marginal margins is technically demanding; further Enneking-appropriate en bloc resection can have significant morbidity. The goal of this study is to identify prognostic variables for local recurrence and mortality in surgically treated patients diagnosed with a primary osteosarcoma of the spine. A multicenter ambispective database of surgically treated patients with primary spine osteosarcomas was developed by AOSpine Knowledge Forum Tumor. Patient demographic, diagnosis, treatment, perioperative morbidity, local recurrence, and cross-sectional survival data were collected. Tumors were classified in 2 cohorts: Enneking appropriate (EA) and Enneking inappropriate (EI), as defined by pathology margin matching Enneking-recommended surgical margins. Prognostic variables were analyzed in reference to local recurrence and survival. Between 1987 and 2012, 58 patients (32 female patients) underwent surgical treatment for primary spinal osteosarcoma. Patients were followed for a mean period of 3.5 ± 3.5 years (range 0.5 days to 14.3 years). The median survival for the entire cohort was 6.7 years postoperative. Twenty-four (41 %) patients died, and 17 (30 %) patients suffered a local recurrence, 10 (59 %) of whom died. Twenty-nine (53 %) patients underwent EA resection while 26 (47 %) patients underwent EI resection with a postoperative median survival of 6.8 and 3.7 years, respectively ($p=0.048$). EI patients had a higher rate of local recurrence than EA patients ($p=0.001$). Patient age, previous surgery, biopsy type, tumor size, spine level, and chemotherapy timing did not significantly influence recurrence and survival. Osteosarcoma of the spine presents a significant challenge, and most patients die in spite of aggressive surgery. There is a significant decrease in recurrence and an increase in survival with en bloc resection (EA) when compared with intralesional resection (EI). The effect of adjuvant and neoadjuvant chemotherapeutics, as well as method of biopsy, requires further exploration.

Reference

Dekutoski MB, Clarke MJ, Rose P, et al. Osteosarcoma of the spine: prognostic variables for local recurrence and overall survival, a multicenter ambispective study. J Neurosurg Spine. 2016;25(1):59–68.

Reference

Makhdoomi K, Kursheed N, Ramzan A, et al. Primary osteosarcoma of the cervical spine. Neurosurg Q. 2010;20(4):250–2.

Myelopathy Due to Spinal Paraganglioma

115

115.1 Definition

Paraganglioma is a rare tumor arising from extra-adrenal paraganglia and accounts for 0.3 % of all neoplasms. Less common sites include the retroperitoneum, the para-arotic region, bladder, filum terminale, skull, larynx and others. According to Zileli et al. 2008, paragangliomas are tumors that arise from the paraganglia cells of the autonomic nervous system, ultimately derived from the neural crest. The majority of paragangliomas are nonfunctional and benign; however, they may produce excess catecholamines or have malignant potential. Paragangliomas arise within or near the carotid bod or the glomus jugulare in 80–90 % of cases. Other locations are the middle ear, thyroid, GI tract and pancreas. In the CNS paragangliomas have been seen in the pineal region, the petrous ridge, and the sella turcica. Paragangliomas of the spine are uncommon and usually present as intradural tumors within the cauda equina, thoracic tumors are even more rare.

115.2 Incidence

Spinal paragangliomas are rare. According to Rosai (2011), spinal paragangliomas are rare and most reported cases occurred in the cauda equina or filum terminale. A series of 30 spinal cases were reported by Marcin et al. 1997, of which 19 were in the lumbar region, six in the cauda equina, two in the filum terminale, two in the thoracic region and two in the cervical spine. For pheochromocytoma and functional paraganglioma, please see Roman 2004.

According to Houten et al. 2002, paragangliomas of the spinal canal are rare, approximately 80 cases have been reported. The vast majority of the tumors are intradural in the cauda equina and most of them are gangliocytic paraganglioma, a

Abstracted from Lehmen et al. (2010) and Falavigna et al. (2010)

I.M. Eltorai, *Rare Diseases and Syndromes of the Spinal Cord*,
DOI 10.1007/978-3-319-45147-3_115

distinctive histiologic entity. It is suggested that these tumors arise from the sympathetic trunk (Cybulski et al. 1991). Extradural tumors are rare and were found mostly in the thoracic spine and some are extension from intradural tumors. They may cause vetebral erosion. Intraosseous paragangliomas are rare. Only the primary intraosseous paragangliomas have been reported in the sacral bone (Falavigna et al. 2010) and they added one more case. Metastatic paraganglioma have been reported from the carotid body and para-aortic paraganglioma (Falavigna et al. 2010)

115.3 Etiology

According to Rosai (2011), paragangliomas are neuroectodermal tumors of the autonomic paraganglioma, derived from the chromaffin cells of neural crest origin. Spinal gangliomas are presumably derived from paraganglionic cells, normal paragangliomas are associated with blood vessels or from residual peripheral neuroblasts, which can give rise to either chemoreceptors or ganglia cells. According to Falavigna et al. (2010), the paraganglia are widely spread collection of specialized neural crest cells that arise in association with segmentation of collateral autonomic ganglia throughout the body. According to S. Roman, "Fewer that 30 % of patients with paragangliomas have catecholamines excess… As many as 40 % of paragangliomas are familial. Mutations in the succinate dehydrogenase complex iron sulfur subunit D (SDHD) have unit C gene (SDHC) and subunit B gene (SDHB) have been mapped to Chromosome I and II (see details in Roman).

However the pathogenicity of paragangliomas are unclear.

115.4 Pathology

According to Zibilli et al. "the majority of paraganglioas are nonfunctional and benign. However, they may produce catecholamines in excess or may be protein malignant (20–49 %). They occur within or near the carotid bodies or the glomus jugulares in 80–90 % of cases. They occur in other sites as well (see incidence above). Extra-adrenal pheochromocytomas are the paragangliomas, which account for 15 % of total pheochromocytomas. They are rarely functional and 80–90 % as mentioned above are in the glomus jugulares or carotid bodies. Retroperitoneal paragangliomas are higher in malignancy and may be manifested by metastasis. Pheochromocytomas may occur as isolated tumor or as part of familial syndromes, e.g. von Hippel Landau, multiple endocrine neoplasia, von Recklinghausen's disease, and Surge-Weber syndrome; paragangliomas show 14 %. Microscopically: the tumor consists of polyhedral chief cells organized in in nests, surrounded by a delicate fibrovascular stroma. The tumor have a granular eosinophilic cytoplasm and round or ovoid nuclei. There is positive staining for synaptic physin, chromagranin, S-100, tumor-specific antigen. Metastatic spinal lesions represent 35 % of the spinal paragangliomas. According to Falavigna et al. The paraganglion systems are a component of the neuorendrocrine system and comprises the chromaffin-positive cells of the adrenal medulla and the extra-adrenal paraganglion system, which in turn, usually consists of chromaffin-negative and non-secretor cells. According to Ramon, immunopositivity for neuro-endocrine markers Chromagenisis A, synaptic physin, and neuronal specific enolase in chief cells and positive reaction for S-100 protein in sustentacular cells support the diagnosis. Relevant secretory activity of spinal paraganglioma cells e.g. release of catecholamines is a rare phenomenon and can be induced by surgical manipulation of the tumor.

115.5 Clinical Picture

The symptoms vary according to the level of the tumor and whether it is chromaffin positive or negative and whether it is benign, as most cases are or malignant. The tumor is most commonly lumbar intradural extramedullary in relation to the cauda equina and the filum terminale. The cervical region is rarely affected. In the thoracic region the tumor is usually extradural causing cord compression. It is rarely functional. In functional paragangliomas, there is headache, hypertension, palpitation, and flushing. Neurological manifestations are local pain, numbness, parathesia, muscle weakness, and paresis. In malignant cases, there may be metastasis in different parts of the body. The tumor is rarely primary intraosseous.

Neurological exam shows, sensory and motor deficits with a level or saddle fashion anesthesia in cauda equina syndrome. Bowel, bladder, and sexual dysfunction may be noted, especially in the lumbosacral level.

115.6 Diagnosis

Diagnosis is based on

1. History of cord or cauda equina compression
2. Neurological findings
3. In functional paragangliomas, signs of catecholamine secretion
4. Imaging: There is usually well defined mass with low to intermediate signal intensity on T1 weighted-images. Intermediate to high signal intensity on T2 weighted-images compared to the paraspinal intensity. The hypervascular nature of paragangliomas results in punctate areas of flow void, interspinal in a matrix of increased signal intensity, caused by slow flow and tumor cells. This produces a salt and pepper appearance on T2 weighted-images.
5. Biochemical tests:
   - 24-h urinary excretion of total or fractuated metanepherisis and catecholamines
   - urinary VMA
   - plasma metanephrines
6. PET scan

115.7 Management

- Surgery: total resection of the paraganglioma is necessary. Laproscopic surgery can be sone for uncomplicated and benign cases. Cord compression must be releaved.
- Local radiotherapy for the incomplete removal and recurrent cases, as well as malignant cases.

Paragangliomas may turn malignant, primarily after surgery with incomplete removal and metastases (about 50 %) and even as many years post-operatively. For malignancy, chemotherapy is palliative using cyclophosphide, docaihazene, and vicetina.

References

Cybulski GR, Nijensohn E, Brody BA, Meyer PR, Cohen B. Spinal cord compression from a thoracic paraganglioma: case report. Neurosurgery. 1991;28(2):306–9.

Falavigna A, Righesso O, Volquind D, Salgado KB, Teles AR. Intraosseous sacral paraganglioma with extradural extension: case report. Acta Neurochir (Wien). 2010;152(3):475–80.

Lehmen JA, Babbel DM, Mikhitarian K, Choma TJ. Paraganglioma presenting as metastatic lesion in a cervical vertebra. Spine. 2010;35:E152–4.

Roman S. Pheochromocytoma and functional paraganglioma. Curr Opin Oncol. 2004;16(1):8–12.

Rosai J. The origin of neuroendocrine tumors and the neural crest saga. Mod Pathol. 2011;24 Suppl 2:S53-7.

Zileli M, Kalayci M, Basdemir G. Paraganglioma of the thoracic spine. J Clin Neurosci. 2008;15(7):823–7.

116 Plasma Cell Leukemia (PCL)

116.1 Definition

Plasma cell leukemia (PCL) is a leukemic variant of multiple meyloma (MM) 2–4 %, which formed an intraspinal mass compressing the spinal cord leading to paraplegia.

116.2 Incidence

According to Hasmoni et al., they report the first case.

116.3 Etiology

The etiology of the disease as a whole is not clear. The compression of the cord was due to formation of PCL in the spinal canal causing the compression myelopathy.

116.4 Pathology

PCL is a pathological condition in which there is malignant proliferation of the plasma cells in the peripheral blood as well as the bone marrow. It is classified as primary when it presents in the leukemic picture and as secondary when there is leukemia transformation of preexisting multiple myeloma. In the peripheral blood more than 20 % are plasma cells with absolute plasma cell count of more than

Abstracted from Hasmoni et al. (2009)

I.M. Eltorai, *Rare Diseases and Syndromes of the Spinal Cord*,
DOI 10.1007/978-3-319-45147-3_116

$2x10^9$/L. Plasmablasts are found in both peripheral and bone marrow. PCL deposits occur in soft tissues, bones, intracrainially, and in the spinal canal.

116.5 Clinical Picture

The clinical picture of PCL differs according to whether it is primary or secondary, in the former it is more aggressive. There is anemia, thrombocytopenia, renal impairment, and frequent extramedullary involvement. There is also hypercalcemia.

116.6 Diagnosis

Diagnosis is based on hematological studies in addition to chemical, cytological, immunological, and genetic studies, which are beyond the scope of this article (see Hasmoni et al.).

116.7 Management

PCL has a poor prognosis. Management by chemotherapy is the usual course adopted: vincristine, doxorubicin, and dexamethasone. The authors conclude that combination chemotherapy has a higher response rate than that of single agent. Autologus stem cells have shown excellent responses up to 2–3year disease free survival rate.

Reference

Hasmoni MH, Wahid FA, Keng CS. Primary plasma cell leukemia presented as progressive paraplegia: a case report. South Med J. 2009;102(1):101–3.

Pleomorphic Xanthoastrocytoma

117

117.1 Definition

According to Nakamura et al., pleomorphic xanthoastrocytoma (PXA) is a new addition to the 1993 WHO classification of the tumors of the CNS.

117.2 Incidence

There was only one case reported by Kepes et al., and Nakamura et al., case is the second. The tumor usually appears in children and young adults and usually is located in the temporal lobe and less frequently in the cerebellum.

117.3 Etiology

The cause of the tumor is unclear.

117.4 Pathology

The tumor described is cervical and well demarcated from the surrounding nervous tissue, attached anteriorly to the leptomeninges and leading to syringomyelia. Microscopically, the tumor contains fusiform cells in small fascicles with nuclear hyperchromatism and markedly pleomorphic giant cells exuberating xanthomatous changes, no mitosis, but there is vascular necrosis. Granular deposits are seen between the cells and continuous fibers surround the tumor cells, which is characteristic features of PXA.

Nakamura et al. (2006)

I.M. Eltorai, *Rare Diseases and Syndromes of the Spinal Cord*,
DOI 10.1007/978-3-319-45147-3_117

117.5 Clinical Picture

Based on Nakamura's case, a healthy 33-year-old woman complained of numbness of legs. Hyperesthesia and hyperalgesia was detected below L1 level. No motor deficit and the reflexes were normal.

117.6 Diagnosis

MRI showed intramedullary mass in the cervical cord associated with a synrinx between C3-T1. After gadolinium injection heterogeneously enhancing tumor was seen as a loblulated tumor attached to the ventral surface of the spinal cord. Selective angiography showed no stain, which ruled out angioma.

117.7 Management

Exposure of the cord by laminoplasty, duratomy, the cord was swollen and distorted, posterior myelectomy was done. The tumor, which was partially cystic was detected by microsurgery from the surrounding nervous tissue and was completely removed. Post-operatively, the patient had marked neurologic deficit, Frankel C, but eventually recovered except for the numbness and there was no recurrence on the MRI follow-up.

117.8 Update

Zhao et al. 2015.

Supratentorial PXAs are the most common. Lesions of other locations were also reported, such as cerebellum, spine and pineal body. Spinal PXAs are extremely rare. Herpers firstly reported a 66-year-old patient with spinal PXA in 1994. Only six patients were presented in the previous literatures until now. The age distribution was 12.9–66 years old with an average age of 42.0 years old. Most of the lesions were located in cervical or thoracic cord.

Case Presented

A 60-year-old patient of spinal PXA and periventricular tumor presented with waist pain and weakness of double legs for 1 month. Neuroimaging showed that a lesion at the level of L2-L3 and periventricular tumor. Postoperative microscopy indicated that WHO grade II PXA. Photomicrograph of the lesion showed spindle cells, marked nuclear and cytoplasmic pleomorphism, with foamy cytoplasm. Immunohistochemical staining showed that GFAP and S-100 were positive. This is a rare case of synchronous multicentric PXA.

Reference

Zhao X, Jiang X, Wang X. Spinal pleomorphic xanthoastrocytoma companied with periventricular tumor. Int J Clin Exp Pathol. 2015;8(1):1036–40.

Reference

Nakamura M, Chiba K, Matsumoto M, Ikeda E, Toyama Y. Pleomorphic xanthoastrocytoma of the spinal cord. Case report. J Neurosurg Spine. 2006;5(1):72–5.

Primary Intraspinal Primitive Neuroectodermal Tumor (PNET)

118

118.1 Definition

Primative neuroectodermal tumor (PNET) is the generic name used to describe a morphologically celled neoplasm showing the potential for multiple differentiations irrespective of the site origin. In 1993, the WHO classification of brain tumors recommended the use of PNET as the generic term for cerebellar medulloblastoma and the central nervous system (CNS) tumors that are morphologically identical to medullobalstoma.

118.2 Incidence

Spinal PNET is extremely rare. Before primary intraspinal PNET is confirmed the secondary due to "drop," as seedlings through the cerebrospinal fluid (CSF) from intracranial source should be excluded. Kim et al., reviewed 24 cases of primary spinal PNET in the literature and added a case of their own.

Male to female ratio is	1.75:1
Average age	29
Injury level	
Lumbar	11 (44 %)
Thoracolumbar	6 (24 %)
Thoracic	3 (12 %)

Abstracted from Kim et al. (2004)

I.M. Eltorai, *Rare Diseases and Syndromes of the Spinal Cord*,
DOI 10.1007/978-3-319-45147-3_118

Cervical	3 (12 %)
Lumbosacral	1 (4 %)
Sacral	1 (4 %)
Tumor site	
Cauda equina	8 (36 %) which seems to be the predilection
Intradural extramedullary	7 (31 %)
Intramedullary	5 (22 %)
Extradural	2 (9 %)

118.3 Etiology

The tumor was called neuroepithelioma arising from the vestige of the neural crest from totipotent cells. The underlying etiological factors are unknown.

118.4 Pathology

PNET consists of small round cells with hyperchromatic nuclei with neural differentiation features, which typically form Homer-Wright rosettes that may vary sustainability. Some tumors may show abortive rosette formation. Strong immunoreactivity for MIC-2, a neuron specific cell tumor, such as lymphoma, neuroblastoma, and small round cell sarcoma. The tumor tends to spread locally and metastasize.

In the series mentioned above, metastasis was found in eleven cases (44 %):

Brain	2 (18 %)
Leptomeninges	2 (18 %)
Diffused intraspinal	2 (18 %)
Bone and lymph nodes	2 (18 %)
Lung	2 (18 %)
Pleura	1 (9 %)

The PNET tumor is histologically and clinically very malignant.

118.5 Clinical Picture

The tumor is rapid growing with brief duration of symptoms and a rapidly progressive course. It starts with back pain radiating to the legs, lower exteremity weakness, paresthesia, paraparesis, and in cervical tumors tetraparesis, sphincter dysfunction e.g. urinary retention may be an early symptom.

118.6 Diagnosis

Diagnosis based on

1. Clinical exam: signs and symptoms
2. MRI: shows the site, level, and extent of the tumor. The T2-weighted images show the tumor mass usually with high signal intensity cyst like lesion. In general, the tumor shows a low signal intensity. T1-weighted MRI and high signal on T2-weighted images, with varying amounts of tumor calcification, necrosis, and surrounding edema. These signs are more marked in cerebellar PNET. Gadolinium enhancement helps in diagnosis. The tumor should be differentiated from ependymoma when it is intramedullary.

118.7 Management

The optimal treatment for PNET is not yet established. Treatment options are:

- Surgery: usually complete removal is not attained.
- Radiation therapy: local or craniospinal radiation; however, this has its disadvantages in childhood. 5000 cGy has been accepted.
- Chemotherapy: there are several protocos for this treatment. Multi-drug therapy is usually tried vinscristine, lomustine, cisplatin, and cyclophosphamide.
- Adaptive immunotherapy: lymphokine activated killer cells possess several attributes that could make them useful in adaptive immunotherapy. They are highly potent against tumors; require no prior antigen exposure to express their oncolytic effect. Their recognition mechanism is able to distinguish between normal and malignant cells and thereby spare normal tissue and express their oncolytic activity against many tumors.
- The study by Richard et al., is promising against cells of PNET. It consists of intrathecal administration of IL-2 and LAK cells as an adjuvant therapy; eradicate the cells of PNET without damage to normal cells in contrast to the radio-chemotherapy.

However, as mentioned above, the optimal therapy for PNET is still uncertain. The above therapies may extend survival, but the prognosis is very poor, according to Kim et al., eight patients still alive (32 %).

Updates

Abstracted from Meng and He 2015.

Primitive neuroectodermal tumors (PNETs) are rare tumors of uncertain histogenesis that occur predominantly in children and young adults. The current study reports a case of PNET in a 60-year-old female, which presented clinically as an intraspinal tumor, causing symptoms of lower back pain, numbness and pain in the right lower extremity. The patient underwent tumorectomy. Following primary therapy, the symptoms of spinal cord compression were relieved. The patient underwent several courses of radiotherapy following surgery but refused to continue with chemotherapy. After a further 4 months, the tumors recurred and the patient succumbed to the disease.

Since the first description of the condition by Hart and Earle in 1973 (2), <100 cases have been documented. The annual incidence of this condition is estimated to range from 0.2 to 0.4 cases per 100,000 (3), and its concept has been controversial for over a decade, as diagnosis remains difficult and no effective treatment has been identified. PNETs are rapidly growing soft tissue masses, which cause symptoms of nerve compression and pain.

Reference

Meng XT, He SS. Primitive neuroectodermal tumor in the spinal canal: a case report. Oncol Lett. 2015;9(4):1934–6.

Reference

Kim YW, Jin BH, Kim TS, Cho YE. Primary intraspinal primitive neuroectodermal tumor at conus medullaris. Yonsei Med J. 2004;45(3):533–8.

Intramedullary Schwannoma Associated with Neurofibromatosis

119

119.1 Definition

The neurofibromatoses are genetic disorders that cause tumors to grow in the nervous system. The tumors begin in the supporting cells that make up the nerves and the myelin sheath--the thin membrane that envelops and protects the nerves. These disorders cause tumors to grow on nerves and produce other abnormalities such as skin changes and bone deformities.

A shwannoma, also known as neurilemoma or neuroma, is a benign, encapsulated neoplasm in which the fundamental component is structurally identical to the syncytium of Schwann cells; the neoplastic cells proliferate within the endoneurium, and perineurium forms the capsule. The neoplasm may originate from a peripheral or sympathetic nerve, or from various cranial nerves, particularly the eighth nerve; when the nerve is small, it is usually found (if at all) in the capsule of the neoplasm; if the nerve is large, the schwannoma may develop within the sheath of the nerve, the fibers of which may then spread over the surface of the capsule as the neoplasm enlarges. Microscopically, schwannomas are composed of combinations of two cell types, Antoni types A and B, either of which may be predominant in various examples of schwannomas.

119.2 Incidence

According to the authors, there have only been 5 cases of intramedullary schwannoma in NF-1 and 6 cases in association with NF-2. Schwannomas constitute 1.1 % of all the spinal schwannomas. The reviewed of reports of all the intramedullary schwannomas up to 2004 showed 66 cases. Among all 66 cases reviewed,

---

Abstracted and reported by Siddiqui and Shah (2004)

I.M. Eltorai, *Rare Diseases and Syndromes of the Spinal Cord*,
DOI 10.1007/978-3-319-45147-3_119

intramedullary schwannomas were seen in males/female ratio of 1.5. The ages of patients ranged from 9 to 75 years (mean 41.5). Duration of symptoms ranged from 3 months to 20 years (mean 31.5 months) and varied with the location of the tumor. Intramedullary schwannomas were most frequent in the cervical spinal cord (65 %), followed by thoracic region (22 %), and lumbar region (10 %).

119.3 Etiology

There are no biochemical markers of the disorder, but the cloning of both the NF-1 and NF-2 genes makes DNA-based diagnosis possible in some families. Both genes appear to be tumor suppressor genes. Both conditions are autosomal dominant, but the variable penetrance and expressivity and high frequency of new mutations make genetic counseling difficult.

119.4 Pathology

See above definition and also according to Siddiqui and Shah:

- late neoplastic development of ectopic Schwann cells originating from the embryonic neural ridge during development;
- Schwann cells ensheathing aberrant intramedullary nerve fibers;
- Schwann cells extending along the anterior spinal artery;
- neoplastic growth from Schwann cells at dorsal-root entry zone;
- transformation of pial cells of neuroectodormal origin into Schwann cells

119.5 Clinical Picture

All intradural schwannomas, with or without associated neurofibromatosis, constitute 1.1 % of all spinal schwannomas. The tumor is manifested by pain, paresthesia, weakness, eventually anesthesia, analgesia, and paresis, depending on the level i.e., tetraparesis or paraparesis. Neurological exam will reveal sensory loss and motor paralysis of the upper motor neuron type. There will be the manifestation of NF-2 if associated.

119.6 Diagnosis

Diagnosis is based on the following criteria:

MRI is the most useful diagnostic tool of intramedullary tumors. T-1 weighted images of the tumor usually give hypointense signals compared to the spinal cord itself. In T2-weighted images: the tumor usually shows hyperintensive signals with occasional isointense or low signal areas. There is marked enhancement on post gadolinium images with well delineated margins. Occasionally there is associated segmental syringomyelia. Differential diagnosis includes other intramedullary tumors, e.g. ependymoma and astrocytoma.

119.7 Management

Ideal treatment is complete excision, which is neurosurgically challenging. The use of real-time MRI, CO_2-laser combined with somatosensory-evoked potential give precision to completely removing tumor within its capsule using microsurgical techniques only.

Reference

Siddiqui AA, Shah AA. Complete surgical excision of intramedullary schwannoma at the cranio-vertebral junction in neurofibromatosis type-2. Br J Neurosurg. 2004;18(2):193–6.

Secondary Syringomyelia due to Spinal Intramedullary Metastasis

120

120.1 Definition

This is a condition in which syringomyelia cavity results from an intramedullary metastatic lesion.

120.2 Incidence

Intramedullary spinal metastases are relatively rare (1–2.1 %) (Keung et al.) of advanced cancer. According to Surcin et al., the presence of syringomyelia due to an intramedullary metastasis is very rare, in the last 30 years four cases have been reported who added one case of their own; however, the cerebral metastasis account for 20 %. In 1–2 % no primary is found, and the thoracic cord is more involved that the cervical cord.

120.3 Etiology

Intramedullary metastatic causes of syringomyelia as a result of:

- mechanical origin: obstruction, which disturbs the normal cerebral spinal fluid circulation (hydrodynamic factor)
- excessive fluid as an transudate or exudate from the vasculature of the tumor
- exudation from the tumor itself
- a multiplication of factors

Abstracted from Surcin et al. (2001) and Keung et al. (1997)

I.M. Eltorai, *Rare Diseases and Syndromes of the Spinal Cord*,
DOI 10.1007/978-3-319-45147-3_120

120.4 Pathology

Syringomyelia is a neurologic disorder characterized by the presence of a fluid collection in a cavity within the spinal cord. The fluid collects more distal and less proximal to the obstruction. As its tension increases it causes circumferential pressure on the spinal cord tracts and cells. According to Isoya et al., the autopsy study of 627 patients with systemic cancer disclosed thirteen cases with intramedullary spinal cord metastases. The lungs and the brests were the most common primary tumors (54 % and 13 % respectively). The pathology depends on the primary lesion. Statistically: pulmonary carcimoma (branchogenic) 49 %, the breast 14 %, lymphomas 9 %, melanomas 7.5 %, colon carcinoma 7 %, endometrial carcinoma 1.2 % (Surcin et al.). From the primary lesion the spinal cord is involved via the venous plexus and/or the arterial route. Regional involvement: cervical 27 %, thoracic 27 % and lumbar 45 %.

120.5 Clinical Picture

The patient is known to have advanced cancer or had it previously treated. It may manifest cervical myelopathy (Weitzner et al.) or thoracolumbar (Surcin et al.). The manifestations are

- Pain in the back or extremities
- Parathesia, anesthesia
- Motor weakness of upper and lower extremities and eventual paralysis
- Increased muscle tone and exaggerated reflexes.

120.6 Diagnosis

Diagnosis is based on:

1. History of pulmonary malignancy
2. Neurological signs
3. MRI: Intramedullary tumors of the spinal cord, syringomyelia below the tumor, and may be above it as well. Brain performed to rule out brain lesions (25 %)
4. CT: may so the tumor site and the syrinx
5. Scintigraphy for other metastases
6. search for primary tumor
7. CSF may show pleocytosis of white and red cells, erythrocytes, and leukocytes

120.7 Management

The management of the primary tumor by radiation and/or chemotherapy.

Local treatment

- Radiotherapy: in selected cases had good results (Decker et al., Findlay et al.)
- Combination of radiotherapy and steroids (Keung et al.)
- Surgical treatement: usually not effective; however in long life expectancy it can be tried; although no neurological recovery there was no recurrence after surgery for 2 years (Isoya et al., Surcin et al.)

References

Keung YK, Cobos E, Whitehead RP, Roberson GH. Secondary syringomyelia due to intramedullary spinal cord metastasis. Case report and review of literature. Am J Clin Oncol. 1997;20(6):577–9.

Surcin B, Bersani D, Lippa A, Tauzin C, Quenel-tueux N. Intramedullary metastases and syringomyelic cavities. J Radiol. 2001;82(6 Pt 1):673–5.

Spinal Hemangioblastomas in Von Hippel Lindau Disease

121

121.1 Definition

von Hippel Lindau disease (VHL) is an autosomal dominant hereditary disease in which the CNS and retinal hemangioblastomas, renal cell carcinoma, pheocromocytoma, abdominal cystic masses e.g. in the kidney, liver, pancreas, and epididymal cysts may develop. VHL disease manifests itself by 65 years of age. The annual incidence is 1/36,000 live births. In the brain its manifestations are in the cerebellum, brain stem, spinal cord and suprasellar hemangioblastomas and endolymphatic sac tumors.

121.2 Incidence

60–80 % of patients with VHL disease manifest hemangioblastomas in the CNS (cerebellum, brain stem, and spinal cord). Spinal cord hemangioblastoma are most common after the cerebellar hemangioblastoma, accounting for 40 % of VHL-associated CNS lesions.

121.3 Etiology

The causative gene is located in the chromosome 3p25-26 region, also related to the occurrence of sporadic hemangioblastoma of the CNS and also the renal cell carcinoma.

Abstracted from Kanno et al. (2009) and Mehta et al. (2010)

I.M. Eltorai, *Rare Diseases and Syndromes of the Spinal Cord*,
DOI 10.1007/978-3-319-45147-3_121

121.4 Pathology

Hemangioblastoma is a highly vascular tumor composed of neoplastic stromal cells, pericytes and endothelial cells. The neoplastic cell of the origin of CNS hemangioblastoma is the mesoderm-derived, embryologically arrested hemangioblast. There is usually a syrinx, which is asymptomatic but as it enlarges symptoms will be manifested.

121.5 Clinical Picture

The earliest features are those of the cerebellar and/or retinal. Spinal cord features are rare to be the earliest. The clinical features of spinal hemangioblastoma associated with VHL disease are in four grades according to McCormik et al.:

- Grade I: neurologically normal, mild focal deficit not significantly affecting the function of the affected limb, mild spasticity or reflex abnormality. Gait is normal.
- Grade II: Presence of sensorimotor deficit affecting function of involved limb, mild to moderate gait difficulty, severe pain or dysesthetic syndrome impairing patient's quality of life, still functions and ambulates independently.
- Grade III: more severe neurological deficit requires cane/brace for ambulation or significant upper limb impairment, may or may not function independently.
- Grade IV: severe deficit requires wheelchair or cane/brace, bilateral upper limb impairment, usually not independent.

Associated conditions of spinal hemangioblastoma are found in the article e.g. renal cell carcinoma, cystic disease etc. In addition to the intracranial hemangioblastoma, the highest incidence of spinal cord hemangioblastoma is cervical, then thoracic and least in the lumbar region. 86.5 % had syrinx.

121.6 Management

Total resection could be done in 95.7 %; subtotal removal in 2.1 %; partial removal in 4.2 %. The results indicate the spinal cord hemangioblastoma can be removed in the majority of cases without neurological deterioration. VHL patients frequently have multiple spinal cord hemangioblastomas requiring multiple operations. It is recommended to do through removal in the first operation. For the functional outcome after resection of spinal cord hemangioblastoma associated with von Hippel Landau disease. See article by Mehta et al. (2010).

References

Kanno H, Yamamoto I, Nishikawa R, et al. Spinal cord hemangioblastomas in von Hippel-Lindau disease. Spinal Cord. 2009;47(6):447–52.

Mehta GU, Asthagiri AR, Bakhtian KD, Auh S, Oldfield EH, Lonser RR. Functional outcome after resection of spinal cord hemangioblastomas associated with von Hippel-Lindau disease. J Neurosurg Spine. 2010;12(3):233–42.

122 Spinal Artery Steal Syndrome in Paget's Disease of the Bone

122.1 Definition

This a condition of paraparesis or paraplegia in association with Paget's disease of the spine not due to cord compression but due to spinal artery steal syndrome due to blood flow diversion in the bone and it is reversible after medical therapy of the disease (Herzberg and Bayliss).

122.2 Incidence

The great majority of cases appear after 40 years of age. The asymptomatic form has been identified in 0.1–3 % of the population in the US and UK. The incidence of neurological complications is probably more than recognized (Porrini et al.). It is usually due to mechanical factors: enlarged vertebra, collapsed, or fractured vertebrae. Another pathological condition is spinal artery steal syndrome (Herzberg and Bayliss). Slightly more males are involved.

122.3 Etiology

Pathologically speaking the disease is evolved in three phases:

- lytic
- osteogenic
- osteoblastic

Abstracted from Herzberg and Bayliss (1980)

I.M. Eltorai, *Rare Diseases and Syndromes of the Spinal Cord*,
DOI 10.1007/978-3-319-45147-3_122

The resorbed bone is replaced by highly vascularized connective tissue. One of the sequela is hemodynamic change. According to Rablin and Cattran (Pathologic Bones of Medicine) there is vasodilatation in the skin and subcutaneous tissue overlying the involved bone. When there is 1/3 – ½ of the skeleton is affected there is increased blood flow which may be associated with high output cardiac failure.

122.4 Pathology

Due to increased bony hemodynamics there may be deviation of some spinal arteries blood to the bone leading to paresis in absence of bone enlargement or bony compression.

122.5 Clinical Picture

From the case described by Porrini et al.:

62 year-old male presented with paraparesis of the lower extremities, wheelchair bound for 5 years, sensory level at T10, no sphincter dysfunction. X-rays showed typical Paget's disease. With collapse at T8 and L4, bone nuclear scan showed increased uptake in the pelvic bones, dorsolumbar spine, left femur, and the skull. CT scan showed no compression of the cord. Alkaline phosphatase was twenty times the normal level at 820 mu/ml; serum Ca and P and acid phosphatase were within normal. Urinary hydroxyproline was normal.

122.6 Management

Patient received salmon calcitonin 500 MCR[1] per day for 5 days a week and in 2 months his paraparesis was reversed slowly. He was continued on 100 MCR salmon calcitonin twice a week. After 5 years he was completely asymptomatic.

Reference

Herzberg L, Bayliss E. Spinal-cord syndrome due to non-compressive Paget's disease of bone: a spinal-artery steal phenomenon reversible with calcitonin. Lancet. 1980;2(8184):13–5.

[1] MCR is the Volume of biological fluid completely cleared of drug metabolites as measured in unit time. Elimination occurs as a result of metabolic processes in the kidney, liver, saliva, sweat, intestine, heart, brain, or other site.

Intramedullary Teratoma 123

123.1 Definition

Teratomas are lesions composed of a mixture of cell types derived from three germinal layers. On the basis of their histological features teratomas can be classified into:

- Immature
- Mature
- Malignant

They may occur in many locations in the body including the central nervous system.

123.2 Incidence

According to Caruso and Colonnese (2006), 59 cases have been reported. They tend to occur in children, particularly in midline sites e.g. in the pineal, sellar, suprasellar sites and the fourth ventricle, excluding the neonatal sacrococcygeal teratoma. Teratomas of the spinal cord are very rare; accounting for 0.2–0.5 % of all spinal tumors. According to Fernández-Cornejo:

> Intradural spinal teratomas accounts for approximately 0.1 % of all spinal tumors. In 1999, Poeze et al. (1999) published a literature review where only 83 cases of spinal teratomas were found. Thirty-one were intramedullary (37 %), most of them occurring in adults (58 %). In this survey, 42 % of cases were associated with several types of split cord malformations. Diastomyelia, myelomeningocele, tethered cord, and others have been reported in relation to spinal teratomas. Patients are usually young adults and males (2.6:1).

Abstracted and reported by Fernández-Cornejo et al. (2004)

I.M. Eltorai, *Rare Diseases and Syndromes of the Spinal Cord*,
DOI 10.1007/978-3-319-45147-3_123

Diplomyelia reported by Mut et al. In adults spinal cord teratomas are rare only seven cases have been reported and reviewed by Nonomura et al. (2002), and added two cases of their own. In adults cervical spinal intramedullary teratoma is quite rare. According to Arvin et al., in (2009) (Arvin et al. 2009), only five cases were reported and they added the sixth case.

123.3 Pathogenesis

Teratomas are formed from remnants of all three primative germinal layers. The exact pathogenic factor is not known. A traditional theory is that early in the embryogenesis, pyramidal germ cells from the yolk sac become misplaced because of alteration in the cell migration. These cells almost always are found in the middle line structures where they gibe rise to germ cell tumors including teratomas.

123.4 Pathology

Totipotential embryonic cells morphed from the yolk sac form the tumor. Teratomas are of three types as mentioned above:

- Mature or benign: these contain mature tissue e.g. cartilage, squamous epithelium, mucous glands, neural elements—bundles of nerve fibers. Fan et al. (2001) (Fan et al. 2001), have recorded a case of carcinoid in mature teratoma.
- Immature: This contains primitive cells of neurepithelial lineage and sometimes mesenchymal elements. These tend to recur in almost all cases.
- Malignant: The tumor shows the characteristics of malignancy.

Intraspinal teratomas occur posteriorly at cervical or lower thoracic and upper lumbar regions and may develop in the filum terminal, the conus, and the cauda equina. The histological picture depends on the type of tumor whether mature, immature, or malignant. They contain dermal, mesenchymal, and endodermal elements, well differentiated mature, primitive in immature.

123.5 Case Report

Depending on the level of the tumor, neurological symptoms are sensory, motor and sphincteric usually of upper motor neuron type except those of cauda equina. Associated congenital lesions may be present—especially dysraphism, syrinx, tethered cord, etc. Skin stigmata e.g. dimples, may be seen.

123.5.1 Diagnosis

Diagnosis is based on the following criteria:

1. Clinical exam
2. Plain Radiography:
3. erosion of the vertebral body,
4. widening of the intrapedicular space,
5. vertebral anomalies e.g. spina bifida,
6. vertebral body fusion,
7. asymmetry of vertebral bodies, diastomyelia,
8. soft tissue shadows of the tumor with calcification
9. CT scan is useful as long as it shows variable densities and calcification
10. MRI of the spinal cord: very useful because the tumor exhibits high and low signal intensities, indicative of tissues heterogeneity, e.g. bone, fat, muscle, cysts, etc.

123.6 Management

Total excision of the mass is advisable, provided no damage to the neural tissues occur. Subtotal excision is also practiced and recurrence may not develop for many years, since tumor regrowth is very rare. Intramedullary tumors are approached through bilateral laminectomy. If the tumor is not visible posteriorly, intraoperative ultrasound is important for localization not for embryogenic cyst. In children, laminectomy and laminoplasty are recommended. In the cauda equina laminoplasty is recommended. Survival in adults with mature teratoma is good. Immature and malignant teratomas have poor prognosis even with chemotherapy. Incomplete removal of mature teratoma needs close followup with MRI. Surgery for dysraphism can follow later. When the tumor recurs a second surgery will be tried. Chemotherapy is of no benefit.

The operation is conducted under microscopy and somatosensory evoked potentials for monitoring the integrity of the cord. The use of coagulants is routine. According to Caruso and Colonnese total removal of the tumor was only possible in 12 out of 59 reported cases. The difficulty for total resection is due to teratoma adhesions between the tumor and healthy cord parenchyma. The same authors share the opinion with Burduck and with controrre that lateral removal of the tumor is unnecessary risk to the function of the sphincter. The authors believe that the short-term growth of the tumor itself will apple to its remnant. Their two cases lasted 7 years and 6 years without recurrence. In the case of recurrence, the tumor is usually malignant or immature. According to Mut et al., subtotal resection is mandatory if there are gross alterations in the signals of SSEP.

References

Arvin B, Pohl U, David K. Intramedullary cervical teratoma in an adult. Spine J. 2009;9(5):e14–8.

Caruso R, Colonnese C. Intramedullary teratomas: two case reports and a review of the literature. Zentralbl Neurochir. 2006;67(4):213–8.

Fan X, Turner JE, Turner TM, et al. Carcinoid tumor development in an intramedullary spinal cord mature teratoma. AJNR Am J Neuroradiol. 2001;22(9):1778–81.

Fernández-Cornejo VJ, Martínez-Pérez M, Polo-García LA, Martínez-Lage JF, Poza M. Cystic mature teratoma of the filum terminale in an adult. Case report and review of the literature. Neurocirugia (Astur). 2004;15(3):290–3.

Nonomura Y, Miyamoto K, Wada E, et al. Intramedullary teratoma of the spine: report of two adult cases. Spinal Cord. 2002;40(1):40–3.

Poeze M, Herpers MJ, Tjandra B, Freling G, Beuls EA. Intramedullary spinal teratoma presenting with urinary retention: case report and review of the literature. Neurosurgery. 1999;45(2):379–85.

Part VII

Toxic Causes of Myelopathy

Benzene Myelitis

124

124.1 Definition

This is a condition of myelopathy due to chronic exposure to benzene fumes.

124.2 Incidence

One case reported by P Herregods et al.

124.3 Etiology

Benzene (Bz) is the prototype aromatic hydrocarbon, since it is composed of only the benzene ring. As such, and because of its physical properties, it is widely used in the chemical industry as a feedstock for chemical reactions and less commonly as a solvent. So frequent is its use as a constituent of commercial products that most people probably have at least inhaled its fumes. It is a myelotoxin: chronic exposure of humans and experimental animals to high concentrations results in blood dyscrasis including lymphocytopenia, thrombocytopenia, and pancytopenia or aplastic anemia. It is also a carcinogen.

124.4 Pathology

Quoting from Herregods et al.

> The neurotoxicity of benzene can be described as follows. The aromatic hydrocarbons have a particular affinity for nerve tissue because of their high lipid content. The presence of

Abstracted from Herregods et al. (1984)

I.M. Eltorai, *Rare Diseases and Syndromes of the Spinal Cord*,
DOI 10.1007/978-3-319-45147-3_124

benzene in the nerve cells interferes with their normal metabolism, both in the brain as in the spinal cord.

Normal metabolic activity and full functions only return after the complete elimination of the aromatic hydrocarbons. However, this effect occurs slowly because of the high lipid solubility of the hydrocarbons.

The neurotoxicity (Gerarde, 1959; Gerarde, 1960; Hine 1954) of the aromatic hydrocarbons is believed to be a consequence of hemorrhage in the nerve system, principally in the grey matter of the cervical and thoracic spinal cord.

These hemorrhages are believed to be the result of local irritation of endothelial cells of the blood vessels, resulting in permeability changes in the capillaries. This in turn leads to increased diapedesis, edema in the surrounding tissues, petechial and gross hemorrhages. Animal experiments showed paralysis of the extremities with final destruction of the nerve cells. Concerning the toxic effect on the nerve tissues Hine (1954) commented as follows, "on reviewing the literature we were surprised to find no reference to detail studies of central nervous system lesions by benzene."

The authors diagnosed the case as transverse myelitis at C7-C8, T1 due to benzene toxicity.

124.5 Clinical Picture

The patient was a 25 year old male who had chronic exposure to benzene and manifested by pain in the interscapular area, radiated to both arms and progressed to both legs. In a couple of hours he had paresis of the upper limbs and complete paralysis of the lower, i.e. quadriplegic, with hypotonic muscles. Parathesia and sensory distortion developed from T1 down. Bladder and bowel dysfunction was noted. Blood picture and CSF studies were unremarkable. Myelography was negative for tumors and somatosenory evoked potential (SSEP) indicated medullary injury.

124.6 Diagnosis

Diagnosis is based on the following criteria:

1. Patient's history including occupational exposure to benzene
2. exclusion of other conditions: multiple sclerosis, tumors, Guillian-Barré syndrome, viral infection, vascular malformation, syphilis, Pott's disease, hematomyelia, polyarteritis nodosa, arachnoiditis, sarchoidosis, syringomyelia, spondilosis, etc.
3. Abnormally high urine phenol levels, with decreasing levels with improvement of the patient.

124.7 Management

The case was managed conservatively, non-specifically, except the withdrawal from the environment. He was exposed to the benzene fumes for many years. His condition improved and patient could walk without crutch, with some residual urinary symptoms indicating Crédé's technique and some weakness of the feet extensors 7 months after the onset. Phenol levels returned to normal.

Conclusion

This benzene neurotoxicity has been reported only once. More than two million people are exposed to benzene and possibly a case may be encountered in the industrial medical practice. Although very rarely, neurotoxicity affected the spinal cord giving the picture of transverse myelitis confirmed by the urinary phenol levels and by exclusion of other pathologies based on clinical data and laboratory tests. When the inhalation is discontinued recovery is obtained although not quite complete.

Reference

Herregods P, Chappel R, Mortier G. Benzene poisoning as a possible cause of transverse myelitis. Paraplegia. 1984;22:305–10.

Myelopathy due to Flexion Drug Overdose

125

125.1 Definition

This is a condition of cervical myelopathy, developing after prolonged extreme neck flexion in association with profound muscular relaxation.

125.2 Incidence

Although cervical myelopathy may develop after prolonged neurosurgical operations, with the neck flexed in the sitting position for occipital fossa lesions; this condition is a different entity. The cervical myelopathy after prolonged extreme flexion of the neck has been reported twice by Kaye et al. (2001) and Nielsen and Damek (2012).

125.3 Etiology

The first case was caused by acute neck flexion for 18 h with use of an overdose of valporic acid. The second case was psychotic case with suicidal tendency and had overdose of quetiapine fumarate, oxycodone/acetaminophen and chloral hydrate. Prolonged neck flexion may be fixable action by criminals, e.g. robbery or prolonged assault.

Abstracted from Kaye et al. (2001)

I.M. Eltorai, *Rare Diseases and Syndromes of the Spinal Cord*,
DOI 10.1007/978-3-319-45147-3_125

125.4 Pathophysiology

Prolonged neck flexion may result in spinal cord damage, cervical myelopathy as in the first case and thoracic myelopathy as in the second case. The cause is not quite clear, theories include:

- Vascular: the acute flexion of the neck, stretching the arteries, and the veins of the spinal cord, thus altering its autoregulation
- Neuronal or mechanical: the cord is injured by direct mechanical distraction by compression or axial stretching
- Combination
  - The ischemia may account for the central gray damage
  - Mechanical stretching may cause the disruption of the axons in the white matter. In Nielsen and Damek case, there was also thoracic myelopathy.

The first case expired and postmortem cord pathology showed dusky softening at C5-C6 dislocation and softening of the entire cross sections. Microscopic exam showed bilateral degeneration of the ascending tracts including gracilis, tractus cuneatus, spinocerebellar, and spinalthalamic tracts. At C6, there was extensive necrosis of the whole sectional area, with only small residual normal tissue around. There was marked macrophages infiltration; there was degeneration of C7 spinal roots.

125.5 Clinical Picture

The type of patient, psychiatric, or an overdose of certain drugs. Prolonged sitting with the cervical spine, markedly flexed for many hours. Consciousness may be veiled; tetraplegia with sensory-motor deficits, and autonomic dysfunction, reflexes exaggerated, Babinski's sign is positive. There may be signs of pressure on the ischial areas.

125.6 Diagnosis

Diagnosis based on:

1. History of kind of patient: the use of drugs, especially with overdose
2. Neurological exam
3. Laboratory tests: routine hematology, blood chemistry, and pharmacology
4. Spinal radiography
5. MRI abnormal cord signals of the cervical cord C4-C5 and possibly upper thoracic segments. Edema of the cord, with loss of fat planes on T2-weighted images. Images show space occupying lesions.
6. Evoked potential sensory and motor show sensory and motor deficits

125.7 Management

- Early diagnosis is important and keeping this pathology in mind
- The use of IV methylprednisolone to reduce edema, inflammatory reactions, excessive cytokine release, excitotoxic damage. However, it is still controversial; it must be used within 8 h.
- Other promising products include monosialo-tetrahexo-synganglioside (AM-1) and thyrotropin-releasing hormone
- Induced systemic hyperthermia in acute setting of spinal cord injury

Updating

Wang et al. 2012

Case report
A 56-year old male presented unable to move his limbs following drug overdose. Neurological examination revealed C6 ASIA spinal cord injury. The CT of his cervical spine showed no fracture; however MRI showed cord edema extending from C3-C6, as well as posterior paraspinal signal abnormalities, suggestive of ligamentous injury. He underwent a posterior cervical laminectomy and fusion from C3-C7. The authors hypothesize likely due to existing cervical stenosis, in addition to overdose of sedating medication, which resulted in cervical spine vascular and/or neurological compromise producing an irreversible spinal cord injury.

Reference
Wang TS, Grunch BH, Moreno JR, Bagley CA, Gottfried ON. Drug overdose resulting in quadriplegia. Eur Spine J. 2012;21 Suppl 4:S521–4.

References

Kaye KL, Ramsay D, Young GB. Cervical flexion myelopathy after valproic acid overdose. Spine. 2001;26(19):E459–61.

Nielsen AS, Damek DM. Window of opportunity: flexion myelopathy after drug overdose. J Emerg Med. 2012;42(1):36–9.

126 Myelopathy due to Heroin Addiction

126.1 Definition

This is a myelopathy due to cocaine and/or heroin addition, whether by intravenous use or intranasal insufflation or smoking or inhalation.

126.2 Incidence

Sporadic cases are reported periodically abstracted from McCreary et al. (2000). In 2000, McCreary reported a case of acute myelopathy following intranasal insufflation of heroin: a case report.

126.3 Etiology and Pathology

The use of illicit drugs is increasing. The toxic effects are well know to toxicology. We will focus on spinal cord damage (myelopathy). Myelopathy can occur as a result of the following:

- spinal cord ischemia due to infarctions resulting from hypotension
- direct toxic myelopathy
- toxic vasculitis with secondary myelopathy

Fux et al., 2003

I.M. Eltorai, *Rare Diseases and Syndromes of the Spinal Cord*,
DOI 10.1007/978-3-319-45147-3_126

- hypersensitivity causing edema and subsequent ischemia of the nerve cells, similar to what happens in the brain. This is seen in the first use after abstinence. This usually occurs via haptenation[1] of the drug with an in-vivo protein. In myelopathy, this may involve a specific protein to the spinal cord parenchyma causing inflammatory reaction, ischemia, and tissue injury.
- Infarction with septicemia
- combination of two or more factors

Myelopathy may be in the form of transverse myelitis or patchy areas of ischemia and cellular infiltration.

126.4 Clinical Picture

This onset is usually acute and associated with other toxic effects of the drug, e.g. toxic encephalitis, hepatitis, nephritis, myocarditis, myopathy, rhabdomyeloysis, electrolyte imbalances, and coagulopathy. Myelopathy is diagnosed by neurological signs, sensory and motor deficit, and sphincter disturbances.

126.5 Diagnosis

1. History of drug use
2. Toxicology tests
3. hematological and biochemical testing
4. electrophysiological studies
5. CT scan shows cord edema and patchy hyperdensity
6. MRI of the spine: consists of acute transverse myelitis. T2-weighted images show cord swelling with increased signals over most of the transverse diameter. Enhancement is usually patchy. Gadolinium enhancement may occur acutely, consistent with an acute inflammatory process, disrupting the blood cord barriers.

126.6 Management

- Detoxification by antidote Narcan
- Cardiovascular stability
- respiratory care
- fluid and electrolyte balance, transfusion if needed
- corticosteroids
- plasmapheresis or immunopheresis

[1] Hapten is a small separable part of an antigen that reacts specifically with an antibody but is incapable of stimulating antibody production except in combination with a carrier protein.

- hemodialysis if needed
- in paraplegia, a rehabilitation program

Reference

McCreary M, Emerman C, Hanna J, Simon J. Acute myelopathy following intranasal insufflation of heroin: a case report. Neurology. 2000;55(2):316–7.

Myelopathy due to Wasp Sting 127

127.1 Definition

The wasp is an insect of the *hymenoptera* order, which includes 100,000 species of insects, including bees, ants, and wasps. These are known to be well developed in social and colonial life. It is stated that four persons die every year in the UK due to anaphylactic reaction to wasp or bee stings. Myelopathies recorded are mostly due to *Vaspa tropica* stings.

127.2 Incidence

Myelopathy due to wasp sting is rare. Although, allergic reactions to wasp stings are common; neurological complications are rare. However, myelopathy, encephalo-myeloradiculopathy, cerebral infarction, optic neuropathy, polyradiculopathy, encephaloraduloneuritis, and even myesthenia gravis have been reported. The course of the illness may lead to partial or complete recovery, or may be permanent and end fatally.

127.3 Etiology

The etiology of neurologic damage may be due to one or more of the following factors:

- the venom contains no myelin proteins or peptides that cause allergic reactions by producing certain antibodies that cross react with myelin basic proteins

Abstracted from Likittanasombut et al. (2003)

I.M. Eltorai, *Rare Diseases and Syndromes of the Spinal Cord*,
DOI 10.1007/978-3-319-45147-3_127

- phosphalypaise-A activity of the venom may liberate encephalogenic basic proteins or other antigens from the myelin membraines of the central and peripheral nervous systems inducing immune reactions
- vascular thrombosis, possibly due to vasoconsticition, secondary to release of mediators released after wasp sting and possibly by platelet aggregation. The venom also has inflammatory and thrombogenic peptides and amines including histamines, leukatrens and throboxane, the latter two are known to be vasocontstrictors

However, there are possibly other mechanisms, which are not known.

127.4 Pathology

There is edema of the spinal cord with areas of demyelination in the cord and nerve roots sometimes the picture of acute myelitis or acute encephalomyeloneuritis. Patchy areas of gray and white matter demyelination, vascular changes, and cellular infiltration May develop due to vasoconstriction and by platelet aggregation.

127.5 Clinical Picture

History of a sting by a wasp, especially in endemic areas. The onset of symptoms is within minutes or hours in up to 96 % of cases. Local reaction at the site of the sting which varies in degree according to antigenecity and antibody reactions. Occasionally, it develops into an anaphylactic shock. Myelopathy is manifested by Numbness of the extremities, weakness, eventually paralysis (tetraplegia) with loss of sensation and sphincter control. First it is hypo or areflexic and later will be hypereflexic. The picture is modified by the presence of encephalitis and radiculoneuritis, with encephalitis. There is decline of tonic-clonic seizures and cerebral paresis, respiratory distress, hypoxia, and possibly respiratory failure.

127.6 Diagnosis

1. There is hyperglobulinemia, throbocytopenia and high ESR.
2. CSF shows monocytosis
3. IgE antibodies to wasp venom are positive
4. Renal and hepatic function may be low
5. EKG may show cardiac ischemia
6. MRI shows ill-defined scattered lesions in the cervical cord, hypotensive signals in T1-weighted images involving both the gray and white matter of the cervical cord and in case of encephalopathy, the brain and brain stem may be involved.
7. Sensory conduction studies may be altered in radiculopathy and peripheral neuropathy.

127.7 Management

- IV methylprednisolone for 5 days, followed by oral hydrocortisone for 7–10 days, gradually tapered
- IM chlorpheniramine
- Plasma exchange
- IV gelofusine in severe hypotension
- subcutaneous adrenaline

Recovery may be partial, subtotal, or incomplete, depending on toxicity, allergenecity, duration, and treatment. Thus far no antivenom is available.

Reference

Likittanasombut P, Witoonpanich R, Viranuvatti K. Encephalomyeloradiculopathy associated with wasp sting. J Neurol Neurosurg Psychiatr. 2003;74(1):134–5.

Part VIII

Vascular Causes of Myelopathy

Anterior Spinal Artery Syndrome 128

128.1 Definition

Anterior spinal artery syndrome (ASAS) or Spiller's syndrome is named for William G. Spiller who described it 1909, however Preobranshenski was the first to describe ASAS in 1904. ASAS is thrombosis ventral to the spinal cord causing blockage of the anterior spinal artery (ASA) and an infarction of the areas supplied. Outside the spinal cord there are some collateral anastomoses, which may help in vascular obliteration. There are anastomoses between the deep cervical, the vertebral and occipital arteries. In addition, the ascending cervical and muscular branches anastomose. There are also anastomoses between the two vertebrals and the radicular arteries at the lower end of the cord. There are cruciate anastomoses between the artery of Adamkiewicz, the postero-lateral arteries and the branch from the caudal vessels in the thoracic region the anastomosis is scanty so that it is a watershed area. Addressing the venous drainage, the veins that drain the cord correspond to the arteries but they are not exactly alike. The have seven categories based on their size. The medullary veins drain into the spinal and into the radicular veins. These anastomose with the epidural veins and the veins of the vertebral bodies and eventually drain into the vertebral, intercostal, lumbar, and sacral, veins. Ultimately they drain into the jugular, azygos, and hemiazygos veins, thus connecting with the venous system of the chest, abdominal, and pelvic cavities. This is what Batson described in the 1940s when he divided the venous plexus from the occiput down to the sacrum into three groups: extradural, intravertebral, and extravertebral.

128.2 Incidence

Foo and Rossier (1983) reviewed 256 spinal cord injuries and found only thirteen (0.05 %) cases of ASAS. Zantl, et al., report ASAS in 0.2 % in 1000 esophagectomies over a 18 year period. The prevalence of these syndromes ranges from 0.5 % in operations for coarctation of the aorta to as high as 15 % after surgery for thoracoabdominal aneurysms.

I.M. Eltorai, *Rare Diseases and Syndromes of the Spinal Cord*,
DOI 10.1007/978-3-319-45147-3_128

128.3 Etiology

The spinal cord is due to ischemia, although there are several sources of vascularization. Functionally, the vascularization is not always adequate, since the ASA is not a continuous channel and the perimedullary do not anastomose with the intramedullary area. Furthermore, the intramedullary anastomosis has no functional value. If the blood pressure falls below the critical level, an infarction occurs. This depends on the site of artery occlusion and the collaterals. It also depends on the onset of anterior occlusion; a slow onset is more tolerable than that of the acute. The extent of damage depends on the perfusion pressure; a pressure of 30 mmHg will cause hypoperfusion and hypoxia, both of which aggravate the damage to the spinal cord. There are anatomic variations, which modify the ischemic effect.

128.4 Pathology

The result of arterial occlusion is infarction of the spinal cord. This leads to necrosis of the involved tissue. There may be minor hemorrhage, cellular infiltration by enormous numbers of scavengers derived from the microglia and the micropahges. These may be filled with fat globules taken up from the disintegrating myelin. The walls of the vessels around the occlusion may be infiltrated with microglia. The peripheral area or the periumbra may have partial recovery depending on the degree of vascular occlusion and management. Eventually the infracted area will have a glial scar formed by the astrocytes.

128.5 Clinical Picture

The symptoms of ASAS are usually sudden and manifested within minutes or hours of the ischemia. There is local or radicular back pain; the nature of the pain may be burning or lancinating. The pain varies in duration it may only be transient. There is usually diffused deep aching pain in both legs. Burning dysthetic pain may start in the feet and ascend up to the abdomen. Soon after the onset of pain there is weakness of the lags and inability to walk, becoming a disability with in minutes. The syndrome varies according to the level of ASA occlusion. There is loss of pain and temperature sensation below the level of the lesion; in addition, there is loss of bowel and bladder control. There is sacral sparing. Partial touch sensation is preserved, as well as proprioception and vibration sense because of the posterior arterial plexus supplying the posterior columns. The leg paralysis is an upper motor neuron due to a lesion in the lateral corticospinal tract. If ischemia involves only the sulcal branches there is a lower motor neuron deficit.

Sometimes signs are restricted to those of either upper or lower motor neurons or both in a pattern similar to that of amyotrophic lateral sclerosis (ALS). However, the major differences are mod of onset and the lack of progressive worsening of the

ASAS. Sulcal thrombosis of ASA leads to lower motor neuron deficit (amyotrophy). This may be unilateral or bilateral depending on the of the sulcal arteries. There is usually motor weakness without sensory changes. The picture varies according to the level of ischemia.

The spasticity in the lower limbs is due to the lesion involving the corticospinal tract and the flaccidity is due to involvement of the gray matter and the anterior horns.

Transient ischemic attacks (TIA) of the spinal cord and the cauda equine lead to cord or cauda claudication as describe by Déjérine in 1906. It causes transient weakness and/or numbness of one or both lower extremities during walking and parathesia in one or both feet. If the patient continues walking they might get a drop foot due to ischemia of the cord; or may develop spastic weakness and increase or exaggerated reflexes if the cord itself is involved. Whereas the weakness due to the cauda the reflexes will be reduced or absent. The spinal intermittent claudication may precede the spinal cord infarction caused by ASA thrombosis.

128.6 Diagnosis

The acute onset of ASAS with motor weakness and discriminative anesthesia are typical of cord infarction. In typical cases, slow onset over time is usually against ASAS. Atypical cases need to be differentiated from: multiple sclerosis (MS), ALS, poliomyelitis, cord compression, and transverse myelitis. These can be confirmed by radiography, myelography, computed tomography scan, and magnetic resonance imaging. Lumbar puncture may confirm the diagnosis of MS by showing an elevated gamma globulin in the cerebrospinal fluid (CSF). In neoplasms there is an increase of the CSF protein to a very high level. In ASAS there is slight protein content elevation, but the gamma globulin is normal. Associated infarction of the vertebral body is sometimes an important sign for diagnosis. Neurophysiological studies and somatosensory evoked potentials will confirm spinal cord infarction.

128.7 Management

Treatment should be started very early after the onset of the symptoms two things must be corrected the hypotension and the hypoxia. The use of anticoagulants and anti-platelets did not contribute to the improvement of the ischemia. The following drugs have been tried:

1. Nalaxone hydrochloride
2. Calcium channel blockers
3. Steroid therapy (methylprednisolone)
4. Free radical scavengers
5. Barbiturates

For the persistent cord edema hyperbaric oxygen may help resolve the edema. For established paralysis the standard spinal cord rehabilitation programs should be involved.

Reference

Foo D, Rossier AB. Anterior spinal artery syndrome and its natural history. Paraplegia. 1983;21(1):1–10.

Cervical Myelopathy Caused by Bilateral Persistence of the First Intersegmental Arteries

129

129.1 Definition

This is a condition of compression myelopathy due to bilateral persistence of the first intersegmental artery (vertebral artery anomaly).

129.2 Incidence

This is a very rare condition noticed in less than 1 % of angiograms. According to Takahashi et al., only four cases have been operated.

129.3 Etiology

This is a congenital anomaly in which there is anomalous vertebral arteries (VA) can cause upper cervical cord compression.

129.4 Pathology

According to Padget, fenestration of the VA is considered to be a persistence of the intersegmental artery during embryogenesis. Failure of resegmentation of the embryonic scleratoma seems to promote the abnormal development of the intersegmental arteries. Previous reports show that fenestration of the VA at the craniovertebral junction was often associated with osseous anomalies, such as occipitalization of the atlas, Klippel-Feil syndrome, hypoplasia of the atlas, basilar impression, cleft

Abstracted from Yamazaki et al. (2004)

I.M. Eltorai, *Rare Diseases and Syndromes of the Spinal Cord*,
DOI 10.1007/978-3-319-45147-3_129

of C1 posterior arch. The osseous anomalies have been explained as a failure of rearrangement of the embryogenic scleratomas. The resulting longer intradural course forms a longer ventral loop, causing cord compression. Other anomalies may be present e.g. Down's syndrome.

129.5 Clinical Picture

This anomaly may be asymptomatic and may be detected by angiography for other reasons. It affects both genders equally. Age ranged from 38 to 75. Symptoms are usually: cervical pain, occipital neuralgia, accessory nerve palsy, pain in the shoulder and/or the arm. Myelopathy presents with bilateral compression of the dorsal and dorsolateral columns by the abnormal VAs. The pain may be intermittent due to VA pulsations on the dorsal root entry zone (DREZ) of the cervical nerve. Later in life, atheroslecosis, pain hammering style, this may be due to compression of the Lissauer's tract, which lies in front of the DREZ. It decussates on or more segments higher than the DREZ.

129.6 Diagnosis

Diagnosis based on:

1. Confirmation of clinical picture
2. Laboratory tests 3D computed angiography, which will show the abnormal course of Vas at C1-C2 level. The course of the VAs is abnormally long intradurally. The arteries form vascular loops reaching the medullar and compressing the cervical cord.
3. MRI of the spinal cord showed T2 weighted-imges reveals bilateral signal void areas in the postrolateral areas of the spinal cord at C1

129.7 Management

Suboccipital craniotomy and C1 laminectomy give good approach. With microsurgery the VAs are mobilized laterally to relieve pressure on the cord and are anchored laterally to the corresponding side of the dura mater with cortex bands. Other techniques may be opted

Update

Abstract from Ozpinar et al. 2015

Vertebral artery fenestration occurs when the vessel lumen is divided into two separate channels that eventually fuse, forming the primary vessel. Autopsy and angiographic studies suggest that the incidence of vertebral artery fenestration is 0.23–1.95 %. Although fenestration of the vertebral artery can occur either intra- or extracranially, extracranial fenestration at the upper cervical level is more commonly reported. When the vertebral artery is fenestrated, each channel has its own muscularis layer and is lined by a separate endothelium. The term fenestration has been synonymously used with duplication in the literature; however, the two describe different anatomical phenomena.

Fenestration of the vertebral artery is a rare vascular anomaly that has been observed at autopsy and on angiography. It is most commonly seen in the extracranial segments of the vertebral artery. This congenital anomaly can arise during multiple different stages of embryological development of the vertebral artery. The clinical significance is unclear, but multiple studies have reported association with other vascular anomalies. Awareness of vascular anomalies is crucial to avoid iatrogenic injuries during endovascular diagnostic and therapeutic interventions. Here, we present a case of a patient with an intracranial vertebral artery fenestration that was identified during work-up for a foramen magnum mass.

Reference

Ozpinar A, Magill ST, Davies JM, Mcdermott MW. Vertebral Artery Fenestration. Cureus. 2015;7(1):e245.

Reference

Yamazaki M, Okawa A, Aramomi MA, Hashimoto M, Masaki Y, Koda M. Fenestration of vertebral artery at the craniovertebral junction in down syndrome: a case report. Spine. 2004;29(23):E551–4.

Myelopathy in Cobb Syndrome 130

130.1 Definition

Cobb syndrome is a rare non-inherited clinical entity characterized by the combination of vascular cutaneous nerves and an angioma in the spinal canal at the same metamere. Cobb described it, in 1895, as a metameric angiomatosis with segmental involvement of the skin, subcutaneous tissues, vertebral column, dura, and spinal cord, i.e. a cutaneomeningospinal angiamatosis.

130.2 Incidence

Brant, et al., quoted 29 cases from the literature, in 1999; in 2003, Soeda et al. added an additional infant case. In 2008, Clark et al. systematically reviewed the literature and found 39 cases. Statistics cannot be valid since only the symptomatic cases are reported.

130.3 Etiology

According to Brant et al.:

During fetal development, each somite divides into a medial half which forms the vertebral bodies (the sclerotome) and the lateral half which develops the muscles (the myotome). The vertebral bodies create the perichordal tube, and other cells from the sclerotome migrate dorsally and form the posterior elements. The blood supply to the vertebrae and spinal cord for the metameres originates from the

Abstracted and reported by Brant et al. (1999).

I.M. Eltorai, *Rare Diseases and Syndromes of the Spinal Cord*,
DOI 10.1007/978-3-319-45147-3_130

segmental dorsal arteries during fetal development. This may account for the common metameric origin of the pathological vessels that create the cutaneo-meningospinal angiomas.

130.4 Pathology

The disease is usually thoracolumbar in location. It consists of cutaneous hemangiomas associated with vertebral, paravertebral, and intraspinal angimatosis, usually fed by branches from the intercostal vessels. There may be other visceral hemangiomas. Myelopathy is caused by compression due to the bulk of the vascular mass. The cord may show some degree of atrophy. The symptoms may be caused also by venous hypertension and/or blood steal phenomena. However, the vascular pathology varies from case to case; a combination of hemangioma and arterial venous fistula (AVF) is also encountered, in which case subarachnoid hemorrhage is a possibility. Occasionally, spina bifida and cord tethering have been recorded by Brant et al. .

130.5 Clinical Picture

The disease may present itself at any age, usually in late childhood. The onset may be slow or sudden, and the course progressive or rapid. The syndrome is congenital manifested by cutaneous nevus on the back in the thoracolumbar region and crossing the middle line. Cord compression is manifested by spastic paraparesis, tetraparesis, or monoparesis. Headache, pains, pyrexia, menigism, and gluteal or limb hypertrophy have been reported.

130.6 Diagnosis

Diagnosis is based on the following criteria:

1. History of birth nevus
2. Clinical exam: the skin angioma corresponds within 1–2 segments to the intraspinal angioma. The cutaneous nevus varies in size. There may be visceral angiomas as well.
3. Spinal angiography and aortogram
4. MRI: in case reported by Soeda, et al., T1 weighted showed low and high signal intensity.
5. X-rays can reveal widening of the spinal canal
6. CT scans also were used diagnostically

130.7 Management

Management especially, in infants is rather difficult. Primary surgical excision is associated with high risk.

Methods adopted are:

1. Systemic corticosteroids therapy
2. Devascularization of the feeding arteries identified by angiography and excluding spinal cord supply. Usually the angioma feeders are distinct from those of the cord
3. Endovascular embolization using *n*-butyl-2-cyanoacrylate (NBCA)
4. Combination of radiotherapy and surgery
5. Conservative treatment

If all above fails, careful excision of the residual mass should be performed. There are various choices in the series reviewed by Clark et al. , with various opinions, combining one or more of the above mentioned modalities. The management has to be multidisciplinary: neurology, neurosurgery, interventional radiology with decisions based on the pros and cons.

References

Brant AJ, James HE, Tung H. Cutaneomeningospinal angiomatosis (Cobb syndrome) with tethered cord. Pediatr Neurosurg. 1999;30(2):93–5.

Clark MT, Brooks EL, Chong W, Pappas C, Fahey M. Cobb syndrome: a case report and systematic review of the literature. Pediatr Neurol. 2008;39(6):423–5.

Soeda A, Sakai N, Iihara K, Nagata I. Cobb syndrome in an infant: treatment with endovascular embolization and corticosteroid therapy: case report. Neurosurgery. 2003;52(3):711–5. discussion 714-5.

Eale's Disease

131

131.1 Definition

According to Jablonski, a noninflammatory disorder of the peripheral retinal vessels characterized by frequently bilateral periphlebitis, avascular peripheral areas, microaneurysms, rope ladder-like capillary dilatations, tortuosity of adjacent vessels, and spontaneous chorioretinal scars. Neovascularization, hemorrhage, vascular orbliteration, and vascular sheathing may be associated. Neurological complications may include vascular lesions of the brain and demyelination of the optic nerve. Epistaxis and constipation may occur.

131.2 Incidence

Extraoccular manifestations of Eales' disease have been reported in the nervous system only in the brain and spinal cord. Until 1993 only 16 cases of Eale's disease myelopathy have been reported.

131.3 Etiology

The etiology so far is unknown. Dastur and Singhal (1976) have suggested the possibility of vasculopathy with demyelination. Retinomyelopathy occurs as a hypersensitive mechanism in response to an inflammatory agent, either bacterial or viral. This could also apply to the myelopathy of the disease.

Abstracted and reported by Sawhney et al. (1986).

I.M. Eltorai, *Rare Diseases and Syndromes of the Spinal Cord*,
DOI 10.1007/978-3-319-45147-3_131

131.4 Pathology

The condition is that of vasculitis, periphlebitis, peripheral ischemia, microaneurysms, rope-ladder like capillary dilation, and tortuosity of adjacent vessels. Hemorrhages and vascular obliterations may be detected. These vascular changes may apply to the brain, optic nerve, and spinal cord; leading to demyelinating myelopathy. There is selective pyramidal demyelination without any selective level in the cord. There may also be a brain lesion.

131.5 Clinical Picture

The disease occurs in males between 16–40 years old and is of insidious onset, but sometimes acute or subacute. There is unilateral or bilateral blindness of various degrees. It starts by progressive weakness and stiffness of lower extremities with micturition dysfunction. Sensory changes of different degrees are noticed and reflexes are hyperactive.

131.6 Diagnosis

Diagnosis based on:

1. Ocular fundoscopy
2. Neurological exam
3. Myelography is usually negative
4. MRI: shows multifocal white matter abnormalities
5. CSF: may show increased lymphocytes

Differential diagnosis: syphilitic myelitis, tuberculosis meningomyelitis, multiple sclerosis (MS), and hereditary spastic paraplegia.

131.7 Management

1. Steroid therapy and Medical care
2. Rehabilitation
3. Opthalmological care

Partial or no improvement may be expected.

References

Dastur DK, Singhal BS. Eales' disease with neurological involvement. Part 2. Pathology and pathogenesis. J Neurol Sci. 1976;27(3):323–45.

Sawhney IM, Chopra JS, Bansal SK, Gupta AK. Eales' disease with myelopathy. Clin Neurol Neurosurg. 1986;88(3):213–5.

132 Ectopic Choroidal Plexus Tissue

132.1 Definition

This is an unique condition where there is ectopic choroid tissue in the spinal cord causing pressure myelopathy.

132.2 Incidence

This is a single case reported, whereas intracranial cysts containing ectopic choroid plexus or choroid-like tissue has been rarely reported (5 cases).

132.3 Etiology

The choroid plexus develops from the telachoroidal and projects into the lateral ventricle on its medial aspect, roof of the third ventricles and roof of the fourth ventricle. Such tissue or like it has been found in the epithelial linked non-communicating cysts intracranially. The exact causative factor is still unknown. It is considered as a developmental aberration with a theory that the same origin and that the ectopic choroid is formed by metaplasia of the ependymal rest.

132.4 Pathology

The histopathology and the immunohistochemical exam showed a normal choroid plexus consisting of a single layer of choroid epithelium arranged in microvillar patter with a microvascular care. Immunohistochemical staining showed with glia

Abstracted and reported by Dwarakanath et al. (2005)

I.M. Eltorai, *Rare Diseases and Syndromes of the Spinal Cord*,
DOI 10.1007/978-3-319-45147-3_132

fibrillary acid protein and epithelial membrane architecture suggestive of a normal choroid plexus confirming the ectopic choroid plexus nature.

132.5 Case Report

A 30-year-old man complained of progressive descending weakness from the upper to the lower limbs giving the neurological picture of tetraparesis. There was disassociated sensory loss between C2-C4 and sacral sparing

132.6 Diagnosis

Diagnosis is based on the following criteria:

- MRI of the spine: Expansion of the spinal cord; C6-T2, forming intramedullary cystic lesion: hypointense on T1 weighted images and hyperintense on T2 weighted images. More details show holocord syrinx.

132.7 Management

Since the patient had compression myelopathy microsurgery performed was through laminectomy C6-T2, the dura was expanded, opened, the cord distended, paper thin, myelotomy and syringostomy through the cyst, which was dissected and removed with its choroid content. Laminoplasty with miniplates and screws was done with uneventful post-operative course.

Reference

Dwarakanath S, Suri A, Mahapatra AK, Mehta VS, Sharma MC. Intramedullary ectopic choroid plexus: report of a rare case. Neurosurgery. 2005;56:869.

133 Myelopathy due to Fibrocartilaginous Spinal Cord Embolism

133.1 Definition

Fibrocartilaginous embolism (FCE) is a condition in which a fragment of the nucleus pulposa migrating to block spinal cord arterial supply, resulting in ischemic infarction.

133.2 Incidence

Initially, all cases of spinal FCE were diagnosed at autopsy studies. In 1961, Naiman et al., reported the first case of FCE in a young man who developed tetraparesis and respiratory failure after minor trauma while playing basketball. At autopsy a diffused embolic material of the nucleus pulposus in the anterior spinal cord and the basilar arterial systems. Since then nearly 40 autopsy proven cases have been reported. In 1991, a case was reported from the Massachusets General Hospital, who survived. Mateen et al. (2011), reviewed all the spinal cord infarction cases admitted to the Mayo Clinic over a 12 year period (1997–2004). They found out of 164 patients with acute spinal infarction 9 met the inclusion criteria for high likelihood of FCE (6 men and 3 women); median age: 46 years old (21–64); all patients were severely affected (Rankin Scale 4); mean time to evaluation 57 days. One patient also had cerebral infarct. All had no improvement from steroids.

Abstracted and reported by Mateen et al. (2011)

I.M. Eltorai, *Rare Diseases and Syndromes of the Spinal Cord*,
DOI 10.1007/978-3-319-45147-3_133

133.3 Etiology

Patients with FCE have exclusion of the following conditions:

- Aortic dissection
- Hypercoagulability state
- Intracardiac embolic source
- AVF
- Rhematalogic disorders
- Demyelinating disease
- Infections and metabolic conditions of the spinal cord (syphilis, HIV, vitamin B12, or Cu deficiencies)
- Systemic malignancy

Potential precipitating event were marked in 7/9 (78 %) of the cases:

- Motor vehicle accident without recognized back injury (n = 2)
- Heavy lifting (n = 3)
- Physical exertion (n = 1) (valsava's maneuver)
- Bending over (n = 1)

The onset of the symptoms was 6 h after the antecedent. Back pain was a common symptom in six of the patients; with a radicular component in three. Four patients had vascular risk factors.

133.4 Clinical Picture

The onset is sudden characterized by back pain associated with paresthesia of the upper and/or lower extremities, resulting in paraparesis or tetraparesis with sphincter dysfunction. Patient's history should be negative for trauma, anticoagulants, blood dyscrasias, etc.

133.5 Diagnosis

Diagnosis is based on the following criteria:

1. Clinical history and findings.
2. MRI studies in nine patients demonstrate the evolution of MRI findings from herniated disk material on initial imaging to longitudinally extensive infarction on subsequent imaging.
3. CSF analysis was only remarkably showed elevated protein in six patients (53–90 mg/dl)

4. Negative for oligoclonal banding, hyperglycorrhachia, xathochromia, or other markers for inflammatory or infectious diseases.
5. Platelet count, international normalized ratio (INR), activated partial thromboplastin time (aPPT) were all normal.

Differntial Diagonsis include prolonged arterial hypotension, spinal disk prolapse or herniation, thrombo-occlusive aortic disease, vasculitis, systemic lupus erythematous, antiphospholipid antibody syndrome, dissecting aortic aneurysm, sickle cell anemia, infections, etc.

133.6 Management

There is no treatment that has an impact on the patient's symptoms in the acute period. Common treatments include IV steroids, IV heparin, and plasma exchange. The current understanding of FCE is based on case reports, nearly all discovered at autopsy; therefore the prognosis of FCE is overwhelmingly pessimistic.

Reference

Mateen FJ, Monrad PA, Hunderfund AN, et al. Clinically suspected fibrocartilaginous embolism: clinical characteristics, treatments, and outcomes. Eur J Neurol. 2011;18(2):218–25.

134 Intravascular Papillary Endothelial Hyperplasia

134.1 Definition

Also known as intravascular papillary endothelial hyperplasia (IPEH), Masson's vegetant hemangioendothelioma. Benign proliferation of endothelial cells, which presents as slow growing, tender, violaceous cutaneous mass on the head, neck, fingers, or trunk. Deep tumors occur as intramuscular hemangiomas, which may be expansile and compressive. Involvement of CNS is rare, usually on top of hematoma from cavernous hemangioma, also may complicate intracerebral hemorrhage.

134.2 Incidence

Only one case of spinal cord compression (T6) by Porter et al., in 1995 and one other case of cauda equina compression reported by Taricco et al. in (1999). Ali et al., in 1994, had one case of hemangioma infiltrating the spinal meninges, causing cord compression.

134.3 Etiology

Lesion is benign and considered to be a neoplasm by some authors and a benign proliferation of endothelial cells by others. The mass occurs in certain pathological conditions:

- On top of a thrombosis, which is organized
- May develop in normal vessels

Abstracted from Taricco et al. (1999)

I.M. Eltorai, *Rare Diseases and Syndromes of the Spinal Cord*,
DOI 10.1007/978-3-319-45147-3_134

- Vascular lesions include cavernous angioma, hemangioma, pyogenic granuloma
- On top of an organized hematoma
- Endothelial basic fibroblast growth factor secretion, which stimulates endothelial cell proliferation.

134.4 Pathology

The lesion is exclusively intravascular. It may present in different morphologies:

- Vascular channels separated by fibrous septa with single endothelial cell layer
- Large blood spaces filled with papillary structures composed of a cord of connective tissue and single layer of endothelial cells
- Fibrous connective tissue, which narrow vascular channels course and vascular buds bearing a single layer of plump endothelium

Signs of malignancy are necrosis, mitosis, and nuclear pleomorphism are lacking.

134.5 Immunohistochemistry

IPEH reacts to Factor VII, CD34 and CD32 corresponding to the endothelial cells proliferative component

134.6 Clinical Picture

Although many intracranial IPEH have been described, only three cases involving the spinal cord; in the case by Porter et al., at T6 and Taricco et al. (1999), at the cauda equina. Neurological picture depends on the lever of compression, giving sensory, motor, and sphincter dysfunction

134.7 Diagnosis

Diagnosis based on:

1. Clinical picture and physical exam
2. X-ray may not show tumor
3. CT scan with enhancement shows hyperdense tumor inside the spinal cord

4. MRI of the spinal cord: T1 weighted-images show an isointense nural parenchyma with strong homogenous gadolinium enhancement. T2 weighted-images showed increased signal intensity

It should be differentiated from angiosarcoma, hemangioma, Kaposi's sarcoma, etc., seen in immunohistochemistry.

134.8 Management

The management of IPEH is complete surgical excision to prevent recurrence and unnecessary radiotherapy. Verification of pathology after surgery by histochemistry is important to rule our more aggressive sarcomas. The outcome in the three reported cases was favorable.

Reference

Taricco MA, Vieira JO, Machado AG, Ito FY. Intravascular papillary endothelial hyperplasia causing cauda equina compression: case report. Neurosurgery. 1999;45(6):1478–80.

135 Posterior Spinal Artery Syndrome

135.1 Definition

This syndrome is a result of spinal cord infarction involving the posterior section of the cord, viz: posterior arteries, bilateral posterior horns, and posterior segments of bilateral lateral columns.

135.2 Incidence

Only a few cases have been reported, which the authors reviewed in the discussion. So far 30 cases have been reported.

135.3 Etiology

The incidence of spinal cord infarction is much less than the cerebral infarction due to the fact the posterior spinal artery has many autonomic branches and is less liable to atherosclerosis than the cerebral vessels. There are four to ten anterior radicular arteries and ten to twenty-three posterior radicular arteries. Whereas cerebral infarction occurs in the elderly, the spinal category occurs in the young and has better prognosis than the cerebral type. Until 1950s, meningovascular syphilis was the main cause of the syndrome. Other causes are thromboembolism, arteriosclerosis, dissecting aortic aneurysm, and minor indirect trauma to the posterior spinal arteries, intrathecal therapeutic phenol injection. In many cases no occlusion was detected in the posterior spinal artery (PSA). With MRA some acute cases are diagnosable.

Abstracted from Matsubayashi et al. (2013)

I.M. Eltorai, *Rare Diseases and Syndromes of the Spinal Cord*,
DOI 10.1007/978-3-319-45147-3_135

135.4 Pathology

The upper thoracic and cervical spinal cord was much swollen and soft. The gray and white matter were indistinguishable. The lower thoracic limbs and sacral cord were normal. There was demyelination of the posterior columns bilaterally and in all spinal cord segments. The axons were in the affected segments. There was also mild demyelination and lymphocytic infiltration in the lateral columns. There was marked granulation tissue formation. There was mild glial nuclear atypia. There were no changes to the anterior columns or anterior horns. There were no thrombosis or cartilage emboli in posterior or anterior spinal arteries. There was no ateriovenous malformation (AVM) or mass lesions or aortic aneurysm, no hematoma, or neoplasia in the rest of the body.

135.5 Clinical Picture

An 84-year-old Japanese woman presented after a fall with a bruise of the head and neck. Neck pain increased and she developed weakness and sensory loss of the lower limbs. Five days after the fall she developed severe weakness of all extremities and rectovesical dysfunction. Deep tendon reflexes were very weak. No superficial sensory loss. MRI showed on T1-weighted images marked swelling of the spinal cord and on T2-weighted images elongation of the cervicothoracic spinal cord. Cerebral spinal fluid showed high protein content 813 mg/100 ml and glucose 66 mg/100 ml. No atypical cells.

135.6 Management

Intravenous methylprednisolone 1000 mg/day; her neurological status worsened and she developed respiratory failure and died 6 weeks after the onset.

Reference

Matsubayashi J, Tsuchiya K, Shimizu S, et al. Posterior spinal artery syndrome showing marked swelling of the spinal cord: a clinico-pathological study. J Spinal Cord Med. 2013;36(1):31–5.

136 Myelopathy due to Spinal Cord Vasculitis

136.1 Definition

Spinal cord vasculitis is a vascular pathology in the spinal cord leading to myelopathy and it is a part of the central nervous system vasculitis.

136.2 Incidence

According to Salvarani et al., primary CNS vasculitis (PCNSV) is uncomomon disease, which lesions are limited to the brain and spinal cord. The authors retrospectively identified 101 consecutive patients with PCNSV in a series at the Mayo Clinic. Spinal cord involvement was documented in five cases. The spinal cord symptoms developed before the cerebral symptoms in one, concurrently in two and after the cerebral symptoms in two. Of the five cases three were men; the median age was 39. The interval before diagnosis was 1 month or less.

136.3 Etiology

The pathogenesis of the disease is not clear. It was presumed as an inflammatory condition, which responds to corticosteroids. Rare cases have been linked to non-vascular causes, e.g. Hodgkin's lymphoma, Hashimoto thyroiditis, and drug-induced allergenic reactions.

Abstracted from Salvarani et al. (2008)

I.M. Eltorai, *Rare Diseases and Syndromes of the Spinal Cord*,
DOI 10.1007/978-3-319-45147-3_136

136.4 Pathology

From the case reported:

There is vascular wall inflammation and destruction and granulomatous formation. Destruction of the vascular basement membrane was seen by periodic acid-Schiff stain for vasculitis, necrotizing vasculitis, and granulomas were encountered. Cordal or caudal infarcts were seen in two patients. Ropper et al., reported an autopsy case. They described the cerebral pathology, which caused the mortality. In the spinal cord small areas of cavitation, some with hemosiderin loaded with macrophages were seen. Foci of the myelomalacia in other areas and pallor are also seen. Occlusion of the subpial vessels with fibrinous material. Thickened vascular walls with subintimal eccentric proliferation of fibrinous tissue. Other finding included endothelial swelling and disruption, and necrosis of the vessel wall. The infiltrate was composed of CD3 and less of CD8 and hemorrhagic infarcts. Viral tests were all negative.

136.5 Clinical Picture

The condition is subacute. It starts with numbness of the feet, weakness of the lower extremities, which creeps upwards, stumbling, inability to walk, sensory loss, and incontinence. The condition progressed to paraparesis in a few weeks. It may be complicated by cerebral vasculitis. Neurological exam shows weakness or paralysis, spasticity, increased tendon reflexes, and sensory loss. The thoracic cord is most commonly involved; the cauda may be involved as well. There is no history of infection or other know vascular causes

136.6 Diagnosis

Diagnosis is based on:

1. Clinical findings
2. MRI of the spinal cord shows leptomeningeal enhancement
3. MRA shows vasculitis, may be with occlusion
4. Laboratory tests are negative for bacterial and viral diseases, CSF chemistry, cytology, microbiology, or virology

Vasculitis needs to be differentiated form sarcoidosis, connective tissue diseases, etc.

136.7 Management

Medcial treatment consists of:

1. Steroids include methylprednisolone, dexamethasone pulse therapy, oral prednisolone for followup
2. Immunosuppression medications
   (a) Cyclophosphamide
   (b) Azathioprine
   (c) Mycophenolate Mofetil

Plasma exchange, immunoglobulin, surgery are rarely indicated.

Reference

Salvarani C, Brown RD, Calamia KT, et al. Primary CNS vasculitis with spinal cord involvement. Neurology. 2008;70(24 Pt 2):2394–400.

Epidural Varix 137

137.1 Definition

Varices are abnormal persistently dilated, elongated, and tortuous spinal epidural veins. These varices may be asymptomatic, but in rare cases may present as radiculopathy or myelopathy.

137.2 Incidence

Spinal epidural varix causing neurologic compression is a rare entity. Gümbel et al. (1969), reported an incidence of 0.5 % of isolated nerve root compression caused by varices among 1091 cases of sciatica. Wong et al. (2003), reported 2 cases. Pekindril and Yaniz reported a case and reviewed the literature.

As regards to the myelopathy, the condition is extremely rare: Bapat and Metkar (2006), reported the first case of acute tetraplegia. Dickman et al. (1988), reported a case of myelopathy due to epidural varix.

137.3 Etiology

Epidural varicosities are of two categories: primary and secondary.

Primary epidural varices: these are extremely rare and they develop in the absence of a predisposing pathology (see Dickman et al. 1988) Hypothesis:

The epidural venous plexus is a network of veins in the epidural spaces of the whole spine from the cranium down to the sacrum. It is a valveless system which allows effective venous return by allowing reversal of the blood flow during pressure fluctuation with respiration, increased abdominal pressure as effort with

Abstracted from Bapat and Metkar (2006)

I.M. Eltorai, *Rare Diseases and Syndromes of the Spinal Cord*,
DOI 10.1007/978-3-319-45147-3_137

coughing, sneezing, valsalva maneuver, and also increased jugular vein pressure during neck movements and actions. The epidural pressure rises during these efforts to come back down when they are terminated. If these factors persist they may lead to primary varices.

Secondary varices are caused by:

- Congenital spinal anomalies: diastomyelia, AVF, dysplasia
- Spinal trauma leading to scaring
- Spinal stenosis and foramenal stenosis, deformity, stenosis
- Disk prolapse
- Vena cava obstruction or occlusion inferior vena cava (IVC) or superior vena cava (SVC) The details of IVC occlusion have been thoroughly reported by Paksoy and Gormus 2004.
- Abdominal masses compressing the IVC (see Paksoy and Gormus 2004): portal hypertension
  - Pregnancy: obesity and epidural lipomatosis
  - Jugular vein thrombosis or compression
  - Secondary to intracranial hypotension
  - Marfan's syndrome

137.4 Pathophysiology

Myelopathy or radiculopathy are caused by:

- Direct pressure by the ectatic varix as a space occupying lesion. The same varix on the root will cause radiculopathy.
- Venous congestion, especially in cases of IVC occlusion causes radicular pain.
- Hemorrhage from varix causes hematoma leading to pressure
- Intramural thrombosis

Acute irreversible neurologic deficit may occur as a result of variceal bleeding or an acute intramural thrombosis.

137.5 Clinical Picture

137.5.1 Myelopathy

This is a very rare condition. The typical case described by Bapat and Metkar:

Twenty-one year old man with inability to move the four extremities after an uneventful auto-rickshaw ride. He had no neck injury, no neck pain. He came in spinal shock, no cranial injury. Radiography of the spine was normal. MRI showed space occupying epidural lesion over the dura from C7-D1 causing cord compression and edema. The swelling was isointense on T1-weighted images and hypointensive with rim-enhancement on T2-weighted images. Laminectomy C7–D1 showed an epidural varix confirmed pathologically. 3 months later there was no recurrance and no masses, but the patient did not recover. At the site of the mass, there was myelomalacia and cystic degeneration on T1-weighted images. The authors explain the tetraplegia was the result of varix compression and the possibility of venous infarction.

137.5.2 Radiculopathy

Epidural varices involve the lumbar region most, followed by cervicothoracic region. The incidence has been 1–4 %. Gümbel et al. (1969), reported 0.5 % of isolated nerve root compression caused by varices among 1091 cases of sciatica. The pathophysiology is different from arteriovenous malformation AVM, which is intradural and telangiectatic. The condition may be associated with herniated disc, spinal stenosis, spondylolisthesis or spondylosis. Lumbar varices are distinct pathophysiological entity resulting in nerve root and thecal sac compression clinically indistinguishable from herniated disc. The herniated disc may be a causative factor of the varix. In a cadaver study, Hoyland et al., suggested that neural structures in the intervertebral foramen were commonly associated with compression and dislocation of large venous plexus and proposed that venous obstruction might be an important pathogenic mechanism in the development of perineural and intraneural fibrosis. Zimmerman et al., suggested that acute disc herniation might cause endothelial injury and venous thrombosis when resolved give the picture of a disappearing disc.

The symptoms are:

- Low back pain
- Radiation to the lower extremeties (sciatica)
- Muscle weakness
- Sensory changes
- Leg extension test is positive.

The differential diagnosis from disc herniation may be difficult and the two conditions may be combined. Hammer et al. (2003), reported six cases of epidural varices simulating herniated disc and could not be differentiated even by MRI, at surgery they found the varices surrounding the nerve roots. In disc prolapse the pain is intractable. The onset is acute after lifting weight or twisting of the spine. It does not respond much to rest, anti-inflammatory drugs or physical therapy.

With varix the pain in mostly constant and may settle spontaneously. Watanabe et al. 1997, reported a cases of epidural hematoma with disc prolapse accompanied by intermittent claudication. The bleeding was from Batson plexus without varices.

Chun et al., 2002 reported a case of symptomatic enlarged cervical anterior epidural venous plexus in a patient with Marfan's syndrome. They concluded that Marfan's syndrome might predispose the patient to enlargement of the cervical anterior epidural venous plexus secondary to vessel wall abnormality. In these patients spontaneous intracranial hypotension resulting in CSF leakage may be a cause (Albayaram and Yilmaz).

137.6 Diagnosis

Diagnosis is based on:

1. History
2. Neurological findings
3. Electromagnetic and nerve conduction studies
4. Imaging
5. Plain radiography
6. CT scan
7. MRI is difficult to interpret

137.7 Management

For symptomatic varices, coagulation ablation or excision is done through laminectomy. Herniated disc is removed at the same time. In secondary cases e.g. portal hypertension should be treated. Intradural varix has been reported, only one case by Moomis et al., L3–L5 laminectomy and L5 foraminotomy. Patient had complete resolution of back and right leg pain.

References

Bapat M, Metkar U. Epidural varix at the cervicothoracic junction: unusual cause of quadriplegia: a case report. Spine. 2006;31(3):E88–90.

Chun JY, Dillon WP, Berger MS. Symptomatic enlarged cervical anterior epidural venous plexus in a patient with Marfan syndrome. AJNR Am J Neuroradiol. 2002;23(4):622–4.

Dickman CA, Zabramski JM, Sonntag VK, Coons S. Myelopathy due to epidural varicose veins of the cervicothoracic junction Case report. J Neurosurg. 1988;69(6):940–1.

Gümbel U, Pia HW, Vogelsang H. [Lumbosacral vascular anomalies as the cause of ischialgia]. Acta Neurochir (Wien). 1969;20(2):131–51.

Hammer A, Knight I, Agarwal A. Localized venous plexi in the spine simulating prolapse of an intervertebral disc: a report of six cases. Spine. 2003;28(1):E5–12.

Paksoy Y, Gormus N. Epidural venous plexus enlargements presenting with radiculopathy and back pain in patients with inferior vena cava obstruction or occlusion. Spine. 2004;29(21):2419–24.

Watanabe N, Ogura T, Kimori K, Hase H, Hirasawa Y. Epidural hematoma of the lumbar spine, simulating extruded lumbar disk herniation: clinical, discographic, and enhanced magnetic resonance imaging features. A case report. Spine. 1997;22(1):105–9.
Wong CH, Thng PL, Thoo FL, Low CO. Symptomatic spinal epidural varices presenting with nerve impingement: report of two cases and review of the literature. Spine. 2003;28(17):E347–50.

Part IX

Miscellaneous Causes of Myelopathy

Paraplegia of Cerebral Origin 138

138.1 Definition

Paraplegia of cerebral origin is due to insufficient blood perfusion of both paracentral areas.

138.2 Incidence and Etiology

Cerebral paraplegia can be cause by:

1. Bilateral lacunar ischemia, especially with bilateral angioma of the paracentral area
2. Parasagittal or falx angioma or arteriovenous malformation (AVM)
3. Frontoparietal midline depressed fracture
4. Bilateral subdural hematoma
5. Rupture of anterior communicating artery aneurysm (ACoA), according to Mauri et al., one case in 200 intracranial aneurysms. According to Greene et al. , the most frequent location of ruptured intracranial aneurysms in the anterior cerebral artery (ACA) and the ACoA is the most frequent site for rupture ACA distribution aneurysms. Greene et al. , had seven cases of ruptured ACoA aneurysm with subarachnoid hemorrhage, amongst 101 cases of sudarachnoid hemorrage seen at 5 year period. Morioka et al., reported a case of ruptured aneurysm of a third or accessory anterior cerebral artery or the midline artery of the corpus callosum. The etiology of the aneurysms is general. Rupture of ACoA leads to ischemia associated with vasospasm and subarachnoid hemorrhage.

Abstracted from Greene et al. (1995)

I.M. Eltorai, *Rare Diseases and Syndromes of the Spinal Cord*,
DOI 10.1007/978-3-319-45147-3_138

138.3 Pathology

Rupture of ACoA causes defective perfusion and is accompanied by spasm, which leads to ischemia of both paracentral areas with sudden appearance of paraparesis. The subarachnoid hemorrhage may accumulate in the interhemispheric fissure leading to parasagittal ischemia. Pathologically there are laminar neurons in the parasagittal distribution of ACA. Microvascular ischemia results from vasospasm. Pankon et al., suggested that the leaked blood accumulates in the posterior fossa, an upper cervical compression of the pyramidal tracts of the brain stem. With the aneurismal rupture there is massive subarachnoid hemorrhage and hydrocephalus. There may be also parenchymal hemorrhage.

138.4 Clinical Picture

Various clinical manifestations of rupture of ACoA were reported. According to Greene et al. , "although these reported clearly document the acute or subacute onset of leg weakness after ruptured ACA aneurysm no precise clinicopathological description exists." The case starts with headache, frontal or occipital or both, dizziness, veiled consciousness, and paresis of the lower limbs, which continues to paraplegia, usually no sensory or sphincteric trouble. The patient is usually hyporeflexic initially and turns to be hyperreflexic.

138.5 Diagnosis

Diagnosis is based on:

1. Patient history: headache and acute or subacute onset of paraplegia.
2. Neurological exam: areflexic paraplegia usually sensory and sphincter changes are absent initially
3. CT scan of the head: shows a subarachnoid hemorrhage with interhemispheric hematoma which may be seen at the genu and the body of corpus callosum according to Morioka et al., in a case of aneurysm of the median artery of the corpus callosum. Ischemic hypodense areas may be seen in the frontoparietal parasagittal regions.
4. Vessel angiography: shows the aneurysm in the anterior communicating or the accessory anterior cerebral artery (triplicate). For more details see Morioka et al. Spasms of both ACAs is noticeable.
5. CSF: xanthochroma or free blood
6. MRA:

138.6 Management

The offending cause should be dealt with accordingly. Early as possible management with craniotomy, clipping of the neck of the aneurysm, and evacuation of the hematoma. Recovery from paraplegia is expected totally or partially; however, patients tend to have postoperatively, according to Greene et al. , what they called 3-H therapy that is hemodilutional intravascular volume expansion to prevent vasospasms (hemodilution-hypertensive-hypervalemic triple-H). Prevention of DVT is important by compression socks, and low-molecular heparin. Patients tend to have frontal lobe manifestations, e.g. affective disorders and loss of memory, but they resolved with the recovery of motor power slowly in months, but not in all patients.

138.7 Prognosis

Greene et al. , from January 1987 – December 1992, 5 years, reviewed 655 patients admitted to Barrows Neurological Institute with aneurismal subarachnoid hemorrhage (SAH) of these 101 patients had ACoA aneurysm as the source of the bleeding. After workup all medically stable patients who had SAH had craniotomy and aneurysm clipping within 24–48 h of admission. All patients were treated with hemodilutional intravascular volume expansion for prevention of cerebral vascular spasm. When angiography revealed vasospasm hemodilutional-hypertensive-hypervolimic therapy was instituted (triple-H) and was continued for 7–14 days. Amongst the 101 patients with ruptured ACoA had paraplegia or paraparesis they had prophylaxis for deep vein thrombosis (DVT). Hydrocephalus shown by CT was drained externally. After surgery paraparesis persisted; however, consequent follow-up showed progressive resolution of the paresis. In spite of the precautions against DVT seven patients developed DVT resulting in two deaths from pulmonary embolism, of the remaining five two patients completely recovered motor power and two of them had mild spasticity, and one patient had persistent one limb weakness.

Reference

Greene KA, Marciano FF, Dickman CA, et al. Anterior communicating artery aneurysm paraparesis syndrome: clinical manifestations and pathologic correlates. Neurology. 1995;45(1):45–50.

139 Decompression Sickness

139.1 Definition

According to DH Elliott (1994), decompression sickness (DCS) is an illness, which arises from the presence of bubbles formed from gasses that have become dissolved in the tissues of the body during sojourn at raised environmental pressure. There are a number of syndromes, which are considered to be typical of DCS, but this will focus on the spinal cord syndrome. There is an overlap of manifestations and pathogenic mechanism between DCS and the condition of arterial gas embolism (AGE) secondary to decompression damage of the lungs (pulmonary barotrauma).

139.2 Incidence

Spinal cord involvement occurs in 10–30 % of the reported cases of DCS.

139.3 Etiology

DCS normally results from a rapid ascent from depth. Upon the rapid ascent and decompression the gas previously forced under pressure into the blood bubbles back out into the blood stream and tissues – a process equivalent to opening a champagne bottle. The severity of the syndrome depends on the depth and duration of the dive.

Abstracted from multiple sources

I.M. Eltorai, *Rare Diseases and Syndromes of the Spinal Cord*,
DOI 10.1007/978-3-319-45147-3_139

139.4 Patholophysiology

The cause of spinal cord ischemia may be due to:

1. The gas bubbles entering the arterial circulation causing embolic vents in the spinal cord; thus, causing an infarct resulting in neurological symptoms.
2. Venous infarction due to venous congestion.
3. Bubbles dissect the tissue plains to reach areas with sufficient pressure to occlude the blood flow.
4. The theory of space-occupying lesions but experimentally there was no evidence of space occupying lesions in animals and only 0.5 % of the cords studied.

Thus, to date, the precise mechanisms of the spinal cord injury in DCS remains to be elucidated in the neurological dysfunction of the spinal cord resulting from DCS. AGE is a result of pulmonary barotrauma with escape of alveolar air into the circulation. The neurological symptoms may be common to both DCS and AGE. AGE may or may not be associated with manifestations due to extravascular gas of alveolar origin in the pleural cavity, mediastinum, or other soft tissues. The pathology of DCS in man is not fully known because the condition is usually transient and not accurately reproducible in animals. In postmortem of man the bubbles are artifacts. The pathology of the bubble is simply by mechanical expansion or surface activity at the blood gas interface. There is stimulation of platelet aggregation at the surface of the intravascular bubble. Activation of compliment, Hageman factor, and other enzyme groups sometimes lead to shock; the bubbles will cause neurological dysfunction and mechanical block.

139.5 Clinical Picture

The diver gets pain in the back or neck, numbness of the extremities, weakness or paralysis, loss of sensation especially to vibration and position, and loss of bladder and bowel control. There may be evidence of decompression sickness I namely pruritis rash, cutis marmorata, bends, and edema due to lymphatic obstruction. The onset may start with nausea, sickness and even shock manifestations. There may be ear barotraumas; however, pulmonary manifestations and cardiovascular manifestations may be undetectable in the beginning.

139.6 Diagnosis

Diagnosis is base on:

The clinical picture is usually evident. Ultrasound may detect the bubbles in the vessels or the heart. An x-ray of the chest may show a pneumothorax. A MRI will show swollen spinal cord due to edema, hyperintense T2 signal occasionally may show evidence of hemorrhage. In the later stages it shows scarring and atrophy of the cord. Neurophysiological studies will confirm spinal cord deficit.

139.7 Management & Prognosis

Rapid recompression according to the United States Navy tables by a specialist is the key for reversal of DCS. Medicines, such as heparin, asprin, or corticosteroids may be tried following HBO, yet they are not as successful as the widely used method of recompression. Chronic cases should be referred to a spinal cord medicine center. The essential thing is prevention of DCS.

Immediate recompression under supervision of deep-sea diving medicine specialist is very important and may resolve the condition. Any delay will take the case to permanent paralysis.

Reference

Elliott DH. Decompression Sickness. In: Hyperbaric Medicine Practice. Flagstaff: Best Publishing Company; 1994. p. 312–26.

Bibliography

Francis TJ, et al. Arterial gas embolism as a pathophysiologic mechanism for spinal cord decompression sickness. Undersea Biomed Res. 1989;16(6):439–51.
Hills BA, James PB. Spinal decompression sickness: mechanical studies and a model. Undersea Biomed Res. 1982;9(3):185–201.
McCormac J, et al. Spinal myelopathy resulting from decompression sickness: MR findings in a case and review of the literature. Emerg Radiol. 2002;9(4):240–2.
Tournebise H, et al. Paraplegia and decompression sickness. Paraplegia. 1995;33(11):636–9.

Exertional Myelopathy due to Congenital Kyphosis Type II

140

140.1 Definition

Congenital kyphosis of three types:

- Type I is a failure of formation leading to a hemivertebra. This is the most common type leading to the most rapid progression of kyphosis.
- Type II is a less common and is due to failure of segmentation leading to a bar.
- Type III is a mixed form of combined type I and II.

140.2 Incidence

McMaster and Sing reviewed 112 consecutive case and found:

- 68 patients with type I
- 24 patients with type II
- 12 patients with type II
- 8 were unclassified

Khanna, et al., reviewed the literature until 2002 and found no cases of type II showing myelopathy. The most progressive was Type II followed by type I; out of 10 patients with myelopathy 7 were type I.

140.3 Etiology

There is no genetic code as of 2002.

Abstracted from Khanna et al. (2002) and McMaster and Singh (1999)

I.M. Eltorai, *Rare Diseases and Syndromes of the Spinal Cord*,
DOI 10.1007/978-3-319-45147-3_140

140.4 Pathology

Compression myelopathy depends on the type, rate of progression, and the age. In type II the rate of progression is 1° per year, before the age of 10 and 1.5° per year after 10 years of age. The case reported is exertional myelopathy.

140.5 Clinical Picture

Depending on the degree and the progression of the congenital kyphosis, myelopathy may be preceded by trauma; the picture is that of an upper motor neuron paraparesis. The only case described in congenital kyphosis type II by Khanna et al., briefly presented:

A 17 year old boy presenting with 3 year history of progressive worsening mid-thoracic congenital kyphosis. During exercise he noticed numbness of the posterior aspects of the legs and wobbly sensation of the lower extremities, leading him to discontinue his sports activities. After running for ten minutes he developed clumsy wide-based myelopathic gait. Magnetic resonance imaging (MRI) showed the spinal ford draped over the vertebral body T10. This may be explained by mechanical or circulatory compromise caused by exercise. At surgery, indentations in the spinal cord were seen at T9 and T10 and minor disc protrusion were noticed at these levels.

140.6 Management

Until 5 years of age posterior spinal fusion is recommended. After 5 years and a curvature more than 50° circumferential fusion is recommended. Kim et al. (2001) recommended surgery in the following statement:

Congenital kyphosis is a rare spinal deformity that us usually progressive without surgical intervention. Progression of the deformity may lead to paraplegia and cardiopulmonary dysfunction. Therefore prompt recognition and treatment of this deformity is preferred. Early surgical intervention is best in congenital kyphosis.

In cases of myelopathy, anterior decompression and stabilization are required possibly with posterior stabilization depending on the degree of the kyphosis.

References

Khanna N, Molinari R, Lenke L. Exertional myelopathy in type 2 congenital kyphosis. Spine. 2002;27(22):E488–92.

Kim YJ, Otsuka NY, Flynn JM, Hall JE, Emans JB, Hresko MT. Surgical treatment of congenital kyphosis. Spine. 2001;26(20):2251–7.

Mcmaster MJ, Singh H. Natural history of congenital kyphosis and kyphoscoliosis. A study of one hundred and twelve patients. J Bone Joint Surg Am. 1999;81(10):1367–83.

Thoracic Compression Myelopathy due to Facet Joint Osteophyte

141

141.1 Definition

Thoracic compression myelopathy is due to several diseases e.g. trauma, degenerative diseases, spondylolisthesis, and neoplasms primary or secondary. A solitary osteophyte of a faceted joint is a rare cause of compression myelopathy.

141.2 Incidence

The author reports the only case in the literature.

141.3 Etiology

The cause of the osteophyte is unknown, probably a degenerative disease, although it is solitary and it is reported in a 63 year old man.

141.4 Pathology

The osteophyte was arising from the posterior aspect of the facetted joint on the right side of the facetted joint of T9-T10 projecting in a beak-like fashion towards the dura.

Abstracted from Abhaykumar et al. (2002)

I.M. Eltorai, *Rare Diseases and Syndromes of the Spinal Cord*,
DOI 10.1007/978-3-319-45147-3_141

141.5 Histology

No cartilage cap: the picture is that of an osteophyte.

141.6 Clinical Picture

Back pain, may radiate up the neck, muscle weakness and ataxic gait. The patient had no sphincter dysfunction; however, there were exaggerated knee and ankle reflexes.

141.7 Diagnosis

Diagnosis based on:

- Neurological examination
- Plain radiography: an anterior osteophyte at T9-T10 level
- MRI: showed an osteophyte arising from the posterior element of T9-T10 protruding towards the dura.
- CT scan: showed the osteophyte from the T9-T10 facet joint on the right side.

141.8 Management

Laminectomy was done and the osteophyte removed piecemeal down to the facet. Complete recovery was attained.

Reference

Abhaykumar S, Tyagi A, Towns GM. Thoracic vertebral osteophyte-causing myelopathy: early diagnosis and treatment. Spine. 2002;27(14):E334–6.

142 Hysterical Paralysis

142.1 Definition

According to Stedman's Medical Dictionary, hysteria is defined as: a somatoform (psychoneurotic or psychosomatic) disorder in which there is an alteration or loss of physical functioning that suggests a physical disorder such as paralysis of an arm or disturbance of vision, but that is apparently an expression of a psychological conflict or need; a diagnostic term referable to wide variety of psychogenic symptoms involving disorder of function, which may be mental, sensory, motor, or visceral. Other hysterical conversion reactions do occur in different manifestations, unexplained monoplegia, hemiplegia, tetraplegia, seizures, or aphonia.

142.2 Incidence

Hysterical paralysis is very rarely reported. The epidemiology of psychogenetic disorders has not been well studied. It is estimated that 1–9 % of the general population depending on different criteria of diagnosis. According to Letonoff et al., conversion disorder is reported in 5 to 22 per 100,000 individuals in the general population.

142.3 Etiology

Historically Charcot, Frued Gowers, and Head are the pioneer contributors to the knowledge of organic and neurological disorders. According to the American Psychiatric Association's Diagnosic and Statistcal Manual of Mental Disorders, 4th ed., Text Revision, the following criteria must be met to fulfill the diagnosis of conversion disorder:

Abstracted from Letonoff et al. (2002)

I.M. Eltorai, *Rare Diseases and Syndromes of the Spinal Cord*,
DOI 10.1007/978-3-319-45147-3_142

- one or more symptoms affecting voluntary motor or sensory function suggest a medical condition;
- psychological factors are judged to be associated with the symptoms because the initiation or exacerbation is preceded by conflicts or stressors;
- the symptom is not intentionally produced or feigned;
- the symptom cannot, after appropriate investigation, be explained by a medical condition, as direct effects of a substance, or as a culturally sanctioned behavior;
- the symptom causes clinically significant distress or impairment that warrants a medical evaluation;
- the symptom is not limited to pain or sexual dysfunction, does not occur exclusively during the course of a somatization disorder, and is not better accounted for by another mental disorder.

142.4 Clinical Picture

Typically the patient is a young adult; more commonly female (2:1), usually disadvantaged socio-economically with limited education and may experience difficulty in expressing their distress. Most often there is an underlying disorder such as depression, or an overwhelming stressor, which the patient cannot cope with. They may have psychiatric disorder, mood disorder, and chronic pain with use of narcotics. Long-term disorders may be associated with this psychogenic condition. The condition may develop after severe emotional trauma or after a spinal trauma without neurological injury. Sometimes paraplegia is extracted from a paraplegic they know or encountered somewhere.

142.5 Diagnosis

A diagnosis of conversion disorder should be made only after a thorough medical assessment and appropriate laboratory workup to rule out neurological disorder. Hysterical paralysis may develop after surgery, medical procedure, or other medical conditions. One has to keep in mind the medicolegal responsibility and the outcome of the patient's condition. One should not save any investigation modality to rule out organic neurogenic condition. The decision should be made by a team, particularly with a neurologist, psychiatrist, psychologist, and if need be a neurosurgeon, orthopedic surgeon, or medical specialist.

It should also be known that the symptoms of the motor and sensory loss as well as sphincter dysfunction are referred to as pseudoneurological. The criteria for pseudoneurlogic paralysis are:

- Contradictory physical signs such as lack of flaccid muscle tone and normal reflexes in upper motor neuron lesions

- Changing sensory deficit and sensory level
- Patchy nonanatomical sensory loss distribution

However, some motor function may be noticed if the patient is distracted or getting up to be dressed. The patient may panic, showing tachycardia and hyperventilation.

Imaging and neurophysical studies should rule our true neurologic paraplegia, including magnetic resonance imaging (MRI), somatosensory evoked potentials (SSEPs), motor evoked potentials (MEPs), and if needed computed tomography (CT).

One should not be offended since the patient may express dissatisfaction with the medical exam and may ask bizarre questions (such as "Where is your medical license?" or "What is your training?")

Intravenous sodium amytal has been used in difficult cases to confirm the psychogenic diagnosis without equivocation.

With the negative laboratory test, still the patient should not be labeled as a malingerer. Instead remember, the patient is coping unconsciously with a stressful situation in an abnormal way.

142.6 Prognosis

After exclusion of organic neurological disease, the patient will be treated by a psychology team, which will get him or her to a certain degree of recovery. Relapses may occur and the patient should be watched periodically to avoid the suicidal tendencies.

142.7 Management

A definitive plan should be made for the patient. A sympathetic, non-adverse, and non-punitive attitude is necessary in order to have a trusting patient-physician relationship. Team involvement and interest in the patient's condition is essential for recovery. Comorbid psychiatric conditions should be treated to avoid suicidal attempts.

Follow-up visits are important to find the stressful situations that precipitated the paralysis. The patient should be encouraged to cope with his or her condition to avoid frequent visits to the emergency room. In some cases, there is complete resolution especially where the precipitating factors are eliminated. In others, it will be difficult especially with hypochondriacs.

Helpful interventions include:

- Antidepressants
- Stress management

- Cognitive behavioral therapy
- Life style changes
- Rehabilitation
- Social activities
- Relaxation sessions
- Support from family

Therapists and a group are helpful to have the patient develop the belief and assumption that he or she can modify their symptoms.

Follow-up routinely is needed even if the patient does not want to, to avoid recurrence, worsening psychological condition or evaluation of an organic disease.

Reference

Letonoff EJ, Williams TR, Sidhu KS. Hysterical paralysis: a report of three cases and a review of the literature. Spine. 2002;27(20):E441–5.

Differential Diagnosis: Hypermagnesemia

143

Severe hypermagnesemia is rare in individuals with normal renal function and in dialysis patients. Although severe hypermagnesemia may be fatal, two case reports here illustrate severe hypermagnesemia causing quadriparesis, induced by abuse of a laxative and antacids containing magnesium.

143.1 Case Report #1

This first reported case was in 1989 by Castelbaum et al. Briefly the authors had a 56-year-old woman known to have hypertension and diabetes mellitus for years. She developed generalized muscular weakness in the last several months: blood pressure 230/120 mm Hg, was normalized by IV Na nitroprusside. On the third hospital day she became lethargic, bradycardic, and diaphoretic. On the sixth hospital day she passed to respiratory arrest. She became anuric: BUN 97 mg/dL, creatine 7.4 mg/dL. She was put on a ventilator. She was alert with facial diplegia, tetraparesis, and areflexic with positive Babinski's signs.

Laboratory findings:

- Na: 121mEg/L
- Chloride: 86mEg/L
- BUN: 120 mg/dL
- Creatine: 10 mg/dL
- Phosphate: 7.5 mg/dL
- Magnesium: 8.4 mg/dL
- Glucose: 295 mg/dL

Abstracted and reported by Castelbaum et al. (1989)

I.M. Eltorai, *Rare Diseases and Syndromes of the Spinal Cord*,
DOI 10.1007/978-3-319-45147-3_143

Electrophysiological studies suggested myesthesia gravis and she had one plasma volume exchange. Magnesium fell to 2.6 mg/dL on day 8 and she started to improve and her ventilator was discontinued and was discharged. The cause of the hypermagnesemia was the ingestion of high magnesium containing cathartic over a long time, as well as magnesium containing antacids especially with renal insufficiency. The authors explain the pathophysiology that hypermagnesemia impairs the neuromuscular junction transmission by decreasing acetylcholine release from the presynaptic membrane by diminishing the depolarizing action of acetylcholine at the postsynaptic junction and by impairing the postsynaptic junction sensitivity to acetylcholine, as proved by the electrophysiologic studies.

143.2 Case Report #2

Jung et al. (2008) present a case of a 32-year-old woman with end stage renal disease due to diabetic neuropathy and on peritoneal dialysis. She presented with chronic constipation for 1 year, causing abdominal pain. She used a magnesium oxide powder laxative 3 g/day. She could not move extremities on day 8. The muscle strength was reduced to grade 1–2. No sensory changes or abnormal reflexes. Nerve conduction velocity showed severe neuropathy with blocked nerve conduction. She was given calcium gluconate 100 mg IV. Magnesium level was 10.5 mg/dL and peritoneal dialysis continued. Magnesium level dropped to 3.1 mg/dL. Quadriparesis disappeared and nerve conduction studies were normal. Magnesium cathartics were discontinued.

References

Castelbaum AR, Donofrio PD, Walker FO, Troost BT. Laxative abuse causing hypermagnesemia, quadriparesis, and neuromuscular junction defect. Neurology. 1989;39(5):746–7.

Jung GJ, Gil HW, Yang JO, Lee EY, Hong SY. Severe hypermagnesemia causing quadriparesis in a CAPD patient. Perit Dial Int. 2008;28(2):206.

Spinal Epidural Lubricant Grease 144

144.1 Definition

This is a traumatic injury of the neck and chest due to high pressure ejection from a hydraulic machine of a bulldozer. The fluid trickled into the spinal canal causing compression.

144.2 Incidence

One case described by Kalnins et al.

144.3 Etiology

While the patient was repairing a pneumatic device on a hydraulic injection instrument of a bulldozer. This resulted in a wound of the neck and upper right chest through the metal plug. The lubricant trickled through the posterior mediastinum into the epidural space down to the thoracic region.

144.4 Pathology

The lubricant trickled epidurally and caused inflammatory reactions, which subsequently led to compression myelopathy.

Abstracted from Kalnins et al. (2009)

I.M. Eltorai, *Rare Diseases and Syndromes of the Spinal Cord*,
DOI 10.1007/978-3-319-45147-3_144

144.5 Diagnosis

The picture is that of compression myelopathy of delayed onset similar to epidural hematoma. The diagnosis was based on:

1. MRI
2. CT Scan
3. Ultrasonography

144.6 Management

- Management of the neck and chest wounds
- Decompressive laminectomy where the lubricant was evacuated.

Reference

Kalnins AU, Geryk B, Olivero W, Kim TA. Spinal epidural lubricant grease collection mimicking traumatic spinal epidural hematoma. AJNR Am J Neuroradiol. 2009;30(10):1847–9.

145 Myelopathy due to Intramedullary Herniated Nucleus Pulposus

145.1 Definition

This is a case of thoracic myelopathy due to intramedullary herniation of the nucleus pulposus.

145.2 Incidence

This is the first reported case. Intradural herniation of intervertebral disc is extremely rare. Migration of disc fragments in the thoracic region into the dura have been described and usually are asymptomatic. It has been estimated that 15–20 % of the general population will have an incidental thoracic disc herniation on MRI. Symptomatic disc herniations are rare and most often affect females at the third through fifth decade of life. Intradural extramedullary thoracic disc herniations are exceptionally rare. They have high incidence of BSS. The incidence of intradural disc herniation in 7–20 %. Ninety two percent of intradural discs are found in the lumbar spine; 5 % thoracic; and 3 % in the cervical spine.

145.3 Pathology

The herniated nucleus pulposus passed through the posterior longitudinal ligament, through the dura and the pia-arachnoid into the spinal cord. The herniated nucleus pulposus appeared as a pearlescent granular mass; it was avascular, well defined and was adherent to the ventral pia mater. Pathological exam showed nucleus pulposus with cartilage fragments.

Abstracted and reported by Teufack et al. (2012).

I.M. Eltorai, *Rare Diseases and Syndromes of the Spinal Cord*,
DOI 10.1007/978-3-319-45147-3_145

145.4 Clinical Picture

Symptomatic cases usually present with Brown-Séquard syndrome. Compression of the corticospinal tract leading to ipsilateral paresis, compression of the posterior column leading to ipsilateral loss of tactile, vibration, and position senses. Compression of the crossed spinothalamic tract results in contralateral loss of pain and temperature sensations.

145.5 Case Report

A 66-year-old female patient presenting with weakness of both lower limbs, pain more in the right leg, sudden onset after yoga exercises two weeks before pain. Along with pain in the lower back, left lower limb hypesthesia and saddle area as well.

145.6 Diagnosis

Diagnosis is based on the following criteria:

1. Physical exam: difficulty in ambulation; weakness of right iliopsoas 4/5; pain sensation lost below T6 dermatome; reflexes were T2 exaggerated.
2. MRI of the thoracic spine: well defined solitary intramedullary mass (T7–T8) with ring enhancement and probable central necrosis, minimal cord expansion, and cord edema. There is disruption of the posterior longitudinal ligament and the ventral dura. finding air inside the dura on CT scan raises suspicion trans-dural herniation. In intramedullary disc fragment there is enhancement rim with contrast injection.
3. CT scan of chest, abdomen, and pelvis were all negative.

145.7 Management

Laminectomy under neuromonitoring and ultrasound, T6–T9 durotomy, midline myelotomy, gross total removal of the mass and wound repair. Patient recovered totally except some saddle hypesthesia. Post-op MRI showed complete resection of the mass.

Reference

Teufack S, Campbell P, Sharma P, et al. Thoracic myelopathy due to an intramedullary herniated nucleus pulposus: first case report and review of the literature. Neurosurgery. 2012;71(1):E199–202.

Spinal Cord Injury Without Radiologic Abnormality (Sciwora) 146

146.1 Definition

Spinal cord injury without radiographic abnormality (SCIWORA) is a spinal cord injury (SCI) without fractures or bony malalignment on either pain radiographs or computed tomography (CT) scans. SCIWORA is most commonly seen in the pediatric age group.

146.2 Incidence

It is reported with indefinite statistics with the literature varying widely from 4 to 66.7 % of all pediatric spinal cord injuries. SCIWORA is exceedingly rare in adults. In our brief literature search we found fewer than twenty cases up to 2003.

146.3 Etiology

The reasons for negative findings on radiography and CT scans are:

- The ligaments' elasticity and joint capsules
- Horizontal orientation of facet joints
- Anterior wedging of the vertebra bodies
- Relatively heavier head

These allow for excessive intersegment motion in flexion, extension, or distraction, resulting in neural injury without bony or overt ligamentous breaks. Rebound is easier to occur with elasticity of spinal ligaments and joint capsules in children. However, in adults the changes in ligaments and joint capsules makes them less

---

Abstracted from Gupta et al. (1999), Pang (2004)

I.M. Eltorai, *Rare Diseases and Syndromes of the Spinal Cord*,
DOI 10.1007/978-3-319-45147-3_146

elastic and changes in morphology of the vertebrae makes SCIWORA a rarity in the skeletally mature patient. Few reports have been published mostly on the cervical spine, and two in the thoracic spine, in the English literature. As regards to SCIWORA of the cervical spine it usually occurs in patients who have cervical spondylosis resulting in narrowing of the sagital diameter of the cervical spinal canal. In such cases hyperextension, minor trauma, even whiplash may cause SCI, either by pinching the cord between the osteophytes and the bulging of the interlaminal ligaments usually resulting in central cord syndrome. Other cord injuries may result in intramedullary hematoma or a contusion of the cord may be a consequence. In some cases, other changes in the adult spinal cord, such as, ossification of the posterior longitudinal ligament or ligamentum flavum and/or disc protrusion, contribute to injury of the cord with standard radiography negative results. In the adult, ischemia of the spinal cord may result in infarction, which occurs in aged patients and may be caused by very minor trauma, or after suppressed sneezing.

Injury to the thoracic cord without radiologic abnormality may be due to the fact that the thoracic spinal cord is supported by the rib cage. Samsani, et al., suggested that disruption of the spinal cord from T10 downwards was due to spinal hyperflexion injury. They postulated that sudden violent traction forces through the ciatic nerves are transferred proximal to the cauda equina, then to the conus medullaris, then to the fixed segments proximal to the conus. Which in turn disrupts the cord; this type of injury happens at high-speed trauma.

Another cause for SCIWORA may be occasionally due to incomplete radiological examination or misinterpretation of the films.

146.4 Clinical Picture

There is a history of trauma of different types, e.g. motor vehicle accidents, falls, sports injuries, etc. The neurological deficit depends on the magnitude of trauma and its level of injury. SCI may be manifested in the following pictures:

- complete transaction
- central cord syndrome
- incomplete injuries manifested by:
  - Brown-Séquard syndrome
  - Anterior spinal cord syndrome
  - Posterior spinal cord syndrome
  - Cauda equina injury

The symptoms depend on the magnitude and level of injury as well as associated injury to the rest of the body. There may be pain and tenderness at the level of injury. The neurological signs will be loss of sensation and motor power depending on the extent and level of the lesion. Paralysis may be complete or incomplete. Anesthesia, analgesia, thermal anesthesia, position agnosia, bladder and bowel disturbances are present. In the early stages of spinal shock the reflexes are absent, including the bulbocavernosus reflex; after the spinal shock the reflexes are exaggerated.

146.5 Diagnosis

SCIWORA should be followed by magnetic resonance imaging (MRI), CT scan, myelography, and angiography may be needed. MRI should be done in all cases for accurate diagnosis of the cord and its surroundings along with neurophysiological studies.

146.6 Management

Management depends on the level and extent of the injury. The presences or absence of associated injuries and the general condition of the patient should be conducted in specialized trauma centers, especially spinal injury department. Details of management can be consulted in books on SCI, with special emphasis on orthopedics and/or neurosurgery. With more sophisticated imaging techniques future cases of SCIWORA should not be encountered.

References

Gupta SK, Rajeev K, Khosla VK, et al. Spinal cord injury without radiographic abnormality in adults. Spinal Cord. 1999;37(10):726–9.

Pang D. Spinal cord injury without radiographic abnormality in children, 2 decades later. Neurosurgery. 2004;55(6):1325–42.

Surfer's Myelopathy 147

147.1 Definition

This is a novel pathological entity of the spinal cord was first described by Thompson et al. 2004. The condition is non-traumatic and occurs in inexperienced surfers, believed to be related to prolonged hyperextension of the spine in the prone position on a surf board.

147.2 Incidence

Thompson et al., reviewed the cases of surfers' injuries in Straub Clinic and Hospital in Honolulu, Hawaii between June 1998 and January 2003. They analyzed the cases of surfer's myelopathy and found nine patients affected by non-traumatic surfer's myelopathy. In 2007, Avilés-Hernández et al., also added one case from Hawaii. In 2011 Karabegovic et al., reported a case of a 25-year-old man. A case presented by Fessa and Lee in 2012; as well as cases by Shuster and Franchetto in 2011. Takakura et al., in 2013 presented three cases including only the second woman with surfer's myelopathy.

147.3 Etiology and Pathology

This myelopathy is non-traumatic and was found to be beginner surfers and mostly Japanese. According to Fessa and Lee, "The incidence of surfing acute injury is 0.6–1.1 injuries per 1000 surfing hours… Injuries associated with permanent neurological deficits are usually spinal fractures as a result of traumatic contact with the seabed."

Abstracted from multiple sources

I.M. Eltorai, *Rare Diseases and Syndromes of the Spinal Cord*,
DOI 10.1007/978-3-319-45147-3_147

Surfer's myelopathy is not associated with such traumas. Hawaii is a surfing site for decades and perhaps cases of surfing myelopathy were missed in the era before spinal cord imaging. Out of the sixteen cases collected, through thorough literature review, 14 were men and two were women. The age range was 19–37 years. There was no spinal disease in any of them or trauma. The common factor was non-experienced beginners; experienced surfers develop strong musculature of the back and neck as well as the arms. The weakness of these muscles in beginners and in demographic Japanese trainees contributes to hyperextension, which may cause vascular damage of the spinal cord; especially in the water-shed areas of the thoracic cord causing infarction and ischemia which may be reversible if the cause is only vasospasm. Under stress there may be increased blood coagulability, which may be a contributing factor. Complete or incomplete recovery is usually resulted; however, a permanent deficit (paraplegia) was seen in six of the cases.

Thompson et al., postulate that the surfer's myelopathy is due to:

- Arterial thrombosis and embolism leading to infarction
- Venous infarction
- Vasospasm of the Artery of Adamkiewicz
- Torsion of cauda by hyperextension
- Cartilage embolism
- Dehydration and increased coagulability in travelers since most of them were tourists
- Compression of inferior vena cava in prone position/more congestion by valsalva's maneuver due to paddling.

Takakura et al., theorized that a lower body mass index as their three patients were rather slight without a muscular build, with a thin and underdeveloped back musculature leaving them more susceptible to surfer's myelopathy.

147.4 Clinical Picture

Surfer's myelopathy is newly reported; it is difficult to have an annual model and there are pathological reports. The condition develops as a young man unexperienced diver, probably a lean body. They have hyperextended back and neck in the prone position on the surfboard and using their arms for paddling. Without trauma the patients develops pain in the back, followed by numbness of the lower extremities, weakness, sensory changes, paresis, and sometimes paraplegia and urinary changes.

147.5 Diagnosis

Diagnosis is based on the following criteria:

1. Physical exam:

1. Sensory changes up to the lumbar or thoracic levels in the form of hyperethesia, hyperalgesia, anesthesia, analgesia, hyperesthesia.
2. Weakness of the lower extremities in different grades even paraplegia.
3. The reflexes may be exaggerated and Babinski's may be positive.
4. The spine in all cases was within normal limits.
5. Abnormal somatosensory evoked potential was found in some patients

2. The history of inexperienced young healthy patients may be Japanese; his back and neck hyperextended, prone on the surf board, without any trauma, complaining of back pain, numbness, and weakness of the lower extremities.
3. MRI of the spinal cord: within 24-hours, MRI shows edema of the lower thoracolumbar cord with increased T2-weighted signal comparable with ischemia.
4. Plain radiography of the spinal rules out orthopedic pathology.
5. Routine lab test and possibly lumbar puncture.

147.6 Management

According to Thompson et al., most patients recovered spontaneously, except for one remained paraplegic. Thompson et al., are proposing ICU for these cases and MRI, spinal angiography, hemodynamics, hydration, increasing blood flow perhaps by hypertension and steroids

References

Avilés-hernández I, García-zozaya I, Devillasante JM. Nontraumatic myelopathy associated with surfing. J Spinal Cord Med. 2007;30(3):288–93.

Fessa CK, Lee BS. An Australian case of surfer's myelopathy. Clin J Sport Med. 2012;22(3):281–3.

Karabegovic A, Strachan-Jackman S, Carr D. Surfer's myelopathy: case report and review. CJEM. 2011;13(5):357–60.

Shuster A, Franchetto A. Surfer's myelopathy – an unusual cause of acute spinal cord ischemia: a case report and review of the literature. Emerg Radiol. 2011;18(1):57–60.

Takakura T, Yokoyama O, Sakuma F, Itoh R, Romero RR. Complete paraplegia resulting from surfer's myelopathy. Am J Phys Med Rehabil. 2013;92(9):833–7.

Thompson TP, Pearce J, Chang G, Madamba J. Surfer's myelopathy. Spine. 2004;29(16):E353–6.

Trampoline Spinal Cord Injuries in Pediatrics

148

148.1 Definition

Cervical spine injuries from trampoline sport in children are second only to football injuries and result in paraplegia and tetraplegia in approximately 5 % of all trampoline injuries.

148.2 Incidence

According to Brown and Lee, in 1998 trampolines were responsible for over 6500 pediatric cervical spine injuries. 8–12 % of trampoline injuries resulted in neurological damage.

148.3 Etiology

Spinal hyperextension injuries result from a failed backward flip and hyperflexion injury results from a failed forward flip.

148.4 Pathology

Different types of cervical injuries result causing fractures, subluxation, dislocation, and fracture dislocations, disc injuries. These may or may not result in cord injury or facet jumping. These are not prevented by spatters or use of padding because the jumper usually lands in the center of the trampoline mat.

Abstracted from Brown and Lee (2000)

I.M. Eltorai, *Rare Diseases and Syndromes of the Spinal Cord*,
DOI 10.1007/978-3-319-45147-3_148

148.5 Clinical Picture

Depending on the type of injury, generally there is neck pain, which may radiate, restriction of the neck movement, paresis, or complete paralysis, and in rare cases death ensues.

148.6 Diagnosis

Diagnosis is based on the following criteria:

history
neurological examination
x-ray findings

148.7 Management

Depends on the type of injury, from closed reduction to open surgery, halo vests different, or types of callus. In permanent neurogenic damage pediatric rehabilitation programs.

148.8 Prevention

It is recommended to ban trampolines, since even in the presence of spatters, safety harnesses, injuries cannot be prevented totally.

Reference

Brown PG, Lee M. Trampoline injuries of the cervical spine. Pediatr Neurosurg. 2000;32(4):170–5.

149 Traumatic Tethering

149.1 Definition

Tethering is to restrict or bind with or as if with a tether or rope, according to the Reader's Digest Encyclopedia Dictionary. Tethering of the spinal cord is a pathological condition of the cord due to its reliant or bundling the caudal position of the neural tube, most commonly due to occult spinal dysraphism, which encompasses one or more entities such as hypertrophied filum terminale, lipomeningoecle, a fibrotic filum terminale extending from the tip of the conus medullaris to the dura anchoring one to the other causing tethering. Other manifestations of dysraphism are lypomatous mass extending from the center of the spinal cord to the skin through the dystrophic vertebral arch. A common course of tethering is scar tissue formation binding the spinal cord and its roots of a previously operated menigomyelocele or lipomatous hamartoma to the repaired dura or skin.

149.2 Incidence

Developmental anomalies of the distal neural tube are increasingly encountered especially due to modern diagnostic measures. These can be consulted in textbooks of pediatric neurosurgery and orthopedics. The subject of the is presentation is a unique case of tethered cord after traumatic paraplegia resulting in tetraplegia. According to the authors Ragnarsson et al., the only case reported.

Abstracted from Ragnarsson et al. (1986)

I.M. Eltorai, *Rare Diseases and Syndromes of the Spinal Cord*,
DOI 10.1007/978-3-319-45147-3_149

149.3 Etiology

Progressive neurological deterioration after traumatic paraplegia is usually due to a syrinx or arachnoiditis or a second trauma. In absence of these tethered cord should be thought of. Flexion and extension of the neck poses more stretching and adherent cord.

149.4 Pathology

The mechanical effect of traction on the cord as shown by Barry et al. (1957), dissipates within five segments rostral to the point of tethering. In dysraphism the mechanism is due to traction as well as pressure. As a result of traction there is ischemia which leads to cord atrophy. Yamamda et al. (1981), demonstrated experimentally impairment of the mitochondrial oxidative process under traction. After release of the tethering the spinal cord blood flow improves as tested by laser Doppler (Schneider et al. 1993). The ischemic changes lead to atrophy as in the case reported.

149.5 Clinical Picture

The case reported by TS Ragnarsson et al. (1986), showed the following:

A 49 year old man with complete T5 paraplegia of 30 years duration over the last 10 years developed cervical myelopathy. A syrinx and arachnoiditis were ruled out. At operation the cord was found tethered and atrophic. Release of the tethering lead to improvement neurologically.

149.6 Diagnosis

Diagnosis is based on:

1. clinical history
2. radiological diagnosis including CT scan, meylography (MRI was not available at the time)
3. Electrophysiological studies

149.7 Management

Tethering due to dysraphism has different modalities of surgery. In this posttraumatic case the neurosurgeon after laminectomy found the cord by scarring at the old fracture at its distal side was attenuated cystic bag tethered circumferentially by arachnoid sclerosis. Because the patient had a complete T5 injury they transected 1 cm section of the cord from its distal end and the cord receded almost 10 cm. The procedure was monitored by SSEP, which improved postoperatively. The resected segment was diagnosed neural tissue with atrophy.

References

Barry A, Patten BM, Stewart BH. Possible factors in the development of the Arnold-Chiari malformation. J Neurosurg. 1957;14(3):285–301.

Ragnarsson TS, Durward QJ, Nordgren RE. Spinal cord tethering after traumatic paraplegia with late neurological deterioration. J Neurosurg. 1986;64(3):397–401.

Schneider SJ, Rosenthal AD, Greenberg BM, Danto J. A preliminary report on the use of laser-Doppler flowmetry during tethered spinal cord release. Neurosurgery. 1993;32(2):214–7.

Yamada S, Zinke DE, Sanders D. Pathophysiology of "tethered cord syndrome". J Neurosurg. 1981;54(4):494–503.

Conclusion

This text was collected for over four decades from different publications of spinal cord. It was collected in the early days from the Index Medicus and later from Pubmed and other online sources. Each subject in this book is given credit to each author, whose cases are presented exactly from their published reports. This book is intended for many practitioners especially, neurologist, neurosurgeon, rehabilitation, physiatrist, residents, and students of medicine. Each subject is divided into definition, incidence, etiology, pathology, clinical picture, diagnosis, and management. They have been thoroughly researched and updated; further, case details can be obtained from the references. The subjects were collected mostly from English literature, as well as translated from other languages. This book is an adequate reference for the occasionally encountered case of rare spinal cord clinical pathologies and rare curiosities. In order to assure progress in future research in this field, it is important to remember the fundamental medical advances that came from studying rare diseases. It is a hope that this book could serve as a model for future rare spinal cord disease research.

I.M. Eltorai, *Rare Diseases and Syndromes of the Spinal Cord*,
DOI 10.1007/978-3-319-45147-3

MIX
Papier aus verantwortungsvollen Quellen
Paper from responsible sources
FSC® C105338

If you have any concerns about our products,
you can contact us on
ProductSafety@springernature.com

In case Publisher is established outside the EU,
the EU authorized representative is:
Springer Nature Customer Service Center GmbH
Europaplatz 3, 69115 Heidelberg, Germany

Printed by Libri Plureos GmbH
in Hamburg, Germany